New Frontiers in Anti-Cancer Drug Discovery

New Frontiers in Anti-Cancer Drug Discovery

Editor: Sydney Bruce

MURPHY & MOORE
www.murphy-moorepublishing.com

www.murphy-moorepublishing.com

MURPHY & MOORE

Cataloging-in-Publication Data

New frontiers in anti-cancer drug discovery / edited by Sydney Bruce.
p. cm.
Includes bibliographical references and index.
ISBN 978-1-63987-385-2
1. Antineoplastic agents. 2. Drug development. 3. Drugs--Design. 4. Cancer--Treatment.
5. Pharmaceutical chemistry. I. Bruce, Sydney.
RS431.A64 N49 2022
615.798--dc23

Murphy & Moore Publishing,
1 Rockefeller Plaza,
New York City, NY 10020, USA

ISBN 978-1-63987-385-2 (Hardback)

Contents

Preface

This book has been an outcome of determined endeavour from a group of educationists in the field. The primary objective was to involve a broad spectrum of professionals from diverse cultural background involved in the field for developing new researches. The book not only targets students but also scholars pursuing higher research for further enhancement of the theoretical and practical applications of the subject.

The drugs which are used in the treatment of cancerous or malignant diseases are termed anti-cancer drugs. The different categories of anticancer drugs are antimetabolites, alkylating agents, hormones and natural products. There are some drugs which do not fall within these categories but exhibit anticancer properties. The selection of a particular anticancer drug to treat a cancer depends on various factors such as the severity of cancer, the location and the type of cancer. The side effects of the drug and whether radiation therapy or surgery can be used are also reasons which help in the determination of which drugs should be administered. This book attempts to understand the multiple branches that fall under the discipline of anti-cancer drug discovery and how such concepts have practical applications. It presents researches and studies performed by experts across the globe. Researchers and students in this field will be assisted by this book.

It was an honour to edit such a profound book and also a challenging task to compile and examine all the relevant data for accuracy and originality. I wish to acknowledge the efforts of the contributors for submitting such brilliant and diverse chapters in the field and for endlessly working for the completion of the book. Last, but not the least; I thank my family for being a constant source of support in all my research endeavours.

Editor

1

A Combined Molecular Docking and Electronic Structure Study for a Breast Cancer Drug Design

Linda-Lucila Landeros-Martinez,
Daniel Glossman-Mitnik,
Erasmo Orrantia-Borunda and
Norma Flores-Holguin

Abstract

The molecular docking of tamoxifen's metabolites, 4-hydroxy-tamoxifen, N-desmethyl-tamoxifen, and 4-hydroxy-N-desmethyl-tamoxifen, in estrogen and progesterone hormone receptors was studied in aqueous solution. The metabolites 4-hydroxy-tamoxifen, N-desmethyl-tamoxifen, and 4-hydroxy-N-desmethyl-tamoxifen exhibit a binding energy in the estrogen receptor cavity of −10.69 kcal/mol, −10.9 kcal/mol, and −11.35 kcal/mol, respectively, and −1.45 kcal/mol, −9.29 kcal/mol, and −0.38 kcal/mol in the progesterone receptor. This indicates a spontaneous interaction between the metabolites and the active sites in the hormone receptors. Docking has an adequate accuracy for both receptors, and from this calculation the active site residues were defined for the different metabolites and the estrogen and progesterone receptors. Also, the chemical reactivity of the amino acids of the active sites of each metabolite was determined. These reactivity properties were obtained within the framework of density functional theory, using the functional M06 with the basis set 6-31G (d). The results indicate that in the estrogen receptor, the highest charge transfer of the three analyzed metabolites is in the union of the metabolite and the Leu346-Thr347 residue. The progesterone receptor shows minor tendency to react with higher hardness values than the estrogen receptor. The hydrogen bonds are three for the estrogen receptor in two different metabolites, while in progesterone only one is formed with the N-desmethyl-tamoxifen metabolite.

Keywords: molecular docking, tamoxifen, binding energy, charge transfer, hydrogen bond, hormone receptors

1. Introduction

Breast cancer is the leading cause of cancer death in women. A prognosis of breast cancer can be issued because there are parameters that predict the evolution or aggressiveness of the cancer, such as lymph nodes, tumor size, and histological grade of cancer [1–4]. In mammary cells there are hormone receptors (estrogen receptors (ERs) and progesterone receptors (PRs)) that function as "switches," activating or deactivating a particular function in the mammary cell.

Over the last two years a number of drugs have been developed with specific properties for the treatment of breast cancer. Fulvestrant is a steroid-based selective estrogen receptor downregulator (SERD) that antagonizes and degrades ER-α and is active in patients who have progressed to antihormonal agents [5]. Also, the selective ER modulators (SERMs)/SERD hybrids (SSHs) have been used to facilitate the first-line treatment for ER 1 degradation in breast cancer cells [6].

Another important piece of research by Srinivasan et al. presents the discovery of a series of SERDs lacking a prototypical side chain. This absence improves the mechanism called "indirect antagonism" [7]. The latest developments have found the optimal design of antiestrogen cores and side chains with the middle structures of the original SERMs class, such as tamoxifen (TAM), raloxifene, lasofoxifene, and bazedoxifene. Also, current studies of SERDs have been made by GlaxoSmithKline(GSK), Genentech, and AstraZeneca. In these studies the side chain is modified to a simple adamantyl core [8].

In addition, for several years, have been used antibodies as cancer drugs, and some examples are trastuzumab and pertuzumab, which are used in breast cancer as the only component. In fact, efforts have been made to use the antibodies conjugated with a variety of substances with the aim of improving their effect. Research on cancer therapy is still in progress [9].

TAM is a SERM [10, 11] and is used for the treatment of hormone receptors expressing breast cancer [12]. This drug is metabolized in the liver, producing three different metabolites: 4-hydroxy-tamoxifen (4OHTAM), N-desmethyl-tamoxifen (NDTAM), and 4-hydroxy-N-desmethyl-tamoxifen, also known as endoxifen (END) [13, 14]. These metabolites show a range of agonist and partial antagonist activities of ER-mediated effects [15]. In vivo studies have shown that TAM competes against estrogens to dock to the receptors, resulting in an attenuation of the cellular response measured by estrogen [16]. Therefore, the clinical response to TAM therapy will depend on the total effect of the resulting metabolites on the patient, their affinity for receptors, and their agonist/antagonist profile [15].

Recently, a number of theoretical studies on TAM and some of its active metabolites have described its interaction with ERs. Calculations of molecular dynamics have been used to model dynamic fluctuations in structures of ERs (ER-α following the binding to estradiol and the metabolite 4OHTAM) [17]. Recently, in an article written by the authors, the molecular docking of TAM in ER and PR was presented in which the active site of the hormone receptors was determined, as well as the charge transfer of the drug to the amino acids of the active sites of the receptors [18]. Other theoretical studies analyzed the chirality of TAM using density functional theory (DFT) with functional B3LYP and BLYP with a basis set 6-311++G(2d, 2p) [12]. In addition, there was a reported analysis of the amount of charge transfer and the direction of the flow of charge of alkylating drugs in the presence of DNA bases allowing prediction among its bases of which one is the main target of these antitumor drugs [19].

Another technique is molecular docking, which is a computational procedure that attempts to predict noncovalent binding of macromolecules (receptor) and small molecules (ligands) efficiently [20]. In detail, docking consists of an operation in which one molecule is brought into the vicinity of another while calculating the interaction energies of the many mutual orientations and conformations of the two interacting species. A docking procedure is used as a guide to identify the preferred orientation of one molecule relative to the other [21]. This method plays a key role in promoting fundamental biomolecular events such as enzyme–substrate, drug–protein, and drug–nucleic acid interactions [22]; it is also widely used in drug design [23]. Some authors have used the molecular docking of macromolecules to define the energy and bonding affinity in ER-α and ER-β with estrogen [24]. It has also been used in the analysis of a maltogenic amylase of *Bacillus lehensis* G1, which provides a view of the substrate and specificity in the macromolecule [25], and in the DNA docking analysis of natural products such as methyltransferase inhibitors, which have become an alternative for cancer therapies [26].

The objective of this research is to develop molecular docking of the metabolites of TAM with the macromolecules ER and PR, to obtain an active site of the hormone receptors. To perform computational protein–ligand docking experiments, a 3-D structure of the target protein at atomic resolution must be available. The most reliable sources are crystal and solution structures provided by the Protein Data Bank (PDB) [26, 27]. The hormone receptors selected for this work are the 1A52 ER-α ligand-binding domain complexed to estradiol, and the 1A28 hormone-bound human progesterone receptor ligand-binding domain. Both belong to the organism *Homo sapiens* and are present in breast cancer cells. Molecular docking has the advantage of working on a large scale, as well as determining the important sites of the macromolecule (active sites) [27, 28]. Once the active site is defined, an accurate calculation of electronic structure can be developed with methods such as DFT, which is the most popular, efficient, and versatile tool for obtaining precise information of molecular systems. For both receptors, the amino acids (residues) forming the active site were analyzed in an attempt to obtain their electronic properties such as ionization potential, electron affinity, electrophilicity, chemical hardness, chemical potential, and electronegativity. A transfer and charge flow direction analysis was also performed.

2. Computational details

2.1. Molecular docking

Molecular docking is calculated with the specially tailored software AutoDock 4.2 with the Lamarckian Genetic Algorithm (LGA) [28, 29] to explore how ER and PR bond with the metabolites. AutoDock uses a semiempirical free energy force field to predict binding free energies of small molecules to macromolecule targets [29]. The force field is based on a comprehensive thermodynamic model that allows incorporation of intramolecular energies into the predicted free energy of binding. It also incorporates a charge-based method for evaluation of desolvation designed to use a typical set of atom types [30]. The use of LGA allows individual conformations to search their local conformational space, find local minima, and then pass this information to later generations [29]; also LGA can handle ligands with more degrees of freedom and is efficient, reliable, and successful [31].

The water molecules in the receivers are eliminated and only the polar H atoms are added. The docking area is selected by constructing a grid box, size 52 × 36 × 34 points, centered at x, y, and z coordinates of 89.304, 14.745, and 70.512, respectively, for ER, and a grid box, size 20 × 18 × 26 points, centered at x, y, and z coordinates of 36.999, 31.767, and 42.694, respectively, for PR using in both receptors a grid spacing of 0.375 Å in AutoGrid [28, 29]. The docking parameters used for the LGA-based conformational searches are: docking trials—150; population size—150; maximum number of energy evaluations—25,000,000; maximum number of top individuals to survive to next generation—1; rate of gene mutation—0.02; rate of crossover —0.8; mean of Cauchy distribution for gene mutation—0.0; variance of Cauchy distribution for gene mutation—1.0; and number of generations for picking the worst individual—10.

2.2. Electronic structure calculations

The energy calculations of the amino acids that make up the active site on ER, PR, and TAM metabolites are calculated with the functional hybrid meta-GGA M06 [32, 33] developed by the Truhlar Group from the University of Minnesota, combined with the basis set 6-31G (d) proposed by Pople [34] and the conductor-like polarizable continuum model (CPCM) [35] using water as a solvent. All calculations were made using DFT [35–38] with the Gaussian program 09 [39]. The charge distribution for amino acids and metabolites was obtained with the population analysis of Hirshfeld charges [40].

Equations	
$$\eta = \frac{(I - AE)}{2}$$	(1)
$$\chi = \frac{(I + AE)}{2}$$	(2)
$$\omega = \frac{\mu^2}{2\eta}$$	(3)
$$\mu = -\chi$$	(4)
$$\Delta N = \frac{\mu_B - \mu_A}{2(\eta_A + \eta_B)}$$	(5)

Table 1. Global reactivity and charge transfer parameters.

The chemical reactivity descriptors of the studied molecular systems were calculated using the DFT conceptual framework. These parameters include ionization potential (I), electron affinity (EA), chemical hardness (η) [41], electronegativity (χ) [41], electrophilicity (ω) [42], and chemical potential (μ) [42]. The overall interaction between metabolites and the amino acids that make up the active site on ER and PR can be identified by the charge transfer. This parameter determines the behavior of the different molecular systems as a donor or as an acceptor system. In this case, the electrons transferred from the metabolites to the amino acids of the active site of receptors or vice versa. The global interactions between two constituents can been determined using the charge transfer parameter (ΔN) [43].

The equations of the reactivity and charge transfer descriptors are shown in **Table 1**.

3. Results and discussion

3.1. Validation docking

Validation docking was performed for each hormone receptor using the PyMOL program [44]. **Figure 1** shows the structure of the native co-crystallized TAM bond and its metabolites. The root mean square deviation (RMSD) between TAM and the metabolites was calculated for each

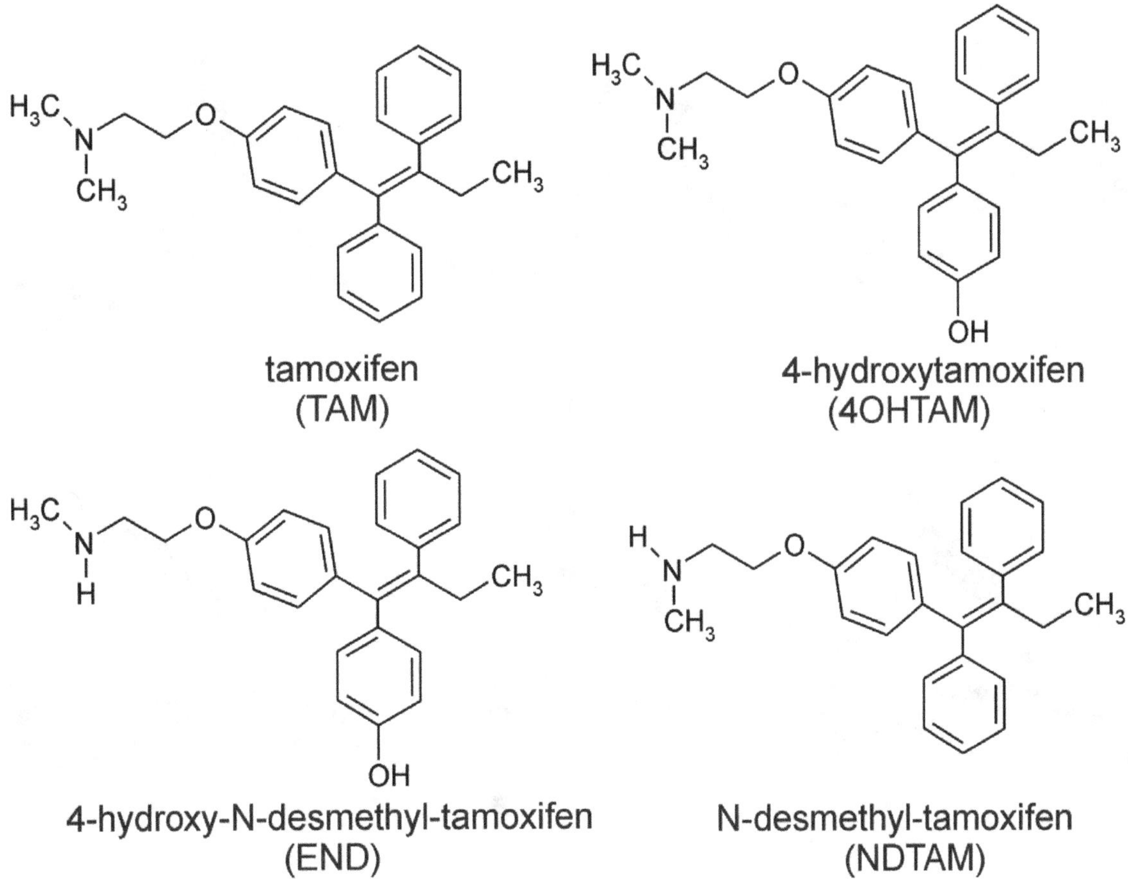

Figure 1. Chemical structures of tamoxifen and metabolites.

of the hormone receptor dockings. An RMSD value is considered a measurement of the accuracy of the docking results. The optimal position is recognized if the RMSD value is less than 2 Å [45]. In the case of metabolite dockings, TAM was used as the template for molecular overlap, as it is known that this drug is metabolized into the metabolites analyzed in this study. The metabolites were aligned by rotation and translation to obtain the RMSD using the "Align" option in PyMOL. Therefore, the RMSD in ER obtained between TAM with 4OHTAM, END, and NDTAM is 0.672, 1.106, and 1.461, respectively. For PR the RMSD obtained between TAM and 4OHTAM, END, and NDTAM is 1.387, 2.006, and 0.953, respectively. **Figure 2** shows the alignment between TAM (black) and 4OHTAM, END, and NDTAM (gray).

3.2. Analysis of the estrogen receptor with the metabolites

An analysis of molecular docking of the metabolites in ER was carried out, revealing the active site of the ER, followed by its description, the analysis of the chemical reactivity parameters of the residues and the metabolites, as well as the description of the hydrogen bonds between the metabolites and the ER active site.

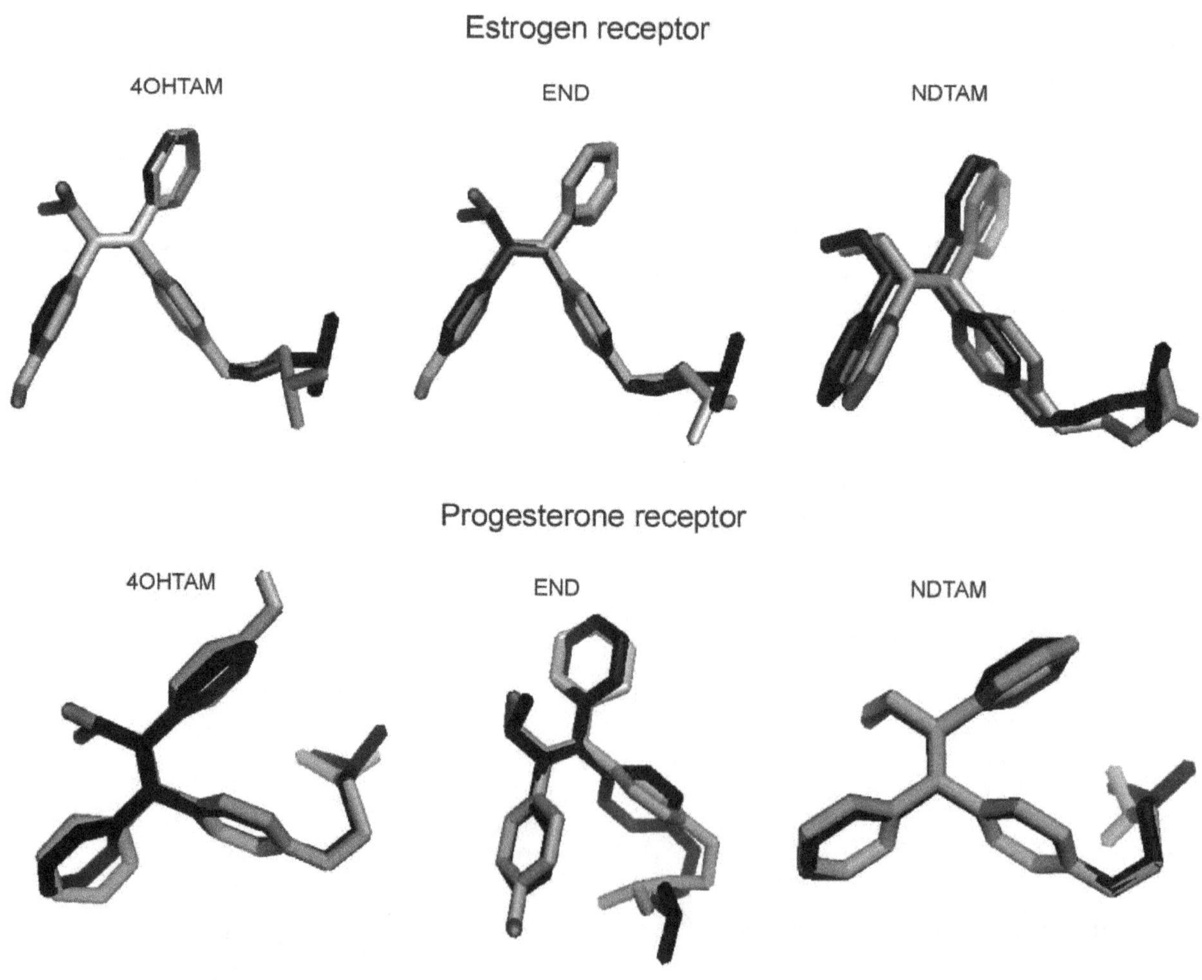

Figure 2. Conformation of tamoxifen and metabolites after docking in hormone receptors.

3.2.1. *Molecular docking*

The binding energy of the metabolites with the ER active site was predicted with molecular docking calculations. The negative value of the binding energy (affinity) in the docking indicates that the system is stable and that there is an interaction between ER and the metabolites in the active site: −10.69 kcal/mol for 4OHTAM, −11.35 kcal/mol for END, and − 10.90 kcal/mol for NDTAM. It was observed that the binding affinity was lower in 4OHTAM; this is due to the effect of the orientation of the metabolite within the active site caused by the influence of the tertiary amine functional group containing the 4OHTAM.

Finally, the binding energy shows that END, which exhibits −11.35 kcal/mol, is the metabolite with the highest affinity with the active site. It even shows a better affinity than TAM at −10.38 kcal/mol [18]. This coincides with previous information reported by Clarke [46] who says that END has an affinity for ERs higher than NDTAM or TAM itself. As can be observed, all the metabolites have a high affinity to the receptor. According with Gareth [47], the greater the affinity of the ligand for the receptor, the more easily it binds to that receptor. This is important because the binding of a drug to a receptor stimulates the physiological response that characterizes the action of the drug, which means that release of a series of biochemical events results in a biological or pharmacological effect [47].

The schematic structure of the active site and the binding energies are shown in **Figure 3**.

3.2.2. *Active site*

The conformational coupling of the active site with each metabolite is described below.

4OHTAM. There are 14 residues in contact with the metabolite 4OHTAM at the active site of the ER. Nine of them are linked forming an amino acids sequence: leucine346-threonine347 (Leu346-Thr347), tryptophan383-leucine384 (Trp383-Leu384), glutamic acid353-leucine354 (Glu353-Leu354), and leucine349-alanine350-aspartic acid351 (Leu349-Ala350-Asp351). The other five are: glycine residue (Gly521)—glycine is the smallest of the amino acids. It is ambivalent, which means that the amino acid can be inside or outside of the protein molecule; lysine529 (Lys529)—this residue contains a protonated amino group that provides a positive charge to proteins as acetyltransferases; histidine524 (His524)—this residue has a positively charged imidazole functional group. This group participates in enzyme-catalyzed reactions; phenylalanine404 (Phe404)—an essential amino acid, it is a derivative of alanine with a phenyl substituent on the β carbon. Due to its hydrophobicity, phenylalanine is nearly always found buried within a protein. The π electrons of the phenyl ring can stack with other aromatic systems and often do so within folded proteins, adding stability to the structure; and finally, methionine388 (Met 388), which has a hydrophobic thiol ether in its lateral chain. According to the results obtained by theoretical calculations, in the metabolite 4OHTAM the active site of estrogen coincides with that reported by Shiau et al. [48].

END. The active site of END is formed by the following residues: leucine346-threonine347 (Leu346-Thr347), leucine387-methionine388 (Leu387-Met388), tryptophan383-leucine384 (Trp383-Leu384), glycine521 (Gly521), and histidine524 (His524). The last two residues are highly hydrophilic.

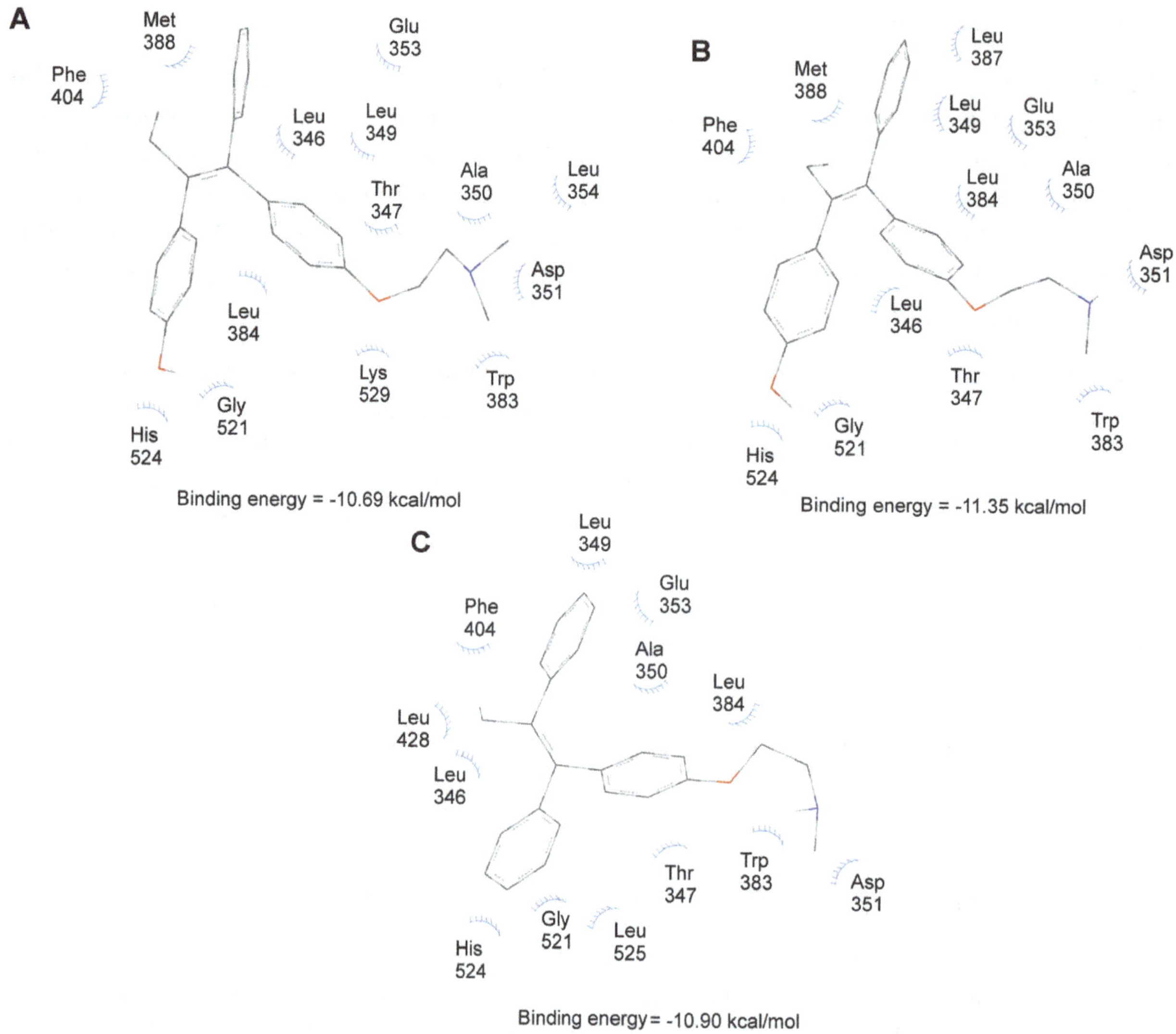

Figure 3. Amino acids of the active site of the estrogen receptor with (A) 4OHTAM, (B) END, and (C) NDTAM.

NDTAM. The active site in NDTAM consists of the following residues: leucine346-threonine347 (Leu346-Thr347), histidine524-leucine525 (His524-Leu525), tryptophan383-leucine384 (Trp383-Leu384), and (Leu349-Ala350-Asp351),and hydrophilic residue glycine521 (Gly521) and hydrophobic residues phenylalanine404 (Phe404), glutamic acid (Glu353), and leucine428 (Leu428).

Most of the residues are situated over the planar core of the ligand. The others surround the functional groups amine and hydroxyl. These interactions contribute to binding energies of up to −10 kcal/mol.

The metabolites act by blocking the activation domain AF-2 of ER found in the ligand bond domain or LBD of the active site. Therefore, the metabolites act as estrogen antagonists over the genes that require only the activation domain AF-2 [49, 50].

The residues for the metabolites in ER are shown in **Figure 3**.

3.2.3. Chemical reactivity

Once the most stable structure of the active site of TAM's metabolites were defined, an analysis of the reactivity of ER residues was performed using descriptors such as ionization potential (I), electron affinity (EA), chemical potential (μ), chemical hardness (η), and electrophilicity (ω). Calculated results for the reactivity parameters of the drug and residues of the ER are shown in **Table 2**.

The electron affinities of the residues fluctuate from 0.21 eV to 0.91 eV. The highest value of electron affinity is for the Trp383-Leu384 residue, which is present in the active site of the three different metabolites analyzed in this work. According to the ionization potential results, the residue with the greatest possibility of losing electrons is Leu346-Thr347 with 7.74 eV. This residue is present in the active site of the three metabolites.

Metabolite	Active site	EA (eV)	I (eV)	hη(eV)	μ = −χ (eV)	ω (eV)
4OHTAM	Gly521	0.21	7.03	3.41	3.62	1.92
	Met388	0.46	6.11	2.82	2.39	1.91
	His524	0.43	6.2	2.89	3.31	1.9
	Lys529	0.83	7.22	3.19	4.02	2.54
	Phe404	0.51	6.4	2.95	3.46	2.03
	Trp383-Leu384	0.91	6.04	2.56	3.47	2.35
	Glu353-Leu354	0.66	5.59	2.47	3.13	1.98
	Leu346-Thr347	0.88	7.74	3.43	4.31	2.71
	Leu349-Ala350-Asp351	0.73	5.79	2.53	3.26	2.1
END	Gly521	0.21	7.03	3.41	3.62	1.92
	His524	0.43	6.2	2.89	3.31	1.9
	Leu387-Met388	0.51	6.25	2.87	3.38	1.99
	Leu346-Thr347	0.88	7.74	3.43	4.31	2.71
	Trp383-Leu384	0.91	5.79	2.53	3.26	2.1
NDTAM	Gly521	0.21	7.03	3.41	3.62	1.92
	Phe404	0.51	6.4	2.95	3.46	2.03
	Glu353	0.2	5.62	2.71	2.91	1.57
	Leu428	0.47	7	3.23	3.73	2.14
	His524-Leu525	0.81	6.1	2.65	3.46	2.25
	Trp383-Leu384	0.91	6.04	2.56	3.47	2.35
	Leu346-Thr347	0.88	7.74	3.43	4.31	2.71
	Leu349-Ala350-Asp351	0.73	5.79	2.53	3.26	2.1

Table 2. Parameters of chemical reactivity of the active site residues of the estrogen receptor.

Chemical hardness ranges from 2.53 eV to 3.43 eV; this parameter measures the resistance to change in the electronic configuration. The Glu353-Leu354 residue with 2.47 eV will react more easily in the presence of 4OHTAM, the Leu349-Ala350-Asp351 residue with 2.53 eV will react more easily in the presence of NDTAM, and the Trp383-Leu384 residue with 2.56 eV will react more easily in the presence of END. The chemical potential ($\mu = -\chi$) represents the average effect between the tendency among molecules to attract and transfer electrons. This parameter is an important part in the description of the charge transfer descriptor. The electronegativity shows that the Leu346-Thr347 residue has the greatest tendency to attract electrons with 4.31 eV. This trend is repeated with the three different metabolites. Electrophilicity ω represents the stabilization energy of the systems when it becomes saturated with electrons coming from the surroundings. In this case, in the active site of 4OHTAM, value decreases in the following order: Leu346-Thr347 > Lys529 > Trp383-Leu384 > Leu349-Ala350-Asp351 > Phe404 > Glu353-Leu354 > Gly521 > Met388 > His524. In END the decreasing order is Leu346-Thr347 > Trp383-Leu384 > Leu387-Met388 > Gly521 > His524 and in NDTAM the decreasing order is Leu346-Thr347 > Trp383-Leu384 > His524-Leu525 > Leu428 > Leu349-Ala350-Asp351 > Phe404 > Gly521 > Glu353.

3.2.4. Charge transfer descriptor

The chemical reactivity descriptors mentioned above are intramolecular parameters, whose values are calculated from the electronic properties of the molecule. To understand a chemical reaction in depth an intermolecular parameter that represents the fractional number of electrons transferred from one system to another should also be considered. This parameter is called charge transfer and is described as Eq. 5 in **Table 1**. In this formula, μA is TAM's metabolites and μB is the chemical potential for the residues of the active site. ηA, ηB represent the chemical hardness of TAM's metabolites and its residues of the active site, respectively [43]. The significance of these kinds of interactions lies in the fact that they are the primary directors of specificity, rate control, and reversibility in many biochemical reactions. Furthermore, it represents a first step in understanding oxidative damage in the active site produced by the TAM's metabolites and leads to identify their functioning and biological activity. Some authors use charge transfer to describe the oxidative damage of DNA bases [51, 52].

The interpretation of the value ΔN is as follows: for $\Delta N < 0$ the charge flows from A to B (A acts as an electron donor). For $\Delta N > 0$ the charge flows from B to A (A acts as an electron acceptor). Therefore, in the presence of Glu353-Leu354, Leu349-Ala350-Asp351, and His524 residues, ΔN of 4OHTAM accepts electrons, while for the rest of the residues it acts as an electron donor. END is an electron acceptor in the presence of the Trp383-Leu384 residue and with the remainder of the residues it acts as an electron donor. Finally, NDTAM acts as an electron acceptor in the presence of Glu353 and Leu349-Ala 350-Asp351 residues, and as an electron donor with the remainder of the residues. The values are shown in **Table 3**.

The charge transfer descriptor is one of the noncovalent interactions that are present in biological systems in a macromolecule–ligand complex. In this case, the highest charge transfer value is in the same residue, Leu346-Thr347, for all the metabolites, which acts as a donor with amounts of −0.080, −0.086, and –0.073 for 4OHTAM, END, and NDTAM, respectively. Therefore, oxidative damage in the active site decreases in the order 4OHTAM > NDTAM > END.

Metabolite	Residue	ΔN
4OHTAM	Gly521	−0.022
	Met388	0.089
	His524	0.004
	Lys529	−0.058
	Phe404	−0.010
	Trp383-Leu384	−0.012
	Glu353-Leu354	0.022
	Leu346-Thr347	−0.080
	Leu349-Ala350-Asp351	0.009
NDTAM	Gly521	−0.016
	Phe404	−0.004
	Glu353	0.047
	Leu428	−0.026
	His524-Lue525	−0.004
	Trp383-Leu384	−0.005
	Leu346-Thr347	−0.073
	Leu349-Ala350-Asp351	0.015
END	Gly521	−0.029
	His524	−0.004
	Leu387-Met388	−0.010
	Leu346-Thr347	−0.086
	Trp383-Leu384	0.001

Table 3. Charge transfer descriptor in the estrogen receptor.

3.2.5. *Electrostatics interactions*

Other noncovalent interactions between the ligand and hormone receptor are the hydrogen bond and π–π interactions. An analysis of these bonds between the ER and each of TAM's metabolites was done. The results are as follows.

4OHTAM. This residue has one hydrogen bond (C=O----O-H) between the donor group (O-H) and the acceptor group (C=O) of the Gly521 residue. Also, there is a π–π interaction between residue Trp383 and the planar core of the ligand.

END. There are two hydrogen bonds: first (C=O----OH) between the acceptor group (C=O) of Gly521 and the donor group (O-H) belonging to one of the rings and second (C=O----HN) between the accepting group (C=O) of Asp351 and the secondary amine (NH). The π–π interaction was found among residue Trp383 and the planar core of the ligand.

NDTAM. In this metabolite was found one hydrogen bond (C=O----HN) between the accepting group (C=O) of Asp351 and the amine group of the ligand. No π–π interactions were found in this ligand–receptor complex.

In all cases the metabolites analyzed followed the Lipinski et al. rule of five, which states: when there are five or fewer hydrogen bonds the drug will not present poor absorption or permeation and will be more active [53]. **Figure 4** shows the metabolites as a ball and stick and the residues of the active site as a tube. The hydrogen bonds are shown as green dots and π–π interactions are the areas marked in yellow.

3.3. Analysis of the progesterone receptor with the metabolites

Analysis of molecular docking between PR and the metabolites is characterized by the active site of PR: the active site was described and the calculation and analysis of chemical reactivity

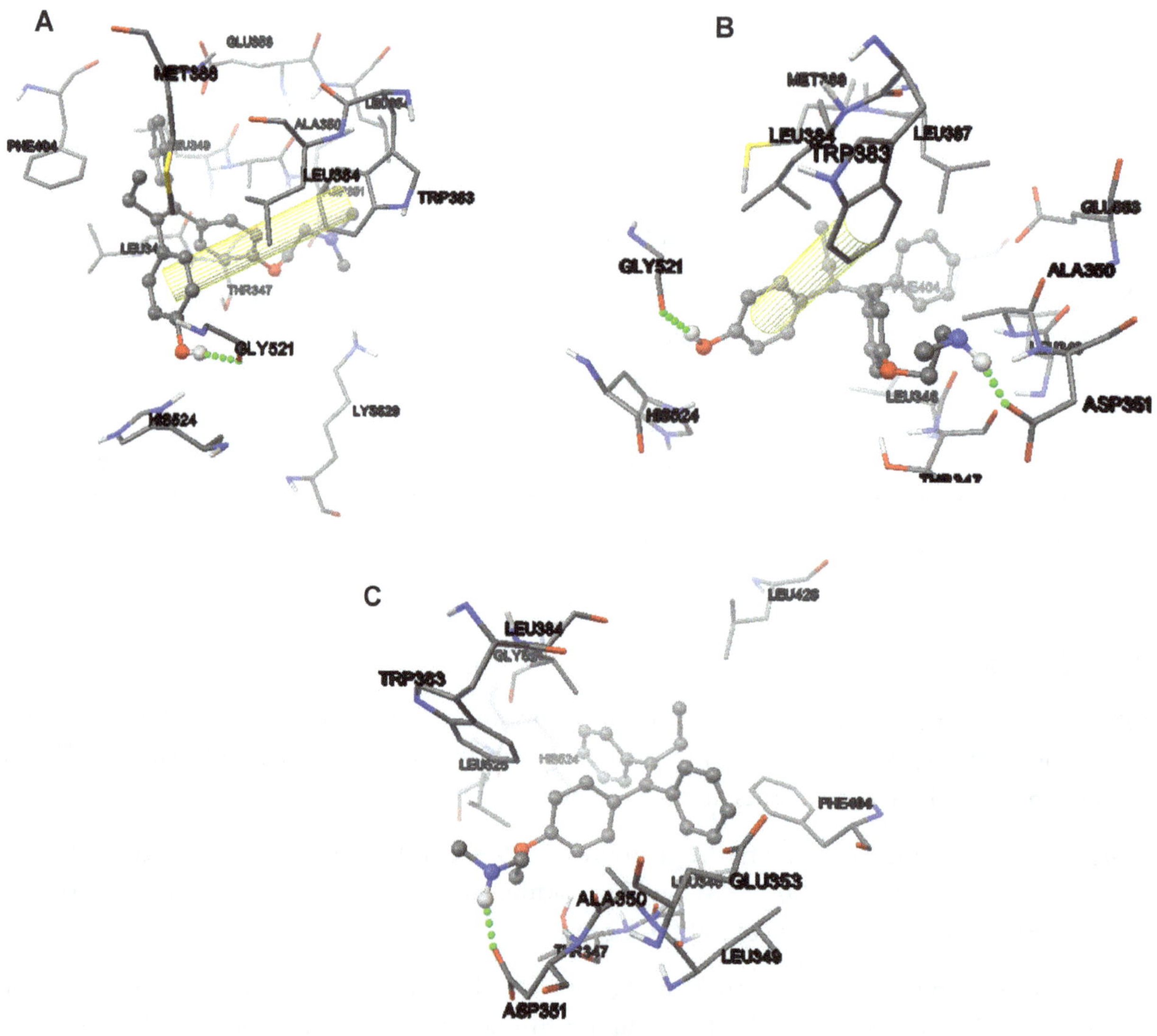

Figure 4. Hydrogen bond (green) and π–π interactions (yellow) at the active site of the estrogen receptor with (A) 4OHTAM, (B) END, and (C) NDTAM.

parameters of the residues and metabolites were carried out, as well as the description of the hydrogen bond formed between the metabolites and the PR active site.

3.3.1. Molecular docking

The binding energy of TAM's metabolites at the active site of PR has been predicted by carrying out molecular docking calculations. The schematic structure of the active site and the binding energies are shown in **Figure 5**. The negative value of the binding energy in the

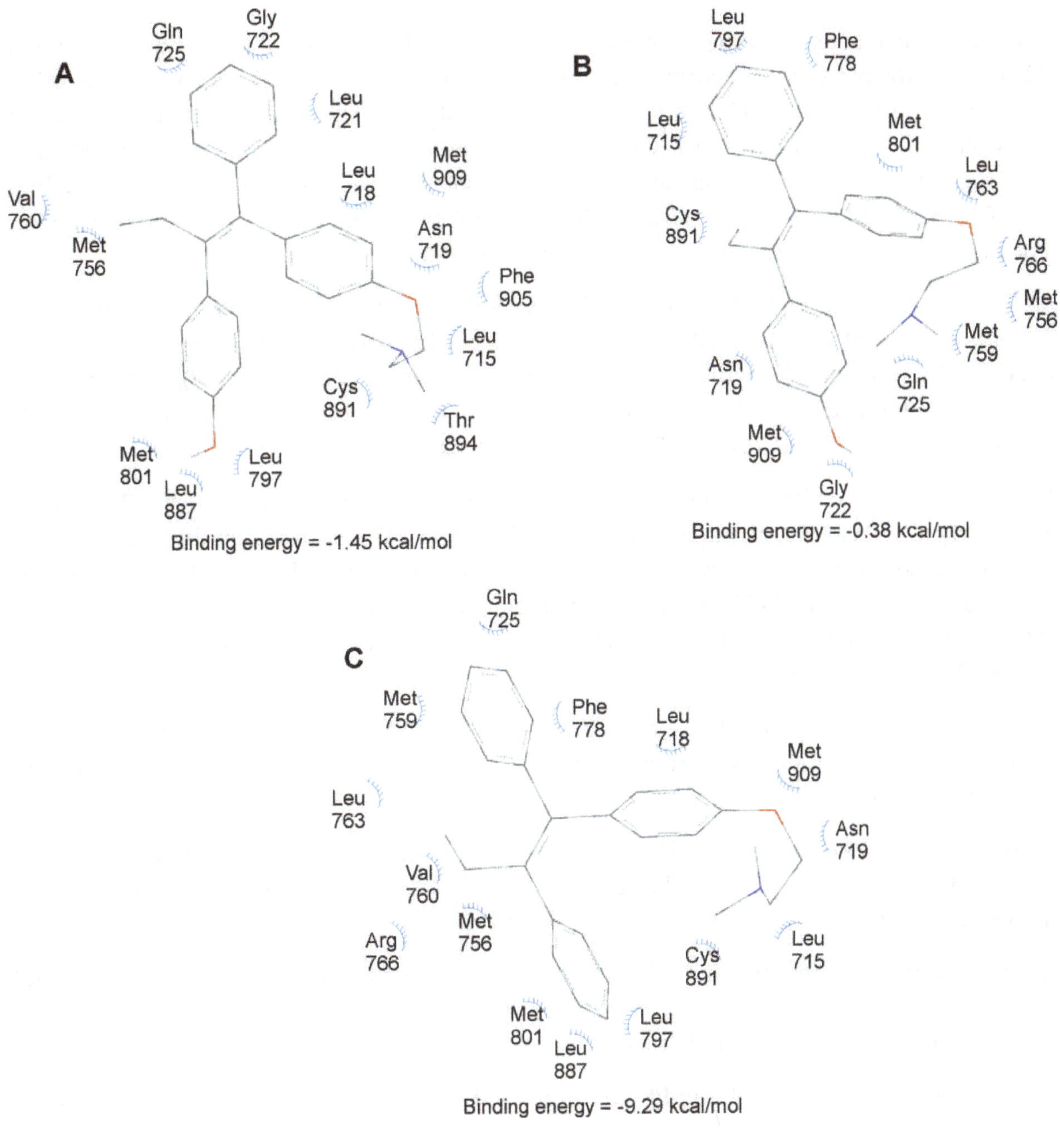

Figure 5. Amino acids of the active site of the progesterone receptor with (A) 4OHTAM, (B) END, and (C) NDTAM.

docking indicates that the system is stable and that there is an interaction between PR and metabolites at the site: –1.45 kcal/mol for 4OHTAM, –0.38 kcal/mol for END, and –9.29 kcal/mol for NDTAM.

Although the metabolites END and 4OHTAM have a negative bond energy, their values remain very low compared to TAM, which has –9.38 kcal/mol [13]. Therefore, these two metabolites will have very low biological activity in PRs.

3.3.2. *Active site*

The active site of PR obtained by theoretical analysis is as follows.

4OHTAM. There are 15 residues in contact with the metabolite 4OHTAM at the active site of PR. Four of them are linked, forming an amino acids sequence, leucine718-aspartic acid719 (Leu718-Asn719) and leucine721-glycine722 (Leu721-Gly722). The other 11 residues are highly hydrophilic: glutamine725 residue (Gln725), cysteine891 (Cys891), threonine894 (Thr894), and phenylalanine905 (Phe905); and seven are hydrophobic residues: methionine756, methionine801, and methionine909 (Met756, Met801, and Met909), valine760 (Val760), and leucine715, leucine797, and leucine887 (Leu715, Leu797, and Leu887).

END. The active site in END is formed by the following residues: glutamine725 (Gln725), cysteine891 (Cys891), glycine722 (Gly722), asparagine719 (Asn19), and arginine766 (Arg766), which are hydrophilic. The hydrophobic residues are phenylalanine778 (Phe778), tryptophan755 (Trp755), methionine756, methionine759, methionine801, and methionine909 (Met756, Met759, Met801, and Met909), and leucine715, leucine763, and leucine797 (Leu715, Leu763, and Leu797).

NDTAM. The active site for NDTAM consists of the following residues: leucine718-aspartic acid719 (Leu718-Asn 719) and methionine759-valine760 (Met759-Val760). Hydrophilic residues are glutamine725 (Gln725), arginine766 (Arg766), and cysteine891 (Cys891). Hydrophobic residues are phenylalanine778 (Phe778), methionine756, methionine801, and methionine909 (Met756, Met801, and Met909), and leucine715, lucine763, leucine797, and leucine887 (Leu715, Leu763, Leu797, and Leu887).

Most of the residues of the active site of 4OHTAM and END surround the planar core of the ligand and over the functional group amine. The steric hindrance of this amine group produces minor binding energy.

When the metabolites bind, there is a conformational change and they are recognized by the amino acids of the active site. This has to do with the coupling energies. In PR, NDTAM has a higher amount of binding energy exceeding –9 kcal/mol.

Even when PR is more labile than ER, the binding energies indicate that the receptor is not sufficiently labile to recognize the metabolites 4OHTAM and END, which present binding energies lower than –1.5 kcal/mol.

The residues for the metabolites in PR are shown in **Figure 5**.

3.3.3. *Chemical reactivity*

As soon as the most stable structure of the active site of TAM's metabolites was obtained, an analysis of the chemical reactivity of progesterone residues was performed by means of the reactivity descriptors. Results for these calculations are shown in **Table 4**.

Metabolite	**Active site**	**EA (eV)**	**I (eV)**	**η (eV)**	**$\mu = -\chi$ (eV)**	**ω (eV)**
4OHTAM	Phe905	0.93	6.58	2.82	3.76	2.50
	Leu797	0.67	6.86	3.09	3.74	2.36
	Leu887	0.43	7.01	3.29	3.72	2.10
	Thr894	0.49	6.57	3.04	3.53	2.05
	Val760	0.76	6.92	3.08	3.84	2.40
	Met756	0.75	6.3	2.77	3.52	2.54
	Leu715	0.60	7.02	3.21	3.81	2.26
	Gln725	0.70	7.10	3.20	3.90	2.38
	Cys891	0.55	6.89	3.17	3.72	2.18
	Met801	0.64	6.27	2.82	3.45	2.12
	Met909	0.50	6.21	2.85	3.36	1.97
	Leu721-Gly722	−0.33	7.13	3.73	3.40	1.55
	Leu718-Asn719	1.06	7.06	3.00	4.06	2.74
END	Arg766	0.21	7.03	3.41	3.62	1.92
	Leu763	0.43	6.2	2.89	3.31	1.90
	Gly722	0.51	6.25	2.87	3.38	1.99
	Met759	0.88	7.74	3.43	4.31	2.71
	Gln725	0.70	7.10	3.20	3.90	2.38
	Trp755	0.86	5.85	2.50	3.35	2.25
	Asn719	0.76	7.16	3.20	3.96	2.45
	Leu797	0.67	6.86	3.09	3.74	2.36
	Met756	0.75	6.30	2.77	3.52	2.54
	Phe778	0.86	6.60	2.87	3.73	2.42
	Leu715	0.60	7.02	3.21	3.81	2.26
	Cys891	0.55	6.89	3.17	3.72	2.18
	Met801	0.64	6.27	2.82	3.45	2.12
	Met909	0.73	5.79	2.85	3.26	2.10
NDTAM	Leu763	0.35	7.17	3.41	3.76	2.07
	Leu797	0.67	6.86	3.09	3.74	2.36
	Leu887	0.43	7.01	3.29	3.72	2.10

Metabolite	Active site	EA (eV)	I (eV)	η (eV)	μ = − χ (eV)	ω (eV)
	Phe778	0.86	6.6	2.87	3.73	2.42
	Leu715	0.60	7.02	3.21	3.81	2.26
	Arg766	0.78	6.70	2.96	3.74	2.36
	Gln725	0.70	7.10	3.20	3.90	2.38
	Cys891	0.55	6.89	3.17	3.72	2.18
	Met756	0.75	6.30	2.77	3.53	2.24
	Met801	0.64	6.27	2.82	3.45	2.12
	Met909	0.50	6.21	2.85	3.36	1.97
	Met759-Val760	1.05	6.26	2.61	3.65	2.56
	Leu718-Asn719	1.06	7.06	3	4.06	2.74

Table 4. Parameters of chemical reactivity of the active site residues of the progesterone receptor.

The electron affinities of the residues fluctuate from −0.33 eV to 1.06 eV. The highest value of electron affinity is for the Leu718-Asn719 residue, which is present in the active site of 4OHTAM, NDTAM, and the Met759 residue of END. The ionization potential results show that the greatest possibility of losing electrons is: Leu721-Gly722 with 7.13 eV in 4OHTAM, Leu763 with 7.17 eV in NDTAM, and Met759 with 7.74 eV in END.

Chemical hardness, the parameter that measures the resistance to change in the electronic configuration, exhibited amounts from 2.50 eV to 3.73 eV. In 4OHTAM, the lowest value and therefore the one that will react more easily in the presence of the metabolites is 2.77 eV for Met756. For END it is 2.50 eV in Trp755 and 2.61 eV in Met759-Val760. Met801 had a value of 2.82 eV in the NDTAM metabolite.

According to chemical potential, Met759 residue at –4.31 eV presents the highest value in END. The electronegativity ($\mu = -\chi$) shows that the Met759 residue has the greatest tendency to attract electrons at 4.31 eV in END. Electrophilicity ω is the measure of the stabilization energy when systems become saturated by electrons from the surroundings. In this case in the active site of 4OHTAM value decreases in the following order: Leu718-Asn719 > Met756 > Phe905 > Val760 > Gln725 > Leu797 > Leu715 > Cys891 > Met801 > Leu887 > Thr894 > Met909 > Leu721-Gly722. In END the decreasing order is Met759 > Met756 > Asn719 > Phe778 > Gln725 > Leu797 > Leu715 > Trp755 > Cys891 > Met801 > Met909 > Gly722 > Arg766 > Leu763 and in NDTAM the decreasing order is Leu718-Asn719 > Met759-Val760 > Phe778 > Gln725 > Leu797 > Arg766 > Leu715 > Met756 > Cys891 > Met801 > Leu887 > Leu763 > Met909.

3.3.4. *Charge transfer descriptor*

Considering the high importance of this parameter in the formation of complexes in biological systems, the highest values in the different metabolites were defined. The charge transfer between metabolites and PR residues was calculated using Eq. 5. The results show that Met909 in 4OHTAM, Met909 and Leu763 in END, and Met909, Met756, Arg766, and Leu763 in NDTAM act as donor acceptors, namely, these residues are oxidized in the presence of the metabolites. The remainder of the residues act as electron acceptors. The values are shown in **Table 5**.

For 4OHTAM and NDTAM the maxima values are in Leu718-Asp719 with −0.064 and −0.057, respectively. For END the maxima value is in Met759 with −0.088. Thus, the calculations

Metabolite	Residue	Δ*N*
4OHTAM	Leu718-Asn719	−0.064
	Leu721-Gly722	−0.002
	Phe905	−0.037
	Leu797	−0.033
	Leu887	−0.03
	Thr894	−0.014
	Val760	−0.043
	Met756	−0.014
	Leu715	−0.039
	Gln725	−0.047
	Cys891	−0.031
	Met801	−0.007
	Met909	0.002
END	Arg766	−0.027
	Leu763	0.001
	Gly722	−0.006
	Met759	−0.088
	Trp755	−0.003
	Asn719	−0.06
	Leu797	−0.04
	Met756	−0.020
	Gln725	−0.058
	Phe778	−0.041
	Leu715	−0.046
	Cys891	−0.037
	Met801	−0.013
	Met909	0.006
NDTAM	Leu763	0.615
	Leu797	−0.027
	Leu887	−0.024
	Phe778	−0.027

Metabolite	Residue	ΔN
	Leu715	−0.033
	Arg766	0.665
	Gln725	−0.041
	Cys891	−0.025
	Met756	0.669
	Met801	−0.001
	Met909	0.008
	Met759-Val760	−0.021
	Leu718-Asn719	−0.057

Table 5. Transfer of charge between metabolites and progesterone receptor residues.

indicate that oxidative damage in the active site decreases in the following order: NDTAM > END > 4OHTAM.

3.3.5. Electrostatics interactions

An analysis of the hydrogen bond and π–π interactions between the active site on PR and TAM's metabolites was performed. In the case of 4OHTAM and END metabolites no hydrogen bonds were generated, nor were there any π–π interactions, whereas with NDTAM only a

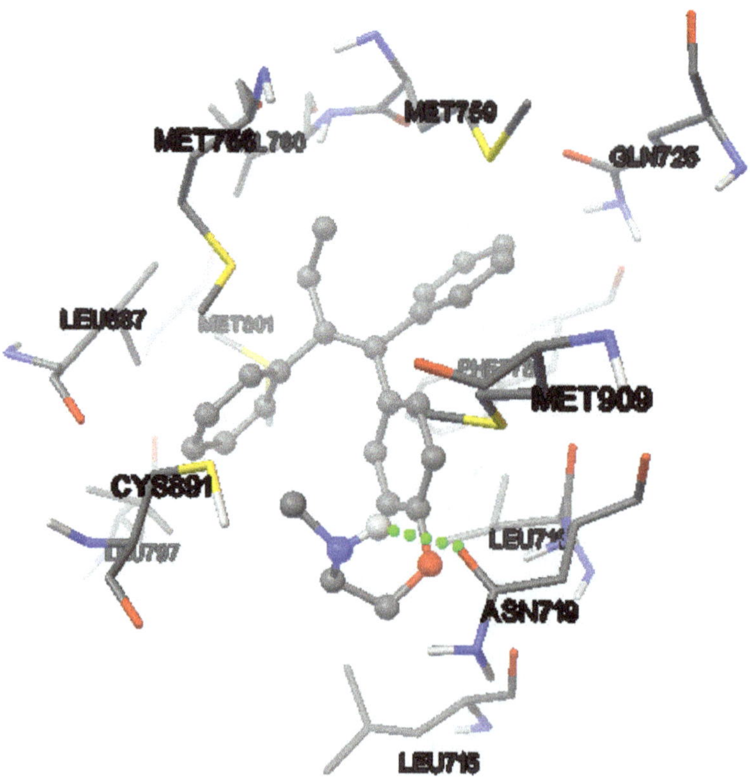

Figure 6. Hydrogen bond (green) at the active site of the progesterone receptor with the NDTAM metabolite.

hydrogen bond (C=O----H-N) was formed between the Asn719 residue and the amino group. The unique electrostatic interaction is shown with green dots in **Figure 6**. Also, it was found that the rule of five by Lipinski et al. [52, 53] was fulfilled.

4. Conclusions

In this chapter the molecular docking of ER and PR with TAM's metabolites, 4OHTAM, NDTAM, and NDTAM, was analyzed. The amino acids sequence of the active site for each ligand–macromolecule complex was examined. The residues that constituted each active site were analyzed separately to find the charge transfer parameter, the hydrogen bond, and the π–π interaction between the ligand and the receptor.

According to the binding energy obtained from docking, ER has greater stability than PR with the metabolites analyzed. However, in both cases there is a coupling between the receptor and the ligand, even when two of the binding energies in PR–ligand coupling are very small.

This coupling plays an important part in avoiding the transcription factor cascade reported by Leehy et al. [54].

This information agrees with the results of the chemical reactivity parameters, where it was found that the average of the chemical hardness values are lowest in active site residues of ER than in PR.

The charge transfer descriptor shows that TAM's metabolites mostly act as electron acceptors in their interaction with the hormone receptors. The hydrogen bonds in ER with END agree with the highest binding energy of this ligand. There are two hydrogen bonds, one π–π interaction, and a ΔN of –0.086. While in PR, there is only one hydrogen bond with NDTAM and the value of ΔN is –0.057.

This work described the successful combination of the methods of molecular mechanics and electronic structure. It also explored the different conformational spaces and binding modes that allow smaller systems to work with them at the electronic level.

In addition to the above a significant conclusion is that the molecular modeling and simulations are an important improvement tool for any laboratory in many industries. Currently, many sectors are moving toward using more modeling and simulations in their laboratories. As Bernard Charlès, Dassault Systèmes CEO, states: "digitalization will mean big changes for everyday lab activities down the road." Two key solutions for all industries (such as pharmaceutical, chemical, life sciences, energy, and consumer goods) are collaboration and the ability to predict using simulation and modeling [55].

Patrick Bultinck et al. in their preface to the book *Computational Medicinal Chemistry for Drug Discovery* [21] wrote: "Nowadays, one can safely state that the computational chemist has become a respectable member of a drug design team." And we can add that the docking tool is essential for most techniques for structure-based drug design.

Author details

Linda-Lucila Landeros-Martinez, Daniel Glossman-Mitnik, Erasmo Orrantia-Borunda and Norma Flores-Holguin*

*Address all correspondence to: norma.flores@cimav.edu.mx

NANOCOSMOS Virtual Lab, Department of Environment and Energy, Advanced Materials Research Center (CIMAV), Miguel de Cervantes 120, Complejo Industrial Chihuahua, Chihuahua, México

References

[1] Weidner N, Cady B, Goodson 3rd W. Pathologic prognostic factors for patients with breast carcinoma. Which factors are important. Surgical Oncology Clinics of North America. 1997;**6**(3):415-462

[2] Veronesi U, Paganelli G, Galimberti V, Viale G, Zurrida S, Bedoni M, et al. Sentinel-node biopsy to avoid axillary dissection in breast cancer with clinically negative lymph-nodes. The Lancet. 1997;**349**(9069):1864-1867

[3] Singletary SE, Allred C, Ashley P, Bassett LW, Berry D, Bland KI, et al. Revision of the American Joint Committee on Cancer staging system for breast cancer. Journal of Clinical Oncology. 2002;**20**(17):3628-3636

[4] Molina M, Reigosa A, Nobrega D, Molina Y. Receptores de estrógeno y progesterona en cáncer de mama. Asociacion con variables clinicopatologicas. Revista Salus Online Facultad de Ciencias de la Salud Universidad de Carabobo (Valencia-Venezuela). 2001;**5**:34-42

[5] Lai A, Kahraman M, Govek S, Nagasawa J, Bonnefous C, Julien J, et al. Identification of GDC-0810 (ARN-810), an orally bioavailable selective estrogen receptor degrader (SERD) that demonstrates robust activity in tamoxifen-resistant breast cancer xenografts. Journal of Medicinal Chemistry. 2015;**58**(12):4888-4904

[6] Wardell SE, Nelson ER, Chao CA, Alley HM, McDonnell DP. Evaluation of the pharmacological activities of RAD1901, a selective estrogen receptor degrader. Endocrine-related Cancer. 2015;**22**(5):713-724

[7] Srinivasan S, Nwachukwu JC, Bruno NE, Dharmarajan V, Goswami D, Kastrati I, et al. Full antagonism of the estrogen receptor without a prototypical ligand side chain. Nature Chemical Biology. 2016;**13**:111

[8] Min J, Guillen VS, Sharma A, Zhao Y, Ziegler Y, Gong P, et al. Adamantyl antiestrogens with novel side chains reveal a spectrum of activities in suppressing estrogen receptor mediated activities in breast cancer cells. Journal of Medicinal Chemistry. 2017;**60**(14):6321-6336

[9] Papageorgiou L, Cuong NT, Vlachakis D. Antibodies as stratagems against cancer. Molecular BioSystems. 2016;**12**(7):2047-2055

[10] Altmeyer C, Karam TK, Khalil NM, Mainardes RM. Tamoxifen-loaded poly(L-lactide) nanoparticles: development, characterization and in vitro evaluation of cytotoxicity. Materials Science and Engineering: C. 2016;**60**:135-142

[11] Khan MM, Wakade C, de Sevilla L, Brann DW. Selective estrogen receptor modulators (SERMs) enhance neurogenesis and spine density following focal cerebral ischemia. Journal of Steroid Biochemistry and Molecular Biology. 2015;**146**:38-47

[12] Gao L, Tu Y, Wegman P, Wingren S, Eriksson LA. Conformational enantiomerization and estrogen receptor α binding of anti-cancer drug tamoxifen and its derivatives. Journal of Chemical Information and Modeling. 2011;**51**(2):306-314

[13] Irarrázaval OME. Tamoxifeno y antidepresivos: ¿Antagonistas en la prevención del cáncer de mama? Revista médica de Chile. 2011;**139**:89-99

[14] Sanyakamdhorn S, Agudelo D, Bekale L, Tajmir-Riahi HA. Targeted conjugation of breast anticancer drug tamoxifen and its metabolites with synthetic polymers. Colloids and Surfaces B: Biointerfaces. 2016;**145**:55-63

[15] Johnson MD, Zuo H, Lee K-H, Trebley JP, Rae JM, Weatherman RV, et al. Pharmacological characterization of 4-hydroxy-N-desmethyl tamoxifen, a novel active metabolite of tamoxifen. Breast Cancer Research and Treatment. 2004;**85**(2):151-159

[16] Beverage JN, Sissung TM, Sion AM, Danesi R, Figg WD. CYP2D6 polymorphisms and the impact on tamoxifen therapy. Journal of Pharmaceutical Sciences. 2007;**96**(9):2224-2231

[17] Ng HL. Simulations reveal increased fluctuations in estrogen receptor-alpha conformation upon antagonist binding. Journal of Molecular Graphics and Modelling. 2016;**69**:72-77

[18] Landeros-Martínez LL, Orrantia-Borund E, Flores-Holguín N. Predicción de la reactividad química de Tamoxifeno en receptores hormonales. Memorias Congreso de Investigación Científica Multidisciplinaria. 2016;**4**(1):24-38

[19] Kumar V, Jain G, Kishor S, Ramaniah LM. Chemical reactivity analysis of some alkylating drug molecules—a density functional theory approach. Computational and Theoretical Chemistry. 2011;**968**(1):18-25

[20] Trott O, Olson AJ. AutoDock Vina: improving the speed and accuracy of docking with a new scoring function, efficient optimization, and multithreading. Journal of Computational Chemistry. 2010;**31**(2):455-461

[21] Bultinck P, De Winter H, Langenaeker W, Tollenare JP. Computational Medicinal Chemistry for Drug Discovery. CRC Press; 2003

[22] Mohan V, Gibbs AC, Cummings MD, Jaeger EP, DesJarlais RL. Docking: successes and challenges. Current Pharmaceutical Design. 2005;**11**(3):323-333

[23] Kitchen DB, Decornez H, Furr JR, Bajorath J. Docking and scoring in virtual screening for drug discovery: methods and applications. Nature Reviews Drug Discovery. 2004;**3**(11): 935-949

[24] DeLisle RK, Yu S-J, Nair AC, Welsh WJ. Homology modeling of the estrogen receptor subtype β (ER-β) and calculation of ligand binding affinities. Journal of Molecular Graphics and Modelling. 2001;**20**(2):155-167

[25] Manas NHA, Bakar FDA, Illias RM. Computational docking, molecular dynamics simulation and subsite structure analysis of a maltogenic amylase from Bacillus lehensis G1 provide insights into substrate and product specificity. Journal of Molecular Graphics and Modelling. 2016;**67**:1-13

[26] Maldonado-Rojas W, Olivero-Verbel J, Marrero-Ponce Y. Computational fishing of new DNA methyltransferase inhibitors from natural products. Journal of Molecular Graphics and Modelling. 2015;**60**:43-54

[27] Berman HM, Westbrook J, Feng Z, Gilliland G, Bhat TN, Weissig H, et al. The Protein Data Bank. Nucleic Acids Research. 2000;**28**(1):235-242

[28] Norgan AP, Coffman PK, Kocher J-PA, Katzmann DJ, Sosa CP. Multilevel parallelization of AutoDock 4.2. Journal of Cheminformatics. 2011;**3**(1):1

[29] Morris GM, Ruth H, Lindstrom W, Sanner MF, Belew RK, Goodsell DS, et al. Software news and updates AutoDock4 and AutoDockTools4: automated docking with selective receptor flexibility. Journal of Computational Chemistry. 2009;**30**(16):2785-2791

[30] Huey R, Morris GM, Olson AJ, Goodsell DS. A semiempirical free energy force field with charge-based desolvation. Journal of Computational Chemistry. 2007;**28**(6):1145-1152

[31] Morris GM, Goodsell DS, Halliday RS, Huey R, Hart WE, Belew RK, et al. Automated docking using a Lamarckian genetic algorithm and an empirical binding free energy function. Journal of Computational Chemistry. 1998;**19**(14):1639-1662

[32] Zhao Y, Truhlar D. The M06 suite of density functionals for main group thermochemistry, thermochemical kinetics, noncovalent interactions, excited states, and transition elements: two new functionals and systematic testing of four M06-class functionals and 12 other functionals. Theoretical Chemistry Accounts. 2008;**120**(1-3):215-241

[33] Zhao Y, Truhlar DG. Density functionals with broad applicability in chemistry. Accounts of Chemical Research. 2008;**41**(2):157-167

[34] Rassolov VA, Ratner MA, Pople JA, Redfern PC, Curtiss LA. 6-31G* basis set for third-row atoms. Journal of Computational Chemistry. 2001;**22**:976-984

[35] Tomasi J, Persico M. Molecular interactions in solution: an overview of methods based on continuous distributions of the solvent. Chemical Reviews. 1994;**94**(7):2027-2094

[36] Hohenberg P, Kohn W. Inhomogeneous electron gas. Physical Review. 1964;**136**:B864-B871

[37] Kohn W, Sham LJ. Self-consistent equations including exchange and correlation effects. Physical Review. 1965;**140**(4A):A1133-A1138

[38] Robert G, Parr YW. Density-Functional Theory of Atoms and Molecules. New York, NY, USA: Oxford University Press; 1989

[39] Frisch MJT, Trucks GW, Schlegel HB, Scuseria GE, Robb MA, Cheeseman JR, Scalmani G, Barone V, Mennucci B, Petersson GA, et al. Gaussian 09; Gaussian, Inc.: Wallingford, CT, USA; 2009

[40] Hirshfeld FL. Bonded-atom fragments for describing molecular charge densities. Theoretica Chimica Acta. 1977;**44**(2):129-138

[41] Pearson RG. Absolute electronegativity and hardness correlated with molecular orbital theory. Proceedings of the National Academy of Sciences of the United States of America. 1986;**83**(22):8440-8441

[42] Parr RG, von Szentpály L, Liu S. Electrophilicity index. Journal of the American Chemical Society. 1999;**121**(9):1922-1924

[43] Padmanabhan J, Parthasarathi R, Subramanian V, Chattaraj P. Electrophilicity-based charge transfer descriptor. Journal of Physical Chemistry A. 2007;**111**(7):1358-1361

[44] DeLano WL. The PyMOL molecular graphics system. DeLano Scientific; Palo Alto, CA, USA; 2002

[45] Samanta PN, Das KK. Prediction of binding modes and affinities of 4-substituted-2,3,5,6-tetrafluorobenzenesulfonamide inhibitors to the carbonic anhydrase receptor by docking and ONIOM calculations. Journal of Molecular Graphics and Modelling. 2016;**63**:38-48

[46] Clarke R, Liu MC, Bouker KB, Gu Z, Lee RY, Zhu Y, et al. Antiestrogen resistance in breast cancer and the role of estrogen receptor signaling. Oncogene. 2003;**22**(47):7316-7339

[47] Thomas G. Fundamentals of Medicinal Chemistry. Weinheim, Germany; 2003

[48] Shiau AK, Barstad D, Loria PM, Cheng L, Kushner PJ, Agard DA, et al. The structural basis of estrogen receptor/coactivator recognition and the antagonism of this interaction by tamoxifen. Cell. 1998;**95**(7):927-937

[49] Dávila JT, Garrán ADT. Moduladores selectivos de los receptores estrogénicos (SERMs): bioquímica, farmacología y aplicación clínica en ginecología. Ginecología y Obstetricia de México. 2005;**73**(08):424-435

[50] Hall JM, McDonnell DP. The estrogen receptor β-isoform (ERβ) of the human estrogen receptor modulates ERα transcriptional activity and is a key regulator of the cellular response to estrogens and antiestrogens. Endocrinology. 1999;**140**(12):5566-5578

[51] Wan C, Fiebig T, Schiemann O, Barton JK, Zewail AH. Femtosecond direct observation of charge transfer between bases in DNA. Proceedings of the National Academy of Sciences. 2000;**97**(26):14052-14055

[52] Kanvah S, Schuster GB. The sacrificial role of easily oxidizable sites in the protection of DNA from damage. Nucleic Acids Research. 2005;**33**(16):5133-5138

[53] Lipinski CA, Lombardo F, Dominy BW, Feeney PJ. Experimental and computational approaches to estimate solubility and permeability in drug discovery and development settings. Advanced Drug Delivery Reviews. 2001;**46**(1-3):3-26

[54] Leehy KA, Truong TH, Mauro LJ, Lange CA. Progesterone receptors (PR) mediate STAT actions: PR and prolactin receptor signaling crosstalk in breast cancer models. Journal of Steroid Biochemistry and Molecular Biology. 2018;**176**:88-93

[55] Tulsi BB. A new generation. Lab Manager 2016;**11**(1):1-100

2

Potential Anticancer Drugs Targeting Immune Pathways

Satyajit Das, Jaydip Biswas and

Soumitra Kumar Choudhuri

Abstract

Studies on the tumor microenvironment reveal that infiltration or induction of tumor-associated immune regulatory populations at the local tumor site is strongly associated with severe immunosuppression as well as worse prognosis of patients. Despite major advances in cancer immunotherapy, most of the therapeutic agents often fail to break negative immunosuppressive network to trigger anticancer immunity, leading to tumor progression and metastasis. Therefore, emergence of potent immunostimulatory agents is of great clinical importance. Emerging evidence suggests that metal chelates of Schiff bases hold the promise to overcome tumor-associated immunosuppression by inhibiting or subverting suppressive immune population toward pro-immunogenic type and thus can be used clinically for immunotherapy of different types of cancers.

Keywords: immunosuppression, tumor microenvironment, antitumor response, reactive oxygen species (ROS), tumor-associated macrophage (TAM), myeloid-derived suppressor cells (MDSC), regulatory T cell (Treg)

1. Introduction

To attain malignant phenotype, the tumor cells overcome the deadly encounter of immune system through a process known as immune editing and thus create an immunosuppressive environment [1]. This phenomenon is evident in clinical scenarios where patients with malignant tumor quite often possess a blunt immune system [2]. Thus the immune system has an impact in the progression and severity of the disease. For most of advanced malignancies where chemotherapy is considered the treatment modality of choice often rely on the strategy to target and destroy rapidly dividing cancer cells, neglecting the possibility that immune system may contribute to the efficacy of treatment. In recent years, extensive research in the context of cancer immune system has led to the development of cancer immunotherapy field that may prove to be a powerful weapon in the treatment of cancer through modulating the immune system. The suppressive roles played by immune cells of tumor microenvironment in promoting tumor progression indicate that these cells can serve as novel therapeutic targets in the treatment of cancer [3]. Emerging evidence in recent time indicates that metal chelates of Schiff base can be used as a potent anticancer agent that imparts their cytotoxic effect through generation of reactive oxygen species (ROS) in cancer cells [4]. Recent study also highlights the role of those metal chelates as immune-stimulating agents [4] that possess the ability to inhibit or subvert immunosuppressive phenotype toward proimmunogenic type and thus associated with tumor regression. In search of novel immune-stimulatory or modulatory agents, we had synthesized a number of metal chelates of a Schiff base namely N-(2-hydroxy acetophenone) glycinate (NG). Among these, copper and manganese complexes of NG, e.g., copper N-(2-hydroxy acetophenone) glycinate (CuNG) and manganese N-(2-hydroxy acetophenone) glycinate (MnNG) exhibit immunomodulatory properties [4]. Other such metal chelates of iron, nickel, and zinc formed with the same organic moiety (NG) lack the property of immunomodulation [4]. This chapter deals with the major negative regulator of immune system during cancer, as well as the key aspects of how the immune system can be controlled or manipulated by the application of novel Schiff base metal chelates to enhance anticancer immunity.

2. Negative regulator of immune system and cancer

The failure of the immune system to completely eliminate the tumor cells results in the selection of tumor cell variants that are able to resist, avoid, or suppress the antitumor immune response, leading to the escape phase [5]. The escape phase of cancer immunoediting process is activated by the simultaneous alteration of both tumor intrinsic mechanisms enabling them to hide from immune attack to avoid recognition and extrinsic mechanisms that rely on disabling or eliminating immune attack by creating suppressive environment [1, 2]. The mechanisms, at the level of tumor, that evades immunity includes the loss of tumor antigen expression, downregulation of antigen presentation through major histocompatibility complex (MHC), defects in IFN-γ receptor signaling pathway, upregulation of antiapoptotic molecules (e.g., Bcl-XL, FLIP), expression of inhibitory cell surface molecules (e.g., PD-L1, FasL), and secretion of various tumor-derived soluble factors that encourage tumor outgrowth [1, 2]. The extrinsic factor of tumor immune escape mechanism is generated by the interferences of the progressing tumor with the host immune system through the induction and/or recruitment of potent immunosuppressive cells in tumor microenvironment that ultimately hinder the induction of protective antitumor immune activity [2]. In recent years, such immune cells have gained special attention, possibly due to their ubiquitous appearance and clear association with disease progression.

Despite being considered as a major weapon of antitumor immunity, the activation, phenotype, and optimal function of T cells are regulated by a complex immunosuppressive network of tumor microenvironment [6]. Due to the weak immunogenic nature of tumor antigen, most of the tumor-specific T cells are deleted in thymic selection, resulting in low frequency of T cells with a low TCR affinity [3]. Furthermore, the presence of immunosuppressive cells in the tumor site often renders insufficient priming and boosting of T cells [3]. Over past decades, evidence implicated the fact that tumor microenvironment is dominated by Th2-type immune response than homeostatic tissue where Th1 type is prominent. Th1-type immunity promotes the expression of type 1 cytokines (TNFα, IFN-γ, and IL-2) and activates cell-mediated responses that are antitumor in nature [7]. On the other hand, Th2-type microenvironment favors the expression of type 2 cytokines (IL-4, IL-10, and TGF-β) that initiate tissue remodeling, angiogenesis, and occasional humoral immunity fostering a protumorigenic state [8]. The Th2 programming in the tumor microenvironment can be attributed by the presence of various immunosuppressive cells notably tumor-associated macrophages (TAMs), regulatory T cells (Tregs), and immature myeloid cells including the myeloid-derived suppressor cells (MDSCs) and immature dendritic cells (iDCs) that form an inhibitory network which suppresses local immunity [3]. Thus strategies involving the inhibition or subversion of suppressive immune population in tumor microenvironment hold the premise to effectively blunt Th2 programming and thereby, tilt the balance back toward Th1-based immune programs that would eventually impede tumorigenesis.

2.1. Tumor-associated macrophages (TAMs) and cancer

Macrophages are well distributed innate immune cells, known for their versatility and plasticity by exerting different functional properties in response to diverse environment stimuli. Originating from blood monocytes, macrophages are recruited into peripheral tissue where they differentiate into distinct mature macrophages by the expression of particular markers [9]. In mice, macrophages are known to exhibit phagocytic activity and express CD11b, F4/80, and colony-stimulating factor-1 receptor (CSF-1R; CD115) marker [9]. In humans, phagocytosis, CD68, CD163, CD16, CD312, and CD115 are the major characteristic features of this lineage [9]. Diverse immunological signals in tumor microenvironment lead macrophages to undergo polarized activation [10]. Such a polarization includes the "activated" macrophage (M1 macrophages) and "alternatively activated" macrophages (M2 macrophages). M1 macrophages that are activated following stimulation with Th1 cytokine IFN-γ alone or in combination with LPS or TNF-α or through engagement of Toll-like receptors (TLRs) are characterized by elevated expression of class II major histocompatibility complex (MHC), expression of interleukin (IL-12) and tumor necrosis factor α (TNF-α), generation of reactive oxygen species and nitric oxide (NO), and the ability to kill pathogens and cells [11]. Early in tumorigenesis M1 macrophages, generally characterized by an IL-12^{high} IL-10^{low} phenotype, support immune response to the nascent tumor by the secretion of large amounts of IL-12, IL-1α, IL-1β, IL-6, and TNF-α, and IFN-γ by Th1 lymphocytes. Furthermore, the induction of nitric oxide (NO) and ARG1 expression by M1 macrophages increases CTL cytotoxicity on tumor cells. In contrast, the "alternatively activated" macrophages (M2 macrophages) that differentiate in response to IL-4, IL-13, M-CSF/CSF-1, IL-10, and TGF-β1 are associated with inducing Th2-type responses, including humoral immunity and wound healing [11]. Interestingly in the context of tumor immune response, reports highlights that macrophages in tumor microenvironment are biased away from the M1 to M2 type macrophages and known as tumor-associated macrophages (TAMs) [12]. During late-stage tumor progression, TAMs exhibit an IL-12^{low} IL-10^{high} phenotype with low tumoricidal activity [12] in TME. Growing body of literature has well established the fact that TAMs have been known to provide a favorable microenvironment for tumor growth, tumor survival, and angiogenesis [11].

2.1.1. Tumor-associated macrophages (TAMs) and immunosuppression

TAMs are the major components of infiltrating immune cells in the tumor site of virtually all types of malignancies. The abundant nature of TAMs within the tumor microenvironment enables them to maintain severe immunosuppression and has been often associated with worst prognosis. During the process of tumor progression, the secretion of tumor-derived soluble factors that support the development of TAM in the local tumor sites includes M-CSF, IL-10, IL-4, and IL-13. Several studies have reported that TAM-derived secreted mediators such as TGF-β, IL-10, arginase 1, prostaglandins, and indoleamine dioxygenase (IDO) make a significant contribution to immunosuppression [13]. Poor antigen presenting capacity of TAMs reduces the tumor-specific T-cell proliferation and response by releasing the immunosuppressive factors, IL-10 and TGF-β [10]. Several studies have reported that the maturation of dendritic cells (DCs) in situ is halted by IL-10 derived from TAM but increases the differentiation of macrophages toward TAM with defective antigen presenting machinery [9, 14]. In contrast, proinflammatory cytokine IL-12 is crucial for the development of CD4+ Th1 response as CD4+ Th1 cells are a major source of IFN-γ. However, autocrine production of IL-10 by TAM is, in part, responsible for the defective LPS/IFN-γ response and reduced expression of IL-12; thereby impaired the cell-mediated immunity in tumor site [15]. Furthermore, TAMs also severely downregulate the expression of other proinflammatory cytokines such as TNF-α, IL-6, CCL3, and IL-1β, upon activation with lipopolysaccharides (LPS) [12]. Immunosuppressive cytokine TGF-β derived from TAMs promotes the development of Th2 cells, and induction and infiltration of $CD4^+CD25^+FoxP3^+$ T cells (Treg) at the tumor site [13] are also regulated by TAMs through secretion of TGF-β and IL-10. Alteration of nutrient starvation of tumor microenvironment is another strategy of tumor-associated myeloid population. Depletion of L-arginine in the tumor microenvironment is also an important mechanism of TAM-mediated T-cell suppression [12]. Metabolization of L-arginine that depends on the activity of two crucial enzymes, nitric-oxide synthase (NOS) and arginase I (ARGI), has been shown to be differentially regulated by macrophages. The expression of iNOS is upregulated by Th1 cytokines, whereas induction of arginase depends on the Th2 cytokines. Thus, in late stage of tumor, high expression of arginase is found to be associated with TAMs. Metabolism of L-arginine by ARGI to urea and L-ornithine is necessary for tumor as L-ornithine is the precursor molecules of many tumor growth factors. Furthermore, depletion of L-arginine from extracellular space inhibits the re-expression of the CD3 ζ chain, which is required for a proper T-cell activity. TAMs display a defective and delayed NFkB activation signaling, which probably provides a molecular mechanism for altered TAM functions, including defective iNOS expression [12].

2.1.2. TAMs as promising therapeutic targets in cancer therapy

Accumulated evidence has demonstrated that immunosuppressive nature of TAM favors tumor cells during tumor development and invasion, suggesting TAM as a target for clinical therapy. TAM-targeting cancer therapy involves on the strategy either by inhibition of TAM recruitment at local tumor site or by modulation of their behavior from protumorigenic M2 to antitumor M1 phenotype. The inhibition of recruitment of TAMs at tumor site can be achieved by targeting chemokine and their receptors as well as selective killing of TAM. Treatment of Met-CCL5 (receptor antagonist of CCL5) significantly reduces the number of macrophage infiltration at tumor site and promotes tumor regression [16]. The pharmacological inhibition of CCL2 with bindarit significantly reduces infiltration of macrophage and suppresses tumor growth [17]. Some studies have also shown that antitumor drug trabectedin exerts cytotoxicity on TAMs without hampering lymphoid subsets [13]. Combination of zoledronic acid with sorafenib dramatically decreases macrophage population, resulting in the enhancement of antitumor effect [16]. A number of other drugs that have also known to inhibit macrophage infiltration include thalidomide, pentoxifylline, and genistein [16]. Furthermore, inhibition of CSF-1R signaling by antibody is also associated with TAM infiltration and tumor regression [18]. Reprogramming of M2 like TAMs toward M1 type macrophage is another potential therapeutic approach. Several studies have shown that activation of TLR signaling stimulates M1 polarized macrophage response [19]. Restoration of IKKβ/NF-kβ pathway is another promising strategy to restore M1 macrophage-mediated intratumoral cytotoxicity [20]. Studies in this direction reveal that combination of CpG plus an anti-IL-10 receptor antibody switched infiltrating macrophages to M1 through restoration of NF-kβ activation thereby promote inflammatory functions [19]. These data suggest that switching the TAM phenotype from M2 to M1 during tumor progression may promote antitumor activities.

2.1.3. Novel approach for modulation of TAM behavior by CuNG

The first study that reveals CuNG as strong immunomodulator is associated with almost complete regression of drug-resistant tumor [21, 22]. CuNG treatment induces gradual reversal of immunosuppression as evident by restoration of lymphoproliferative response in drug-resistant tumor-bearing animal model. CuNG treatment in vivo increased the number of IFN-γ producing $CD4^+$ and $CD8^+$ cells but decreased the number of T regulatory marker-expressing T cells in tumor sites. Although no direct cell-mediated cytotoxicity was observed, robust expression of apoptogenic cytokines viz. IFN-γ and TNF-α at tumor site as well as peripheral and spleen mononuclear cells were sufficient enough to resolve many drug- and radiation-resistant tumors [21, 22]. This is particularly substantial as local cytokine milieu in tumor microenvironment profoundly affects the functional plasticity of macrophages, which plays a key role in skewing suppressive Th2 response toward Th1 type [11, 23]. The evocation of Th1 response largely depends on the critical level of the two regulatory cytokines, IL-10 and IL-12. IL-10 inhibits important aspects of cell-mediated immunity, whereas IL-12 induces type 1 cytokine production and effective antitumor cell-mediated response [3, 6].

Numerous therapeutic strategies involving TAM relies on reeducation or polarization of TAM suggesting that it could be possible to convert them toward nonsuppressive and antitumorigenic type by creating appropriate cytokine microenvironment [23]. Previously it was shown that in the presence of IL-12, TAMs rapidly alter their functional phenotype from tumor supportive and immunosuppressive to antitumorigenic type [24]. Our study in this direction showed that CuNG owns the potential to alter the immunosuppressive phenotype of TAMs toward proinflammatory by evoking a robust IL-12 and decreased IL-10 and TGF-β production by TAMs and thereby polarize its functional phenotype toward inflammatory both in vitro and in vivo [25]. CuNG-mediated cytokine alteration in TAMs is associated with the establishment of beneficial cytokine in tumor microenvironment that skewed the unresponsive $CD4^+$ T-cell population toward Th1 type in contact in an independent manner. The critical balance between elevated IL-12 and reduced IL-10 in CuNG treated TAMs is significant; because in one hand presence of IL-12 results in hugely elevated levels of IFN-γ [3], which limits T-cell survival and shortens Th1 response [26], on the other hand small amount of IL-10 limits the self-killing mechanism of Th1 cells and thereby prolonged its persistence [27]. Interestingly, CuNG-treated TAMs maintained a stable balance between IL-10 and IL-12 production, where IL-12 levels were higher than IL-10. This critical balance between these two cytokines was sufficient enough to induce Th1 response. Further study disclosed that in vitro treatment of CuNG significantly reduces the immunosuppressive cytokines and augments IL-12 generation in the blood monocytes of patients with metastatic cancers. Therefore, abrogation of immune suppression in tumor microenvironment through CuNG is principally due to the reprogramming of TAM in terms of their cytokine profile [25].

To decipher the underlying mechanisms of phenotypic conversion of TAM immunosuppressive ($IL\text{-}12^{low}$, $TGF\text{-}\beta^{high}$) to proimmunogenic ($IL\text{-}12^{high}$, $TGF\text{-}\beta^{low}$) type, our study in this direction reveals that CuNG induces ROS generation by TAMs, which is associated with the activation of two mitogen-activated protein kinases (MAPKs) (p38MAPK and ERK1/2), and also causes upregulation of intracellular GSH in TAMs [28]. Earlier reports showed that LPS-induced IL-12 production in normal macrophages is regulated by the activation of p38MAPK signaling [29], and activation of ERK1/2 in macrophages is associated with the production of IL-10 and TGF-β and negatively regulates IL-12 production [30–32]. CuNG-mediated ROS generation leads to the activation of p38MAPK that upregulated the initial IL-12 production and to the activation of ERK1/2 pathway along with GSH upregulation separately, found responsible for IFN-γ production by TAMs. It is important to note that GSH/oxidized GSH plays a crucial role in regulating IFN-γ-mediated augmentation of IL-12 production by macrophages and DCs. CuNG-mediated activation of ERK1/2 signaling and GSH upregulation are independently associated with IFN-γ augmentation in TAMs. This IFN-γ, further, increased the GSH production that, in turn, prolonged IL-12 production and downregulated TGF-β production, thereby plays the decisive role in CuNG-mediated reprogramming of regulatory cytokine production by TAMs. Although ROS-mediated cytokine modulation in TAMs toward proimmunogenic ($IL\text{-}12^{high}$, $TGF\text{-}\beta^{low}$) type has also been found by application of other Schiff base metal, e.g., ZnNG and FeNG [28], unlike CuNG, their effect were found to be temporary. Therefore, inclusion of copper within NG scaffold provides the compound with a unique characteristic to skew and maintain a sustained proimmunogenic phenotype in TAM.

2.2. Role of myeloid-derived suppressor cells (MDSCs) in immune regulation in cancer

2.2.1. History, origin, and phenotype

The descriptions of myeloid suppressor cells were first reported more than 20 years back in normal and tumor-bearing mice as well as in patients with cancer. Initially they were known as natural suppressor (NS) cells due to induction of tolerance to foreign antigens by inhibiting various activities of the immune system [33]. Recent evidence has disclosed that these suppressive cell populations significantly differ from normal myeloid precursors. In healthy individuals, normal hematopoiesis give rise to common myeloid progenitor cells in bone marrow, which, in turn, convert to immature myeloid cells (IMC) that ultimately differentiated into mature granulocytes, macrophages, or dendritic cells (DCs) [34]. However, in pathological conditions such as cancer, sepsis, trauma, and various infectious diseases, the differentiation of IMCs are partially blocked and thus resulting in the expansion of MDSCs [34]. Based on the origin and biological function, the term MDSCs has been suggested [35].

MDSCs are a heterogeneous group of myeloid population comprising granulocyte, monocyte, and dendritic cells, which have been prevented from fully differentiating into mature cells and are capable of suppressing the immune response [34]. They do not express the cell-surface markers that are exclusive for monocytes, macrophages, or DCs and are comprised of a mixture of myeloid cells with a morphology similar to both granulocytes and monocytes. In healthy mice, around 20–30 of cells represent this phenotype and approximately 2–4% of cells are present in the spleen, although the frequency of these cells in tumor-bearing mice is largely enhanced. In mice, MDSCs are characterized by the co-expression of the myeloid lineage differentiation antigens Gr1 and CD11b (also known as αM-integrin) [34]. Since Gr-1 antigen consists of two separate epitopes, Ly6G and Ly6C, the establishment of Ly-6C- and Ly-6G-specific mAbs has led to the identification of two MDSC subsets in the spleens of tumor-bearing mice: $CD11b^{+}Ly\text{-}6C^{low}Ly\text{-}6G^{+}$ MDSCs with granulocytic morphology (PMN-MDSCs) and $CD11b^{+}Ly\text{-}6C^{high}Ly\text{-}6G^{-}$ MDSCs with a monocytic phenotype (MO-MDSCs) [36]. The Ly6G molecule is expressed primarily by granulocytes, whereas Ly6C is highly expressed by monocytes. Although the pattern of PMN-MDSC and MO-MDSC subsets differs between tumors and organs, over 80% of MDSCs are PMN-MDSCs, whereas less than 10% of MDSCs are MO-MDSCs in most of experimental models [36]. However, it is difficult to discriminate PMN-MDSCs from neutrophils as neutrophils also express both CD11b and Ly6G.

In humans, identification of MDSCs is very difficult due to the absence of a good marker such as Gr-1 and fewer opportunities to obtain samples. However, several studies have identified PMN-MDSCs ($CD11b^{+}CD14^{-}CD15^{+}$ cells with a PMN morphology) and MO-MDSCs (being $CD11b^{+}CD14^{+}HLA\text{-}DR^{low/-}$ and secreting TGF-β) [34] in the peripheral blood of patients with cancer. Other studies have shown that PMN-MDSCs are usually defined as $CD14^{-}CD11b^{+}$ or, more narrowly, as cells expressing the common myeloid marker CD33, but lack expression of markers of mature myeloid and lymphoid cells and of the MHC class II molecule HLA-DR [34, 37]. MO-MDSCs have also been identified within a $CD15^{+}$ population in human peripheral blood [34]. In healthy individuals, IMCs represents about 0.5% of peripheral blood mononuclear cells [37]. Nevertheless, information on each human MDSC subset is much less specific than it is for mice and warrants further investigations.

2.2.2. MDSC-mediated immunosuppression in cancer

MDSC suppresses immunity by perturbing both innate and adaptive immune responses. MDSC exerts its suppressive activity against T cells through diverse mechanisms [34]. One of such mechanisms is associated with L-arginine metabolism. Expression of inducible nitric oxide synthase (iNOS) and arginase 1 (Arg1) in MDSCs is dependent on the substrate L-arginine. Arg1 and reactive oxygen species (ROS) are upregulated in activated PMN-MDSCs [36, 38], whereas Arg1 and iNOS are highly expressed in activated MO-MDSCs [39]. The upregulation of either Arg1 or iNOS results in L-arginine shortage from the tumor microenvironment, leading to consequent inhibition of T-cell proliferation through multiple mechanisms such as reduction of CD3 ζ-chain expression and IFN-γ/IL-2 secretion by T cells [40]. High levels of ROS in PMN-MDSCs can induce nitrosylation of the T-cell receptor (TCR) during direct cell-to-cell communication, which contributes to the inhibition of antigen-specific T-cell activation [34]. ROS production by PMN-MDSCs is known to be induced by several tumor-derived factors such as TGF-β, IL-6, IL-10, and GM-CSF [41]. The suppressive function of PMN-MDSCs depends on Arg1 and ROS [36, 38], whereas that of MO-MDSCs requires a signal transducer and activator of transcription 1 (STAT1) and iNOS [38]. In activated PMN-MDSCs, STAT3 is highly activated, which results in increased expression levels of ROS through the upregulation of NADPH oxidase (NOX2) but not NO production [38, 39]. On the other hand, STAT1 and iNOS are highly upregulated in MO-MDSCs, resulting in increased levels of NO but not ROS production [34]. In addition, STAT6 signaling pathway is involved in the upregulation of Arg1 and TGF-β through activation of IL-4 and IL-13, leading to immunosuppressive activity [40]. However, the immunosuppressive mechanisms overlap between G-MDSCs and M-MDSCs in human cancers. iNOS is also upregulated in PMN-MDSCs in a variety of human cancers [42–44]. $CD14^{+}HLA\text{-}DR^{-/low}$ MO-MDSCs express NADPH oxidase component gp91 (phox) and produce high level of ROS in human non-small cell lung cancers [45]. These MO-MDSCs inhibit T-cell proliferation and IFN-γ secretion in a cell-contact-dependent manner.

Another mechanism of MDSC-mediated T-cell suppression is associated with cysteine deprivation from local environment [46]. Cysteine is the essential component required for T-cell activation, differentiation, and proliferation, which they cannot synthesize; rather dependent on antigen-presenting cells. Dendritic cells and macrophages can deliver cysteine to T cells by converting methionine and cystine to cysteine [47]. Like the APCs, MDSCs also import extracellular cystine for converting it to cysteine, but unlike APCs, they do not export cysteine, leading to lack of cystine from local environment for dendritic cells and macrophage [46].

The potential suppressive property of MDSCs can also be reflected on the innate immunity. Studies have shown that MDSCs impair NK-cell development, IFN-γ production, and cytotoxicity against tumor cells. This suppression is mediated by membrane-bound TGF-β1 and through downregulation of NKG2D (the primary activating receptor for NK cells) [48]. Cytotoxic activity of NK cell and their apoptogenic cytokine secretion is also disrupted by $CD14^{+}HLA\text{-}DR^{-/lo}$ MO-MDSCs secretion in a cell-contact-dependent manner in human hepatocellular carcinoma [48]. The inhibition of NK cells is independent on arginase activity. The similar inhibitory mechanism of NK-cell development and functions by IL-1β-induced PMN-MDSCs have been also demonstrated in a mouse model [49]. Furthermore, MDSCs can skew macrophage-derived cytokine profiles from type 1 to type 2 putatively through Toll-like receptor 4 signaling pathway [49]. This effect is amplified by macrophages that increase the MDSC production of IL-10. Indeed, increased MDSC levels in peripheral blood and tumor are closely associated with the infiltration of CD163$^+$ M2 macrophages in human esophageal cancer [50].

2.2.3. Therapeutic strategies against MDSCs

Several strategies that are currently being tested against MDSCs to break the immunosuppressive network can broadly be categorized into four groups.

A first strategy would be promoting the differentiation of MDSCs into mature, non-suppressive cells. A number of agents, e.g., all-trans retinoic acid (ATRA), have been identified as a candidate agent that possesses this ability, which favors MDSC differentiation into mature DC, macrophages, and granulocytes [51]. Treatment of ATRA on mouse or human MDSCs results in the induction of myeloid cell differentiation both in vitro and in vivo and thereby improves antitumor immune responses [51]. However, ATRA was also shown to induce the development of CD4$^+$ regulatory T cells (Tregs), by upregulating expression of the T cell cell-fate regulatory transcription factor FoxP3 [52]. Thus, ATRA is not an ideal candidate for MDSC depletion, as simultaneous Treg induction induced by ATRA treatment could further contribute to tumor development. Another promoter of MDSCs differentiation is 25-dihydroxyvitamin D3, which has been reported to drive myeloid progenitor cell differentiation both in vitro and in vivo [52, 53]. Treatment in patients with head and neck squamous cell carcinoma resulted in reduction of the circulating CD34$^+$ MDSCs with increased levels of plasma IL-12 and IFN-γ and T-cell proliferation. However, in another study, 25-hydroxyvitamin D_3 alone has failed to improve the clinical outcome [52, 53].

Second promising approach is to inhibit or block the expansion of MDSCs. Many tumor-derived factors can induce the development and expansion of MDSCs from hematopoietic precursors. Several neutralizing antibodies or inhibitors against tumor-derived factors or those receptors such as GM-CSF, GMCSF receptor (GM-CSFR), M-CSF, M-CSF receptor (MCSFR), G-CSF, VEGF-A, or stem cell factor (SCF or KI) [52–54], and MMPs have been reported to inhibit MDSC expansion or mobilization. However, anti-VEGFA monoclonal antibody, bevacizumab, could not reduce the accumulation of MDSCs in human renal cell cancer [53].

Thirdly, MDSCs can be selectively depleted in pathological settings by employing certain chemotherapeutic agents such as sunitinib, cimetidine, gemcitabine, and 5-fluorouracil (5-FU) [53]. Application of such drugs in tumor-bearing hosts resulted in a dramatic decrease in the number of MDSCs and a marked improvement in the antitumor response. Treatment with 5-fluorouracil (5-FU) selectively induced apoptosis in MDSCs, resulting in delayed tumor growth with concurrent T-cell-dependent antitumor responses. As compared to gemcitabine, 5-FU induced a more potent apoptosis-mediated MDSC depletion in vitro and in vivo. However, one study shows that a combination of gemcitabine and capecitabine does not affect the levels of MDSCs in patients with advanced pancreatic cancer [52]. Furthermore, 5-FU treatment was not curative in this tumor model because of Nlrp3 inflammasome induction, which led to MDSC-derived IL-1β secretion and angiogenesis [53]. Attempts have also been made to deplete Gr-1$^+$ MDSCs by using anti-Gr-1 antibody that result in delayed tumor growth in mice [53]. However, this antibody also targets neutrophils, thus lacking the necessary specificity for clinical use.

Fourthly, another attractive way to control MDSC function would be interrupting the underlying signaling pathways that are responsible for the production of suppressive factors by these cells. The molecules that can be effectively targeted for this purpose include cyclooxygenase 2, arginase 1, iNOS, and indoleamine 2,3-dioxygenase [52]. Since ARG1 and iNOS are the primary enzymes responsible for MDSC immunosuppression, these enzymes are the most likely targets for novel therapeutic interventions. Various different drugs including nitroaspirin, COX-2 inhibitors, and phosphodiesterase-5 (PDE5) inhibitors have been shown to profoundly inhibit both ARG1 and iNOS activity in MDSC. By removing MDSC suppressive mediators, these drugs exhibited a potent ability to restore antitumor immune responses and delayed tumor progression in several mouse models [52–54]. Interestingly, in addition to inhibiting MDSC function, COX2 inhibitors also blocked the systemic development of MDSC as well as CCL2-mediated accumulation of these cells in the tumor microenvironment in a mouse model of glioma [52, 54].

2.2.4. Novel therapeutic strategies against MDSCs

Although various agents such as chemotherapeutic drugs, vitamin derivative, and mAb are widely applied against MDSCs, only few of them are known to exhibit their inhibitory effect directly on MDSCs. Moreover, restricted use of these drugs on certain conditions or cancer patients often opens the possibility to apply emerging agents that bear direct inhibitory effect on MDSCs.

Earlier investigations reveal CuNG as a strong immunomodulator that successfully induce the conversion of immunosuppressive TAMs toward proimmunogenic type, enhancing Th1 response sufficient to resolve drug-resistant cancer in animal model. Interestingly, the effect of CuNG is not exclusive to TAMs; rather it also targets MDSCs which happens to be another strong negative regulator of tumor immunity [55]. Treatment with CuNG in drug-resistant mice severely abrogates the accumulation of MDSCs in spleen as well as tumor site. Further study discloses that this reduction was associated with enhanced Th1 responses (evident from increase in IFN-γ production) and diminished Th2 responses (decrease in IL-4 production) as well as decline in Foxp3$^+$Treg numbers [55]. Detailed investigation reveals the underlying mechanism that is associated with Fas-FasL interaction between MDSCs and CD4$^+$T cells. Treatment of CuNG increases the FasR expression in MDSCs and FasL in CD4$^+$T cells. Although FasL expression is enhanced, FasR expression in CD4$^+$ T cells was not observed following the treatment that determines the specificity of CuNG [55].

Another study that deals with metal chelate of Schiff's base is associated with the immunomodulation of tumor microenvironment. Metal chelate of manganese (MnNG) can have a number of valence states and possess the ability to modulate the immunosuppressive TME by reducing the number of tumor-associated MDSCs in drug-resistant tumor-bearing mice. A closer look at MnNG-mediated action reveals that it promotes MDSC differentiation into dendritic cells but not toward macrophages [56]. Additionally, it helps in the proliferation of T cells that ultimately skew Th2 immunity toward protective Th1 response. Thus MnNG may help in the differentiation of immunosuppressive MDSCs toward dendritic cells and with the upregulation of costimulatory molecules, namely CD80 and CD86, enabling them to act as better antigen-presenting cells (APCs) that ultimately generate protective antitumor immunity [56]. However, the plausible molecular mechanism underlying MnNG-mediated differentiation of MDSCs in TME is still elusive and warrants further investigations.

2.3. T-regulatory cells in cancer

The tumor escape of immune surveillance is also achieved by the recruitment of immunosuppressive $CD4^+CD25^+FoxP3^+$ Tregs into the tumor microenvironment. The phenotype and functional properties of Tregs are similar in mice and human. They include both natural Treg (nTreg) and locally induced Treg (iTreg) cells [57, 58]. nTreg cells are derived from thymus without specific antigenic stimulation and represents a small fraction (5–6%) of total $CD4^+$ T cells. They are characterized by the expression of CD25, FoxP3, and GITR [3]. $CD4^+$ or IL-10 expressing iTreg cells are also known to express high levels of Foxp3 and GITR [58]. Induced Tregs are emerged from naive T cells by specific modes of antigenic stimulation, especially in a particular cytokine milieu [57, 58]. Both subsets possess a strong capacity to suppress the immune system, although they differ in a distinct suppressive mechanism. A large number of $CD4^+CD25^+FoxP3^+$ Treg cells are found in both the circulation and tumor site of different cancer-bearing patients and their number inversely proportional to the survival of the patients. They are either naturally occurring or locally induced Treg population [58]. Experimental observation reveals that chemokine CCL2 produced by tumor and its associated macrophages facilitate the recruitment of thymus-derived Treg cells in tumor microenvironment [3]. Defective myeloid DCs also induced $IL\text{-}10^+$ regulatory T cells in vitro and in vivo in patients with cancer. Conversion of Treg from $CD4^+CD25^-$ T cells depends on local cytokine milieu. Immunosuppressive cytokines such as TGF-β and IL-10, which are present at high levels in the tumor microenvironment, might mediate induction and differentiation of iTreg cells [58]. Recent studies also highlighted the role of MDSCs to facilitate the de novo development of Tregs through TGF-β dependent and independent pathways [34].

2.3.1. Tregs and immunosuppression

Tumor-associated Tregs suppress both the innate and the adaptive immune responses. The suppressive function of tumor-induced Tregs depends on the antigen-specific stimulation of these cells. Once activated, they efficiently suppress $CD4^+$ and $CD8^+$ T cells in an antigen non-specific manner [58]. This suppressive potential of Tregs depends on the cell-cell contact and soluble mediators (e.g., TGF-β and IL-10) released by Tregs. Recent evidence suggests that Treg exerts immunosuppressive function by lowering the endogenous TAA-specific T-cell immunity, thereby contributing to tumor progression [3]. Furthermore, the progressive infiltration and induction of Treg tilt the balance between Treg cells and effector T cells toward immunosuppression. This is, in part, mediated by competition for IL-2 between Tregs and conventional T cells. IL-2 promotes the differentiation of T cells into effector T cells. Interestingly, it also promotes the differentiation of immature T cells into regulatory T cells. Therefore, competitive consumption of IL-2 is also indirectly related to suppressive mechanism for Tregs in established tumors [59]. Another effective way to suppress T-cell activation and promote tolerance is to reduce the availability of tryptophan, which is performed by the IDO+ APC in the tumor microenvironment. CTLA4+ Tregs help inducing the expression of IDO in APCs through CTLA4 to mediate their suppressive activity [60]. Furthermore, Tregs also downregulate the expression of CD80 and CD86 through CTLA-4 and induce immunosuppressive costimulatory molecule B7-H4 on DCs by IL-10 and thus hamper activation of other T cells by DCs [61]. Additionally, Treg-mediated suppression of natural killer (NK)-cell function is associated with TGF-β in tumor-bearing mice [62].

2.3.2. Therapy against Tregs

Tregs within tumor site are crucial components for tumor immunosuppression. Therefore depletion or functional inhibition could be a promising strategy for inducing antitumor immunity. Selective depletion of Tregs can be achieved by anti-CD25 antibody, which significantly improves T cell-mediated tumor regression [58, 62]. CTLA4 is another potential target. Administration of CTLA4-specific antibody with cancer vaccine effectively reduces Tregs and improves immunity [58, 62]. However, blocking of CTLA4 is strongly associated with the induction of autoimmune manifestation [58, 62]. Furthermore, this antibody fails to induce depletion of peripheral Tregls. An alternative therapeutic approach for the depletion of Tregs is the use of denileukin diftitox (Ontak®), which is a ligand toxin fusion consisting of full-length IL-2 fused to the enzymatically active and translocating domains of diphtheria toxin. The complex inhibits protein synthesis, leading to apoptosis of Tregs [3]. A recent study indicates that treatment with this complex significantly reduces the absolute number of peripheral Tregs and increases effector T-cell activation in different cancer patients. However, this requires further detailed investigation.

2.3.3. CuNG-mediated Treg modulation

Another promising approach for blocking the infiltration or functional modulation of Treg includes the application of novel metal containing drug, e.g., CuNG that might have therapeutic advantages. Previously, it was found that a sizable proportion of CD4+ cells of drug-resistant tumor-bearing mice exhibited T-regulatory markers (CD25 and Foxp3). After in vivo treatment of CuNG, only a few CD25+Foxp3+ cells were observed in tumor-bearing mice [22, 25]. Moreover, CuNG-treated TAMs could modulate TGF-β producing CD4+CD25+ T cells toward IFN-γ producing T cells with concomitant decrease in the level of FoxP3 expression, indicating that Treg can be reprogrammed toward Th1 phenotype. However, this approach requires further investigations.

3. Conclusion

Cancer is a major problem worldwide and is the most common cause of death in many countries. Although treatment with conventional chemotherapy is widely successful, it fails to induce potent antitumor immune response. Emerging evidence indicates that treatment with metal-containing agents destroy cancer cells through ROS generation and also shows the way to cure cancer through inhibition or subvertion of immunosuppressive network toward proimmunogenic type. Strategies to target these molecular pathways by novel, cost-effective, redox-active molecules may usher a new era in immune therapy.

Author details

Satyajit Das, Jaydip Biswas and Soumitra Kumar Choudhuri*

*Address all correspondence to: soumitra01@yahoo.com

Department of In Vitro Carcinogenesis and Cellular Chemotherapy, Chittaranjan National Cancer Institute, Kolkata, India

References

[1] Kim R, Emi M, Tanabe K, Arihiro K. Tumor-driven evolution of immunosuppressive networks during malignant progression. Cancer Res. 2006,**66**:5527–5536. DOI: 10.1158/0008-5472.CAN-05-4128

[2] Finn OJ. Immuno-oncology: understanding the function and dysfunction of the immune system in cancer. Ann Oncol. 2012,**23**:viii6-9. DOI: 10.1093/annonc/mds256.

[3] Zou W. Immunosuppressive networks in the tumour environment and their therapeutic relevance. Nat Rev Cancer. 2005,**5**:263-74. DOI:10.1038/nrc1586

[4] Ganguly A, Chakraborty P, Banerjee K, Choudhuri SK. The role of a Schiff base scaffold N-(2-hydroxy acetophenone) glycinate-in overcoming multidrug resistance in cancer. Eur J Pharm Sci. 2014,**51**:96-109. doi. 10.1016/j.ejps.2013.09.003

[5] Dunn GP, Old LJ, Schreiber RD. The three Es of cancer immunoediting. Annu Rev Immunol. 2004,**22**:329–60. DOI: 10.1146/annurev.immunol.22.012703.104803

[6] Smyth MJ, Godfrey DI, Trapani JA. A fresh look at tumor immunosurveillance and immunotherapy. Nat Immunol. 2001,**2**:293–299. DOI: 10.1038/86297

[7] Knutson KL, Disis ML. Tumor antigen-specific T helper cells in cancer immunity and immunotherapy. Cancer Immunol Immunother. 2005,**54**:721-728. DOI: 10.1007/s00262-004-0653-2

[8] Ruffell B, Denardo DG, Affara NI, Coussens LM. Lymphocytes in cancer development: polarization towards protumor immunity. Cytokine Growth Factor Rev. 2001,**21**:3–10. DOI: 10.1016/j.cytogfr.2009.11.002

[9] Qian BZ, Pollard JW. Macrophage diversity enhances tumor progression and metastasis. Cell. 2010,**41**:39-51. DOI: 10.1016/j.cell.2010.03.014

[10] Mantovani A, Sica A. Macrophages innate immunity and cancer. balance tolerance and diversity. Curr Opin Immunol. 2010,**22**:231–237. DOI: 10.1016/j.coi.2010.01.009

[11] Gordon S, Taylor PR. Monocyte and macrophage heterogeneity. Nat Rev Immunol. 2005,**5**:953–964. DOI: 10.1038/nri1733

[12] Biswas SK, Mantovani A. Macrophage plasticity and interaction with lymphocyte subsets. cancer as a paradigm. Nat Immunol. 2010,**11**:889–896. DOI: 10.1038/ni.1937

[13] Allavena P, Sica A, Garlanda C, Mantovani A. The Yin-Yang of tumor-associated macrophages in neoplastic progression and immune surveillance. Immunol Rev. 2008,**222**: 155–161. DOI: 10.1111/j.1600-065X.2008.00607.x

[14] Ben-Baruch A. Inflammation-associated immune suppression in cancer: the roles played by cytokines chemokines and additional mediators. Sem Cancer Biol. 2006,**16**: 38–52. DOI:10.1016/j.semcancer.2005.07.006

[15] Sica A, Saccani A, Bottazzi B, Polentarutti N, Vecchi A, van Damme J, Mantovani A. Autocrine production of IL-10 mediates defective IL-12 production and NF-kappa B activation in tumor-associated macrophages. J Immunol. 2010,**164**:762–767. DOI: 10.4049/jimmunol.164.2.762

[16] Hao NB, Lü MH, Fan YH, Cao YL, Zhang ZR, Yang SM. Macrophages in tumor microenvironments and the progression of tumors. Clin Dev Immunol. 2012,**2012**:948098. DOI: 10.1155/2012/948098

[17] Gazzaniga S, Bravo AI, Guglielmotti A, van Rooijen N, Maschi F, Vecchi A, Mantovani A, Mordoh J, Wainstok R. Targeting tumor-associated macrophages and inhibition of MCP-1 reduce angiogenesis and tumor growth in a human melanoma xenograft. J Invest Dermatol. 2007,**127**:2031–2041. DOI: 10.1038/sj.jid.5700827

[18] Kubota Y, Takubo K, Shimizu T, Ohno H, Kishi K, Shibuya M, Saya H, Suda T. M-CSF inhibition selectively targets pathological angiogenesis and lymphangiogenesis. J Exp Med. 2009,**206**:1089–1102. DOI: 10.1084/jem.20081605

[19] Krieg AM. Therapeutic potential of Toll-like receptor 9 activation. Nat Rev Drug Discov. 2006,**5**:471–484. DOI: 10.1038/nrd2059

[20] Greten FR, Eckmann L, Greten TF, Park JM, Li ZW, Egan LJ, Kagnoff MF, Karin M. IKK beta links inflammation and tumorigenesis in a mouse model of colitis-associated cancer. Cell. 2014,**118**:285–296. DOI: 10.1016/j.cell.2004.07.013

[21] Mookerjee A, Basu JM, Dutta P, Majumder J, Bhattacharya S, Biswas J, Pal S, Mukherjee P, Raha S, Baral RN, Das T, Efferth T, Sa G, Roy S, Choudhuri SK. Overcoming drug resistant in cancer by a newly developed copper chelate through host protective cytokine mediated apoptosis. Clin Cancer Res. 2006,**12**:4339–4349. DOI: 10.1158/1078-0432.CCR-06-0001

[22] Mookerjee A, Basu JM, Majumder S, Chatterjee S, Panda GS, Dutta P, Pal S, Mukherjee P, Efferth T, Roy S, Choudhuri SK. A novel copper complex induces ROS generation in

doxorubicin resistant Ehrlich ascites carcinoma cells and increases activity of antioxidant enzymes in vital organs in vivo. BMC Cancer. 2006,**6**:267–277. DOI: 10.1186/1471-2407-6-267

[23] Stout RD, Jiang C, Matta B, Tietzel I, Watkins SK, Suttles J. Macrophages sequentially change their functional phenotype in response to changes in micro environmental influences. J Immunol. 2005,**175**:342–349. DOI: 10.4049/jimmunol.175.1.342

[24] Watkins SK, Egilmez NK, Suttles J, Stout RD. IL-12 rapidly alters the functional profile of tumor-associated and tumor-infiltrating macrophages in vitro and in vivo. J Immunol. 2007,**178**:1357–1362. DOI: 10.4049/jimmunol.178.3.1357

[25] Chatterjee S, Mookerjee A, Mookerjee-Basu J, Chakraborty P, Ganguly A, Adhikary A, Mukhopadhyay D, Ganguli S, Banerjee R, Ashraf M, Biswas J, Das PK, Sa G, Chatterjee M, Das T, Choudhuri SK. A novel copper chelate modulates tumor associated macrophages to promote anti-tumor response of T cells. PLoS One. 2009,**4**:e7048. DOI:10.1371/journal.pone.0007048

[26] Murphy KM, Reiner SL. The lineage decision of helper T cells. Nat Rev Immunol. 2002,**2**:933–944. DOI:10.1038/nri954

[27] Oral HB, Kotenko SV, Yilmaz M, Mani O, Zumkehr J, Blaser K, Akdis CA, Akdis M. Regulation of T cells and cytokines by the interleukin-10 [IL-10]-family cytokines IL-19 IL-20 IL-22 IL-24 and IL-26. Eur J Immunol. 2006,**36**:380-388. DOI:10.1002/eji.200425523

[28] Chakraborty P, Chatterjee S, Ganguly A, Saha P, Adhikari A, Das T, Chatterjee M, Mookerjee-Basu J, Choudhuri SK. Reprogramming of TAM toward proimmunogenic type through regulation of MAP kinases using a redox-active copper chelate. J Leukoc Biol. 2012,**91**:609–619. DOI:10.1189/jlb.0611287

[29] Dobashi K, Aihara M, Araki T, Shimizu Y, Utsugi M, Iizuka K, Murata Y, Hamuro J, Nakazawa J, Mori M. Regulation of LPS induced IL-12 production by IFN-γ and IL-4 through intracellular glutathione status in human alveolar macrophages. Clin Exp Immunol. 2001,124:290–296. DOI: 10.1046/j.1365-2249.2001.01535.x

[30] Otsuka M, Goto K, Tsuchiya S, Aramaki Y. Phosphatidylserine specific receptor contributes to TGF-β production in macrophages through a MAP kinase ERK. Biol Pharm Bull. 2005,**28**:1707–1710. DOI:10.1248/bpb.28.1707

[31] Mathur RK, Awasthi A, Wadhone P, Ramanamurthy B, Saha B. Reciprocal CD40 signals through p38MAPK and ERK-1/2 induce counteracting immune responses. Nat Med. 2004,**10**:540–544. DOI:10.1038/nm1045

[32] Feng GJ, Goodridge HS, Harnett MM, Wei X Q, Nikolaev AV, Higson AP, Liew FY. Extracellular signal-related kinase (ERK) and p38 mitogen-activated protein (MAP) kinases differentially regulate the lipopolysaccharide-mediated induction of inducible nitric oxide synthase and IL-12 in macrophages. Leishmania phosphoglycans subvert macrophage IL-12 production by targeting ERK MAP kinase. J Immunol. 1997,**163**:6403–6412.

[33] Strober S. Natural suppressor (NS) cells neonatal tolerance and total lymphoid irradiation: exploring obscure relationships. Annu Rev Immunol. 1984,**2**:219-237. DOI:10.1146/annurev.iy.02.040184.001251

[34] Gabrilovich DI, Nagaraj S. Myeloid-derived suppressor cells as regulators of the immune system. Nat Rev Immunol. 2009,**9**:162–174. DOI:10.1038/nri2506

[35] Gabrilovich DI, Bronte V, Chen SH, Colombo MP, Ochoa A, Ostrand-Rosenberg S, Schreiber H. The terminology issue for myeloid-derived suppressor cells. Cancer Res. 2007,**67**:425-426. DOI:10.1158/0008-5472.CAN-06-3037

[36] Youn JI, Nagaraj S, Collazo M, Gabrilovich DI. Subsets of myeloid-derived suppressor cells in tumor-bearing mice. J Immunol. 2008,**181**:5791–5802. DOI: 10.4049/jimmunol.181.8.5791

[37] Almand B, Clark JI, Nikitina E, van Beynen J, English NR, Knight SC, Carbone DP, Gabrilovich DI. Increased production of immature myeloid cells in cancer patients: a mechanism of immunosuppression in cancer. J Immunol. 2001,**166**:678-689. DOI: 10.4049/jimmunol.166.1.678

[38] Movahedi K, Guilliams M, Van den Bossche J, Van den Bergh R, Gysemans C, Beschin A, De Baetselier P, Van Ginderachter JA. Identification of discrete tumor-induced myeloid-derived suppressor cell subpopulations with distinct T cell-suppressive activity. Blood. 2008,**111**:4233-4244. DOI:10.1182/blood-2007-07-099226

[39] Mazzoni A, Bronte V, Visintin A, Spitzer JH, Apolloni E, Serafini P, Zanovello P, Segal DM. Myeloid suppressor lines inhibit T cell responses by an NO-dependent mechanism. J Immunol. 2002,**168**:689–695. DOI: 10.4049/jimmunol.168.2.689

[40] Bronte V, Zanovello P. Regulation of immune responses by L-arginine metabolism. Nat Rev Immunol. 2005,**5**:641–654. DOI:10.1038/nri1668

[41] Sauer H, Wartenberg M, Hescheler J. Reactive oxygen species as intracellular messengers during cell growth and differentiation. Cell Physiol Biochem. 2001,**11**:173–186. DOI:10.1159/000047804

[42] Liu CY, Wang YM, Wang CL, Feng PH, Ko HW, Liu YH, Wu YC, Chu Y, Chung FT, Kuo CH, Lee KY, Lin SM, Lin HC, Wang CH, Yu CT, Kuo HP. Population alterations of l-arginase- and inducible nitric oxide synthase-expressed $CD11b^{+}/CD14^{-}/CD15^{+}/CD33^{+}$ myeloid-derived suppressor cells and $CD8^{+}$ T lymphocytes in patients with advanced-stage non-small cell lung cancer. J Cancer Res Clin Oncol. 2010,**136**:35–45. DOI:10.1007/s00432-009-0634-0

[43] Jiao ZJ Gao JJ, Hua SH, Chen DY, Wang WH, Wang H, Wang XH, Xu HX. Correlation between circulating myeloid-derived suppressor cells and Th17 cells in esophageal cancer. World J Gastroenterol. 2012,**18**:5454-61. DOI: 10.3748/wjg.v18.i38.5454

[44] Lechner MG, Megiel C, Russell SM, Bingham B, Arger N, Woo T, Epstein AL. Functional characterization of human $Cd33^{+}$ and $Cd11b^{+}$ myeloid-derived suppressor cell subsets

induced from peripheral blood mononuclear cells co-cultured with a diverse set of human tumor cell lines. J Transl Med. 2001,**9**:90. DOI:10.1186/1479-5876-9-90

[45] Huang B, Pan PY, Li Q, Sato AI, Levy DE, Bromberg J, Divino CM, Chen SH. Gr-1+CD115 + immature myeloid suppressor cells mediate the development of tumor induced T regulatory cells and T-cell anergy in tumor-bearing host. Cancer Res. 2013,**66**:1123–1131. DOI:10.1158/0008-5472.CAN-05-1299

[46] Srivastava MK, Sinha P, Clements VK, Rodriguez P, Ostrand-Rosenberg S. Myeloid derived suppressor cells inhibit T-cell activation by depleting cystine and cysteine. Cancer Res. 2010,**70**:68–77. DOI:10.1158/0008-5472.CAN-09-2587

[47] Angelini G, Gardella S, Ardy M, Ciriolo MR, Filomeni G, Di Trapani G, Clarke F, Sitia R, Rubartelli A. Antigen-presenting dendritic cells provide the reducing extracellular microenvironment required for T lymphocyte activation. Proc Natl Acad Sci U S A. 2002,**99**:1491–1496. DOI:10.1073/pnas.022630299

[48] Li H, Han Y, Guo Q, Zhang M, Cao X. Cancer-expanded myeloid-derived suppressor cells induce anergy of NK cells through membrane-bound TGF-beta 1. J Immunol. 2009,**182**: 240-249. DOI: 10.4049/jimmunol.182.1.240

[49] Bunt SK, Clements VK, Hanson EM, Sinha P, Ostrand-Rosenberg S. Inflammation enhances myeloid-derived suppressor cell cross-talk by signaling through Toll-like receptor 4. J Leukoc Biol. 2009,**85**:996–1004. DOI:10.1189/jlb.0708446

[50] Gao J, Wu Y, Su Z, Amoah Barnie P, Jiao Z, Bie Q, Lu L, Wang S, Xu H. Infiltration of alternatively activated macrophages in cancer tissue is associated with MDSC and Th2 polarization in patients with esophageal cancer. PLoS One. 2014,**9**:e104453. DOI:10.1371/journal.pone.0104453

[51] Nefedova Y, Fishman M, Sherman S, Wang X, Beg AA, Gabrilovich DI. Mechanism of all-trans retinoic acid effect on tumor-associated myeloid-derived suppressor cells. Cancer Res. 2007,**67**:11021–11028. DOI:10.1158/0008-5472.CAN-07-2593

[52] Katoh H, Watanabe M. Myeloid-derived suppressor cells and therapeutic strategies in cancer. Mediat Inflamm. 2015,**2015**:159269. DOI:10.1155/2015/159269

[53] Wesolowski R, Markowitz J, Carson WE. Myeloid derived suppressor cells—a new therapeutic target in the treatment of cancer. J Immunother Cancer. 2013,**1**:10. DOI:10.1186/2051-1426-1-10

[54] Di Mitri D, Toso A, Alimonti A. Molecular pathways targeting tumor-infiltrating myeloid-derived suppressor cells for cancer therapy. Clin Cancer Res. 2015,**21**:3108-3112. DOI:10.1158/1078-0432.CCR-14-2261

[55] Chakraborty P, Das S, Banerjee K, Sinha A, Roy S, Chatterjee M, Choudhuri SK. A copper chelate selectively triggers apoptosis in myeloid-derived suppressor cells in a drug-resistant tumor model and enhances antitumor immune response. Immunopharmacol Immunotoxicol. 2014,**36**:165-75. DOI:10.3109/08923973.2014.897727

[56] Das S, Banerjee K, Roy S, Majumder S, Chatterjee M, Majumdar S, Choudhuri SK. Mn complex-mediated enhancement of antitumor response through modulating myeloid-derived suppressor cells in drug-resistant tumor. In Vivo. 2014,**28**:909-918.

[57] Sakaguchi S, Setoguchi R, Yagi H, Nomura T. Naturally arising Foxp3-expressing CD25 +CD4+ regulatory T cells in self-tolerance and autoimmune disease. Curr Top Microbiol Immunol. 2006,**305**:51–66. DOI:10.1038/ni1178

[58] Zou W. Regulatory T cells tumour immunity and immunotherapy. Nat Rev Immunol. 2006,**6**:295-307. DOI:10.1038/nri1806

[59] De la Rosa M, Rutz S, Dorninger H, Scheffold A. Interleukin-2 is essential for CD4+CD25+ regulatory T cell function. Eur J Immunol. 2004,**34**;2480–2488. DOI:10.1002/eji.200425274

[60] Fallarino F, Grohmann U, Hwang KW, Orabona C, Vacca C, Bianchi R, Belladonna ML, Fioretti MC, Alegre ML, Puccetti P. Modulation of tryptophan catabolism by regulatory T cells. Nat Immunol. 2003,**4**:1206–1212. DOI:10.1038/ni1003

[61] Misra N, Bayry J, Lacroix-Desmazes S, Kazatchkine MD, Kaveri SV. Human CD4+CD25+ T cells restrain the maturation and antigen-presenting function of dendritic cells. J Immunol. 2004,**172**:4676–4680. DOI:10.4049/jimmunol.172.8.4676

[62] Shevach EM. CD4+ CD25+ suppressor T cells: more questions than answers. Nat Rev Immunol. 2002,**2**:389–400. DOI:10.1038/nri821

3

Aurora Kinases: New Molecular Targets for the Therapy of Aggressive Thyroid Cancers

Enke Baldini, Chiara Tuccilli, Salvatore Sorrenti,
Domenico Mascagni, Stefano Arcieri,
Angelo Filippini and Salvatore Ulisse

Abstract

Epithelial thyroid carcinomas (TC) account for more than 90% of all endocrine malignancies and represent one of the most frequent cancers in women. They include the well-differentiated TC (DTC), comprising the papillary (PTC) and follicular (FTC) histotypes, the poorly differentiated (PDTC), and the undifferentiated or anaplastic TC (ATC). Both PDTC and ATC are aggressive human neoplasms with a dire prognosis due to the absence of effective therapies, which makes mandatory the identification of novel therapeutic strategies. Intrinsic chromosomal instability (CIN, an increased rate of gain or losses of chromosomes during cell division) is a common feature of solid tumors and represents a major driving force in thyroid cancer progression, thought to be responsible for the acquisition by malignant cells of novel functional capabilities. Different mitotic kinases, whose expression or function has been found altered in human cancer tissues, are major drivers of thyroid tumor aneuploidy. Among these are the three members of the Aurora family (Aurora-A, Aurora-B and Aurora-C), serine/threonine kinases that regulate multiple aspects of chromosome segregation and cytokinesis. Over the last few years, several small molecule inhibitors targeting Aurora kinases were developed with promising antitumor effects in preclinical and clinical studies against different human cancers, including TC. Here, we will focus on the Aurora mitotic functions in normal cells; we shall then describe the main implications of their overexpression in the onset of genetic instability and aneuploidy. We will finally describe the consequences of Aurora kinase inhibition on TC cell growth and tumorigenicity.

Keywords: thyroid cancers, Aurora kinases, mitosis, therapy, Aurora kinase inhibitors

1. Introduction

The incidence of thyroid cancer (TC) has increased from about five new cases per 100,000 persons observed in the early 90s to 15 new cases per 100,000 persons recorded in 2012 [1]. This increase is mainly due to the improved ability to detect malignancy in small thyroid nodules [2, 3]. TC represents about 96% of all endocrine malignancies and one of the most frequent cancers in women [1]. Based on histological and clinical criteria, TC are classified as well-differentiated TC (DTC), which includes the papillary (PTC) and follicular (FTC) histotypes, poorly differentiated TC (PDTC), and anaplastic TC (ATC). The PTC accounts for about 86% of all epithelial TC. It appears as a mass of branching papillae covered by cells with eosinophilic cytoplasm and enlarged nuclei and typically metastasizes via lymphatic vessels to local lymph nodes [4]. The FTC accounts for approximately 9% of all TC. It resembles the normal microscopic pattern of the thyroid and is characterized by hematogenous spread producing lung and bone metastases [4]. The less differentiated and more aggressive PDTC and ATC, each of which accounts for 1–2% of all TC, are thought to develop from the dedifferentiation of DTC, according to the multistep model of thyroid carcinogenesis [4–8]. The PDTC was included as a separate entity in the WHO classification of TC in 2004. PDTC retains sufficient differentiation to produce scattered small follicular structures and some thyroglobulin but generally lacks the usual morphologic characteristics of DTC, showing an intermediate clinical behavior between DTC and ATC. In addition, it is characterized by high-grade features such as widely infiltrative growth, necrosis, vascular invasion, and numerous mitotic figures [6, 9]. The ATC is composed of disseminated fleshy masses with areas of necrosis and hemorrhage. The cells have an undifferentiated phenotype with marked cytological atypia and high mitotic activity, and they are negative for thyroglobulin [4].

Established risk factors for TC include radiation exposure, family history of TC, lymphocytic thyroiditis, reduced iodine intake, and female gender [10]. All of them are thought to induce chromosome instability (CIN) in thyrocytes through still poorly defined direct and indirect mechanisms [10–13]. Actually, number and frequency of chromosomal abnormalities increase from DTC to PDTC and ATC [13]. CIN is also sustained by alterations in cell cycle regulators, frequently encountered in TC [10]. In particular, a deregulated control of the G1/S transition, following either an increased expression of promoting factors (cyclin D1 and E2F) or the downregulation or presence of loss-of-function mutations of factors inhibiting the G1/S transition (retinoblastoma, p16INK4A, p21CIP1, p27KIP1, and p53), has been documented in TC [10]. In addition, the aberrant expression of mitotic kinases, such as the polo-like kinase and the three members of the Aurora kinase family, is held co-responsible for abnormal cell divisions and the establishment of aneuploid TC cells [14, 15].

About 80% of PTC are characterized by mutually exclusive activating somatic mutations of genes encoding for proteins involved in the mitogen-activated protein kinase (MAPK) signaling pathway [4, 16]. These include rearrangements of the *RET* (rearranged during transformation) (RET/PTC) and neurotrophic tyrosine kinase receptor 1 (*NTRK1*) genes, and activating point mutations of the three *RAS* oncogenes (*HRAS*, *KRAS*, and *NRAS*) and *BRAF* [16]. In addition, mutations of genes encoding key players of the phosphoinositide 3-kinase

(PI3K) pathway, such as *PTEN*, *PIK3CA*, and *AKT1*, have been reported in PTC at lower frequencies [16]. Genetic alterations encountered in FTC include activating point mutations of *RAS*, present in about 45% of FTC; rearrangement of the paired-box gene 8 (*PAX-8*) with the peroxisome proliferator-activator receptor-γ (PAX8-PPARγ), observed in 35% of FTC; loss-of-function mutations of the tumor suppressor *PTEN* gene, encountered in about 10% of FTC; activating mutations or amplification of the *PI3KCA* gene, present in about 10% of FTC [17, 18].

Progression of DTC to PDTC and ATC implies tumor acquisition of novel genetic alterations, which are absent or present with low frequency in DTC tissues. Among these are mutations of the tumor suppressor gene *p53*, thought to be a gatekeeper of TC progression from the indolent DTC to the aggressive PDTC and lethal ATC [19]. In fact, *p53* mutations are rarely encountered in DTC (5–9% of cases), while increase in the PDTC (17–38% of cases) and ATC (67–88% of cases) [10, 20, 21]. A similar trend regards the *CTNNB1* gene, encoding the β-catenin, involved in cell adhesion and in the wingless (Wnt) signaling pathway [10]. In particular, *CTNNB1* gene mutations are not found in DTC, while they are present in PDTC (25% of cases) and ATC (66% of cases) [22, 23]. The conversion of early-stage TC to more aggressive and invasive malignancies occurs through an epithelial-to-mesenchymal transition (EMT), which implies the loss of cell-cell contacts, remodeling of cytoskeleton, and the acquisition of a migratory phenotype [24, 25]. Reduced expression of E-cadherin and abnormal expression of integrins, Notch, MET, TGFβ, NF-kB, PI3K, TWIST1, matrix metalloproteinases, components of the urokinase plasminogen-activating system and p21-activated kinase, all of them involved in the EMT, have been identified in TC progression [24–29].

Total thyroidectomy followed by adjuvant therapy with radioactive iodide (^{131}I) is the treatment of choice for the majority of patients affected by DTC [30]. Although the prognosis of these patients is favorable, with 10-year survival rate around 90%, about one-third of them face the morbidity of disease recurrence and TC-related deaths [30]. The worst outcomes are observed in patients with PDTC and ATC, in which the reduced expression of the thyroid-specific gene natrium/iodide symporter (NIS) renders ^{131}I treatment useless [31–33]. In particular, patients affected by ATC have a dismal prognosis with a mean survival time of few months from the diagnosis [32]. Outcome of ATC patients is not influenced by current anticancer treatments (i.e., palliative surgery when possible, chemotherapy, and radiotherapy), and in the majority of cases, death occurs following tumor airway obstruction [34]. Thus, the identification of novel therapeutic approaches capable of improving PDTC and ATC patients' outcome is very much needed.

2. The Aurora kinases

The Aurora kinases belong to a family of serine/threonine kinases having in the Ipl1p (Increase in ploidy 1) gene, subsequently named Aurora gene, the founding member discovered in the budding yeast *Saccharomyces cerevisiae* during a genetic screening for mutations causing defective chromosomal segregation [35–38]. In mammals, the Aurora kinase family includes three proteins: Aurora-A, Aurora-B, and Aurora-C [39]. Structurally, they are characterized by three domains: a N-terminal domain with little similarity among the three Aurora kinases, instrumental in determining their different intracellular localizations, substrate specificity and functions; a catalytic domain, containing the activation loop and highly related in sequence among the three proteins; and a short C-terminal domain of 15–20 residues (**Figure 1**). Aurora kinase expression is tightly regulated during cell cycle, being low in the G1/S phase and maximal in the G2/M phase.

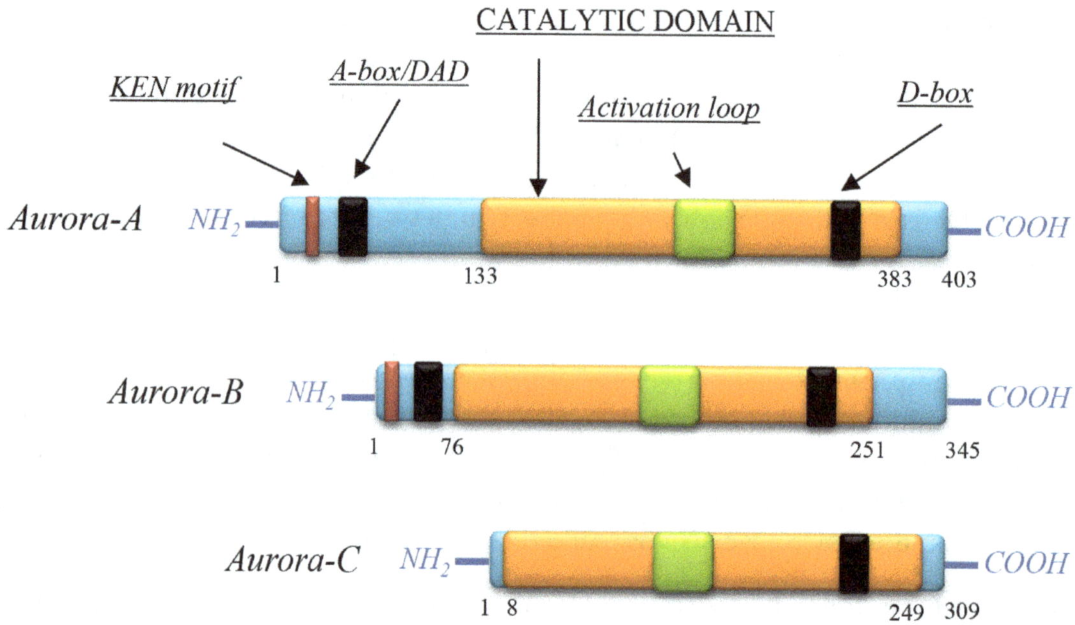

Figure 1. Schematic representation of Aurora kinase proteins. D-Box, destruction box; DAD, D box activating domain; KEN motif, amino acidic K-E-N, which serves as targeting signal for the Cdh1–anaphase promoting complex (adapted with permission from Ref. [14]).

2.1. Aurora-A

The Aurora-A is encoded by the *AURKA* gene located on the chromosome 20q13.2 and containing 11 exons (Gene ID: 6790). The *AURKA* promoter contains a putative TATA box at −37 to −14 and two CCAAT boxes at −101 to −88 and at −69 to −56 [Eukaryotic Promoter Database, Swiss Institute of Bioinformatics]. Two distinct cis-regulatory elements have been identified [40]. Of these, one positively regulates *AURKA* gene transcription, while the other is a cell cycle-dependent transcriptional repressor [40]. The former, essential for the gene expression, is a 7-bp sequence located at −85 to −79 that binds the transcription factor E4TF1. The second is formed by two repressor elements: a cell cycle-dependent element (CDE) located at −44 to −40, and a cell cycle gene homology region (CHR) located at −39 to −35 [40]. Over the last few years, a number of transcription factors capable of repressing or inducing *AURKA* gene expression have been identified. These include the p53, the HIF-1, and the INI1/hSSNF5, all reported to regulate negatively the activity of the *AURKA* promoter [41–43]. Conversely, other transcription factors have been shown to induce *AURKA* expression, among which the ΔEGFR/STAT5, the oncogene MYCN, and the MAPK via Ets2 transcription factors [44–47]. The

Aurora-A protein consists of 403 amino acids with a predicted molecular mass of 45.8 kDa (**Figure 1**). In the activation loop, an Aurora kinase signature (xRxTxCGTx) is present in which the autophosphorylation of the Thr288 is required for kinase activation [48]. In addition, the Thr288 is positioned within a protein kinase A (PKA) consensus sequence, and *in vitro* experiments indicated a potential role of PKA in Aurora-A phosphorylation [49, 50]. The phosphatase PP1 has been shown to dephosphorylate and inactivate Aurora-A [16]. The C-terminal located destruction box (D box), containing the motif RxxLxxG, and the N-terminal A-box/D-box-activating domain (DAD), containing the motif RxLxPS, play an essential role in Aurora-A degradation by the anaphase promoting complex/cyclosome (APC/C)-ubiquitin-proteasome pathway. Aurora-A degradation occurs in late mitosis/early G1 phase, when the D box is targeted by Fizzy-related proteins that transiently interact with the APC, and it is dependent from the APC/C activator protein Cdh1 [49–52]. In the N-terminal region the amino acidic sequence K-E-N, known as KEN motif, is also present, which serves as targeting signal for Cdh1-APC-mediated degradation of several mitotic proteins such as Nek2 and B99 [53]. However, this does not seem to be crucial for Aurora-A degradation [53]. Phosphorylation of the serine residue (Ser51) in the DAD domain has been shown to prevent Aurora-A degradation [54, 55].

2.2. Aurora-B

The Aurora-B is encoded by the *AURKB* gene mapped to chromosome 17p13.1, and consisting of nine exons (Gene ID: 9212). Its promoter contains three putative CAAT boxes at −99 to −86, at −66 to −53, and at −30 to −17 [Eukaryotic Promoter Database, Swiss Institute of Bioinformatics]. As above described for the *AURKA* promoter, also the *AURKB* promoter possesses the CDE and CHR elements, thought to be responsible for the regulation of gene expression throughout the cell cycle [54]. *AURKB* promoter activity is positively increased by transcription factors such the ETS2 *via* ETS-binding sites present in its sequence [46, 47]. The 1.4 kb transcript encodes a protein of 345 amino acids with a predicted molecular mass of 39 kDa (**Figure 1**) [39]. As Aurora-A, Aurora-B protein is characterized by a catalytic domain, a C-terminal D box, and an N-terminal A box/DAD [49–53]. However, different from Aurora-A, Aurora-B is not degraded by the same ubiquitin ligase, but following its binding to the human proteasome α-subunit C8 in a proteasome-dependent manner [55].

2.3. Aurora-C

The Aurora-C is encoded by the *AURKC* gene localized at chromosome 19q13.43 and consisting of seven exons (Gene ID: 6795). The *AURKC* promoter is much less characterized with respect to those of Aurora-A and Aurora-B. A CCAAT box is present at −36 to −23 (Eukaryotic Promoter Database, Swiss Institute of Bioinformatics). *AURKC* promoter activity has been shown to be downregulated by the transcription factor PLZF [56]. The 1.3 kb transcript encodes a protein of 309 amino acids with a predicted molecular mass of 35.6 kDa (**Figure 1**) [39]. Different from Aurora-A and Aurora-B, Aurora-C does not contain the KEN and the A box/DAD motifs in its N-terminal region, while the C-terminal D box is present. The mechanism(s) underlying its degradation, however, still remains to be elucidated.

3. Expression, subcellular localization, and functions of the Aurora kinases

The Aurora kinases play a major role during mitosis [49, 50]. As mentioned above, these proteins display distinct intracellular localizations, substrate specificity and functions, and their expression and activity are tightly regulated at the transcriptional or posttranscriptional level, through phosphorylation/dephosphorylation and protein degradation [57].

3.1. Aurora-A

The expression of Aurora-A is cell cycle regulated, being very low during the G1-phase and starting to accumulate at the centrosome in the late S phase to be maximal at the G2-M transition. In this period, it localizes at the spindle poles, and it is degraded before cytokinesis [50, 53]. Aurora-A regulates centrosome separation and maturation, mitotic entry, and bipolar spindle formation. Recruitment of Aurora-A to the centrosome is controlled by the centrosome

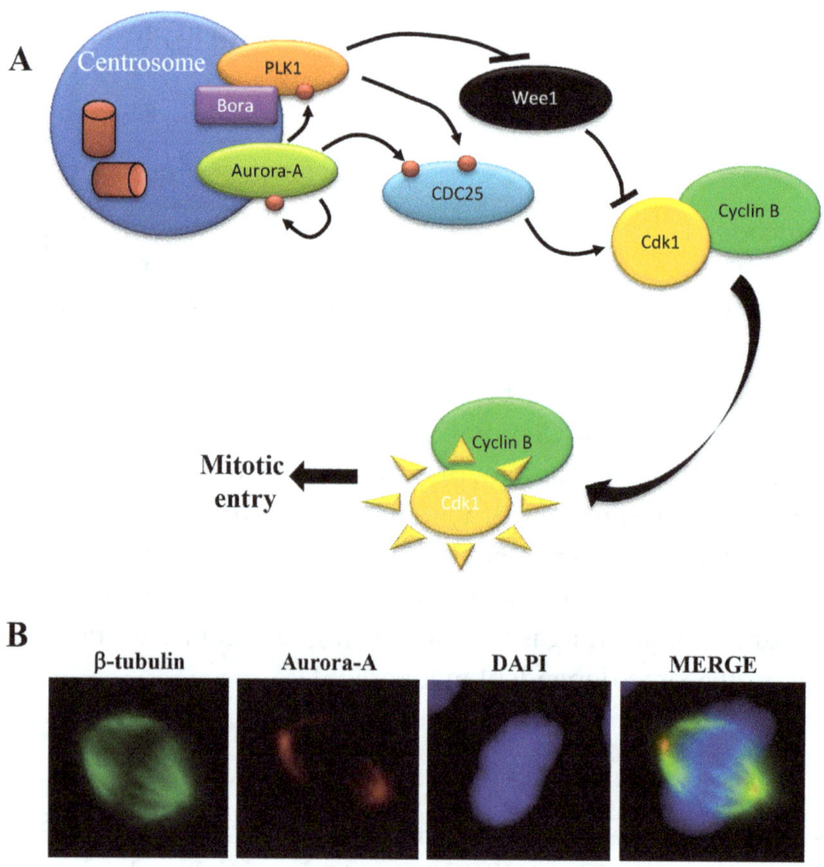

Figure 2. (A) Schematic representation of the pathway induced by Aurora-A to activate the CDK1/cyclin B complex allowing the transition of the cell from the G2 to the M phase. Aurora-A in association with Bora phosphorylates the PLK1. Both Aurora-A and PLK1 phosphorylate CDC25B (cell division cycle 25 B) allowing cyclin-dependent kinase 1 (CDK1)/cyclin B complex activation and thus promoting mitotic entry. PLK1 facilitates this process also by inhibiting the CDK1 inhibitor WEE1. Inactivation of Aurora-A or Plk1 individually shows no significant effect on Cdk1 activation and entry to mitosis, while their simultaneous inactivation produces a marked delay in both Cdk1 activation and mitotic entry, suggesting that the two kinases have redundant functions. (B) Immunofluorescence showing Aurora-A localization at the spindle pole of an anaplastic thyroid cancer cell in metaphase. Adapted with permission from Ref. [14].

protein of 192 kDa/spindle defective 2 (Cep192/Spd-2) [58]. On the centrosome, Aurora-A promotes the concentration in the pericentriolar mass of a number of proteins required for centrosome maturation and function. These include centrosomin, γ-tubulin, large tumor suppressor, homolog 2 (LATS2), transforming acidic coiled coil 3 (TACC3), and nuclear distribution element-like 1 (NDEL1) [50, 53, 59]. A central role of Aurora-A during mitosis is that to support the microtubule-organizer center (MTOC) responsible for the formation of the bipolar spindle. In this context, Aurora-A has been shown to form complexes with TACC1 and TACC3, which in turn, by binding to ch-TOG/XMAP215 proteins, stabilize microtubules at the centrosome [60–62]. In addition, Aurora-A interacts with and phosphorylates TPX2, which is capable of promoting spindle microtubule polymerization [53].

Aurora-A, along with the polo like kinase 1 (PLK1), controls the G2 to M phase transition (**Figure 2**) [63–65]. First, Aurora-A in association with the Bora protein phosphorylates the PLK1, after which both Aurora-A and PLK1 phosphorylate the cell division cycle 25 B (CDC25B), a member of the CDC25 family of phosphatases, which activates cyclin-dependent kinases by removing two phosphate groups, leading to CDK1/cyclin B complex activation and finally promoting mitotic entry [50, 63–66]. PLK1 facilitates this process also by inactivating the CDK1 inhibitor WEE1 (**Figure 2**).

3.2. Aurora-B

Aurora-B protein level peaks at G2/M phase, with the highest kinase activity recorded from metaphase to the end of mitosis [49, 50]. Aurora-B acts in concert with three other proteins, inner centromere protein (INCENP), Survivin, and Borealin/Dasra B, to which it associates forming the chromosomal passenger complex (CPC). In early prophase, the CPC is located on chromosomal condensing arms where it displaces the heterochromatin protein-1 from DNA

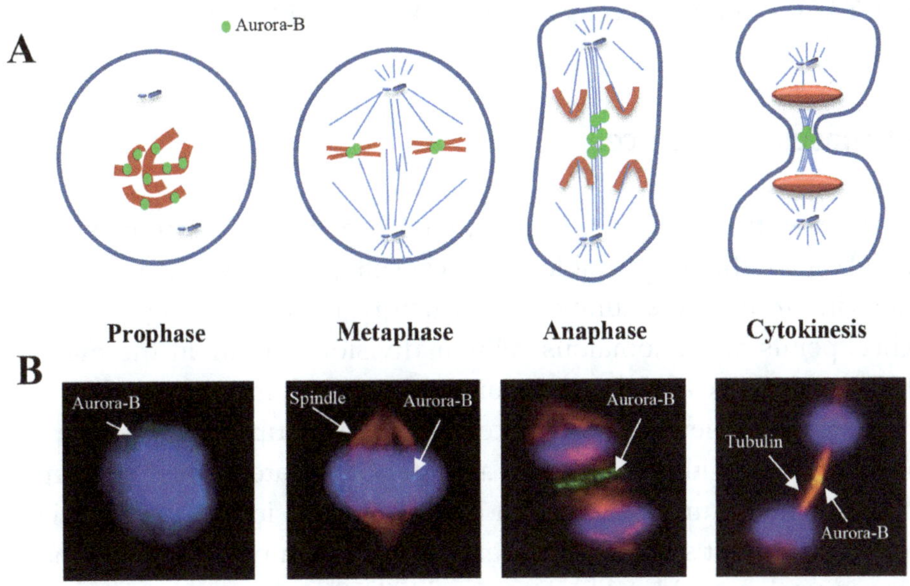

Figure 3. Schematic representation (A) and immunofluorescence images (B) of Aurora-B localization during mitosis in an anaplastic thyroid cancer cell. In (B) Aurora-B is in green, microtubules in red and DNA, stained by DAPI, in blue. Adapted with permission from Ref. [14].

to recruit condensin proteins (**Figure 3**) [67, 68]. From early G2 phase to prophase, Aurora-B phosphorylates histone H3, but its physiological meaning remains unclear. From late prophase to metaphase CPC localizes to the inner centromere, playing a role in formation and stability of the bipolar mitotic spindle, kinetochore assembly, correction of non-bipolar chromosome-spindle attachments, and control of the spindle checkpoint (**Figure 3**). In anaphase, the CPC relocates to the midzone of the mitotic spindle and to the cell cortex, remaining evident in the midbody of telophasic cells where it modulates the activity of several proteins involved in spindle dynamics, cleavage furrow formation and completion of cytokinesis (**Figure 3**) [49, 50, 67–69].

Aurora-B activation requires the auto-phosphorylation and binding to INCENP, while all CPC components are necessary for its proper localization during mitosis. Several kinases, such as BubR1 and Bub1 (checkpoint kinases), monopolar spindle 1 (Mps1), checkpoint kinase 1 (Chkl), Tousled-like kinase-1, Plk1, and TD-60/RCC2 (regulator of chromosome condensation 2), have been shown to be involved in Aurora-B activation. The phosphorylation status and activity of Aurora-B are controlled by PP1 and PP2A phosphatases [69].

3.3. Aurora-C

The expression of Aurora-C is maximal during the G2/M phase. This kinase seems to have a prominent role in the meiotic division, as it is expressed at relative high levels in germ cells during spermatogenesis and oogenesis, and at very low levels in somatic cells. Aurora-C is highly similar to Aurora-B in sequence (61% identity), which may explain why the two kinases display similar localization patterns and share interacting proteins and substrates such as INCENP, Survivin, Borealin, and others [49, 70]. Interestingly, when ectopically expressed in cells depleted of Aurora-B, Aurora-C is capable of rescuing the Aurora-B-dependent mitotic functions [40]. It is also worth to note that Aurora-C has been shown to interact with and phosphorylate TACC1 in thyroid cells in the cytokinetic bridge [71, 72].

4. Aurora kinases and cancer

Chromosomal instability is thought to represent the mean by which premalignant cells acquire novel functional capabilities responsible for cancer cell growth and tumor progression [73]. In fact, aberrations in chromosome number and structure, likely resulting from a combination of ineffective checkpoints and anomalous cellular divisions, occur in the majority of human cancers [74]. Given the crucial tasks of Aurora kinases in all mitotic stages, their dysfunction and/or dysregulation is believed to greatly contribute to aneuploidy. Whether Aurora kinases may have a role in cancer initiation is still a matter of debate. It has been reported that the overexpression of either Aurora-A, Aurora-B, or Aurora-C induces cell malignant transformation [75–77]. In different studies, however, the transforming ability of either Aurora-A or Aurora-B overexpression could not be confirmed [78, 79].

Aurora-A kinase has been often implicated in cancer progression, and its hyperactivation has been demonstrated to induce resistance to microtubule-targeted chemotherapy [80–82]. The

AURKA gene is amplified in many malignancies, and its overexpression has been reported to be significantly associated with a higher tumor grade and a poor prognosis in a number of cancers, including chondrosarcoma, nasopharyngeal carcinoma, breast cancer, glioblastoma, colorectal cancer, gastric cancer, and ovarian carcinoma [83–89]. In addition, somatic mutations located within the catalytic domain of Aurora-A, altering kinase activity and subcellular localization, have been described in human cancer cells [90]. The oncogenic potential of Aurora-A derives from a sum of several spatially and temporally distinct actions. Unlike normal cells, in many cancer cells the expression of Aurora-A becomes constitutive throughout the cytoplasm, regardless of the cell cycle phase; this can trigger a plethora of improper interactions, phosphorylations, and mislocalizations. Aurora-A may also represent the downstream target of mitogenic pathways, such as MAPK/ERK (mitogen-activated protein kinases), and be overexpressed because of their constitutive activation in tumors [81]. The Aurora-A excess interferes with different cell cycle checkpoints, that is, the late G2 checkpoint, which restrains genetically aberrant cells to enter mitosis, the spindle assembly checkpoint, which blocks the metaphase–anaphase transition in cells with defective spindles, and the post-mitotic G1 checkpoint, which arrests cell cycle in aneuploid cells [81, 83]. Centrosome amplification and unrestrained multinucleation, leading to abnormal mitotic spindle, are also observed in Aurora-A overexpressing cells [91]. Moreover, Aurora-A may significantly contribute to tumor progression by interacting with and inhibiting several tumor suppressor proteins such as p53, BRCA1 (breast cancer 1), and Chfr (checkpoint with forkhead and ring finger domains). Interestingly, activation of the MAPK signaling pathways has been found to induce accumulation of Aurora-A kinase in $ER\alpha^{+}$ breast cancer cells, and epithelial-to-mesenchymal transition (EMT) [92, 93]. In these cells, Aurora-A has been shown to promote SMAD5 phosphorylation and nuclear translocation, upregulation of stemness gene SOX-2, and acquisition of a stem cell-like phenotype [92, 93].

Aurora-B plays a less clear role in tumorigenesis. An increased level of Aurora-B in normal cells induces premature chromosome separation and segregation errors, promotes generation of tetraploid/aneuploid cells, and potentiates Ras oncogenic activity [77, 80, 94–96]. Neither amplification nor specific mutations of *AURKB* gene have been shown to occur in human malignancies; nevertheless, Aurora-B overexpression has been demonstrated in several cancer types, including hepatocellular and oral squamous cell carcinomas, where it correlates with poor prognosis [80, 94–96].

At present, very little is known about the role of Aurora-C in cancer progression. Although Aurora-C is almost not detectable in normal somatic cells, it is highly expressed in various tumor cell lines [97–100]. One study has described the transforming potential of overexpressed Aurora-C in NIH-3T3 cells, and a correlation between the level of active kinase and tumor aggressiveness of the cells injected in nude mice [77].

4.1. Aurora kinase inhibitors

The overexpression of Aurora kinases in human cancers and their relevance in controlling the mitotic process have led to the development of small-molecule inhibitors as anticancer drugs. Aurora inhibition results in cytokinesis failure and generation of tetraploid cells, which, depending on the post-mitotic checkpoint activation, may be unable to proceed in a new cell cycle or rather may proliferate and become polyploid. The exit from cell cycle is likely to generate viable quiescent cells, whereas endoreplicating cells have greater tendency to undergo apoptosis. Actually, the functional inhibition of Aurora kinases is considered a promising therapeutic option against those malignancies that do not respond to the available therapies [101–108]. Up to date, about 30 small-molecule inhibitors of Aurora kinases have been developed and some of them, reported in **Table 1**, are being evaluated in Phase I-II clinical trials [101–108]. Of some interest are the preclinical observations showing the ability of different Aurora kinase inhibitors to have additive or synergist effects when combined with other anticancer therapies [109, 110]. At example, among the pan-Aurora kinase inhibitors, the AMG-900 in combination with the HDAC (histone deacetylase) inhibitor vorinostat has been shown to synergistically reduce proliferation and survival of medulloblastoma and prostate cancer-derived cell lines [111, 112]. Similarly, the SNS-314 has been shown to possess additive inhibitory effects on the HCT 116 cell line when combined with either carboplatin, gemcitabine, 5-FU, daunomycin, docetaxel, or vincristine [113]. Also the MK-0457 has revealed additive effects when combined with docetaxel on ovarian cancer cell lines or with cisplatin on the HepG2 cell line [114, 115]. Finally, the pan-Aurora kinase inhibitor CCT 137690 has been shown to sensitize SW620 colorectal cancer cells to radiotherapy [116]. In clinical trials, disease stabilization and, less frequently, partial responses in patients with solid cancers have been witnessed with the majority of Aurora kinase inhibitors, while more encouraging observations have been made in patients with hematological malignancies [101–110]. On-target toxicity observed with these drugs included grade 3/4 neutropenia, leukopenia, and myelosuppression, while off-target effects included hypertension, somnolence, mucositis, stomatitis, proctalgia, and ventricular dysfunction [101–110]. For example, the MK-0457 has been employed in different clinical trials in which patients with advanced solid tumors have been enrolled. In a Phase I dose escalation study, the most common dose-limiting toxicity observed was neutropenia and herpes zoster, and major adverse events include nausea, vomiting, diarrhea, and fatigue [117]. Although no objective tumor responses were observed in this trial, 12 of 27 patients experienced stable disease with a median duration of 75.5 days (range 38–328 days). Of the latter, one patient with ovarian cancer achieved prolonged stable disease for 11 months, and one patient with rectal cancer had stable disease over 7 months [117].

The MK-0457 was found to have off-target inhibitory effects on both wild-type and mutant Abl kinases and showed to be a potent inhibitor of the BCR-ABL T315I mutant, which mediates clinical resistance to imatinib, nilotinib, and dasatinib [118]. On these bases, a phase I/II dose escalation study of MK-0457 was performed in patients with leukemias [119, 120]. Patients with refractory hematologic malignancies received 1–21 cycles of MK-0457, and maximum-tolerated doses were calculated for a 5-day short infusion as 40 mg. Mucositis and alopecia were the most common drug-related adverse events observed in these patients. Forty-four percent (8/18) of patients, positive for the BCR-ABL T315I mutation, affected by chronic myelogenous leukemia (CML) had hematologic responses, and 33% (1/3) of patients with Philadelphia chromosome-positive (Ph+) acute lymphoblastic leukemia (ALL) obtained complete remission [119, 120].

Inhibitor (company) commercial name	Clinical trial
Pan-Aurora inhibitors	
VX-680/MK-0457 (Vertex/Merck) Tozasertib	Phase II (terminated due to severe toxicity)
PHA-739358 (Pfizer/Nerviano) Danusertib	Phase II
PHA-680632(Pfizer/Nerviano)	Phase II
CYC-116 (Cyclacel)	Phase I
SNS-314 (Sunesis)	Phase I
R763 (Rigel)	Phase I
AMG-900 (Amgen)	Phase I
AT-9283 (Astex)	Phase II
PF-03814375 (Pfizer)	Phase I
GSK1070916 (GlaxoSmithKline)	Phase I
Aurora-A inhibitors	
MLN8237 (Millennium)	Phase II
EMD-2076 (EntreMed)	Phase II
MK-5108 (Vertex)	Phase I
Aurora-B inhibitors	
AZD1152 (AstraZeneca)	Phase II

Table 1. Aurora kinase inhibitors in clinical trials (adapted with permission from Ref. [14]).

Another multicenter phase II study evaluated the safety and efficacy of MK-0457 on 52 patients affected by CML or Ph+ ALL with BCR-ABL T315I mutation [121] (Seymour et al. 2014). Patients were treated with a 5-day continuous infusion of MK-0457 administered every 14 days at 40, 32, or 24 mg. The most common adverse events were neutropenia and febrile neutropenia. Eight percent (4/52) of patients achieved major cytogenetic response and 6% (3/52) had a complete or a partial response. Thirteen percent (2/15) of patients with chronic phase CML achieved complete hematologic response. None of the patients with advanced CML or Ph+ ALL achieved major hematologic response [121].

A comprehensive description of clinical trials performed with the different Aurora kinase inhibitors has been recently reported [109, 110].

5. Aurora kinases and thyroid cancers

Normal human thyrocytes express all three Aurora kinases in a cell cycle-dependent manner [98]. The expression of Aurora-A and Aurora-B in these cells is mainly regulated at the transcriptional level, while that of Aurora-C appears to be modulated at the posttranscriptional level [98]. An increased expression of all the Aurora kinases has been shown in various cell lines originating from different epithelial thyroid tumor histotypes, compared with normal thyrocytes, as well as in DTC and ATC tissues, compared with normal matched tissues [60, 98, 122]. In addition, a study aimed to evaluate the gene expression profile in ATC identified *AURKA* as one of the most frequently and most strongly overexpressed genes in these tumors [123]. In fact, gain of chromosome 20q, where *AURKA* is located (20q13.2), is frequently encountered in ATC [124]. Based on these findings, the potential therapeutic value of Aurora kinase inhibition on the proliferation and growth of PTC and ATC cells has been evaluated in preclinical studies [125–130]. In particular, different pan-Aurora kinase inhibitors, including the MK-0457 (VX-680), the SNS-314 mesylate, and the ZM447439 have been evaluated *in vitro* [126–129]. These molecules were found to inhibit proliferation of ATC cells in a time- and dose-dependent manner and to impair cancer cell colony formation in soft agar. Cell cultures exposed to pan-Aurora inhibitors revealed an accumulation of tetra- and polyploid cells because of endoreplication events followed by the activation of caspase-3 and accumulation of a sub-G0/G1 cell population, both indicative of apoptosis [126–129]. Treated cells showed mitotic alterations consistent with the inhibition of Aurora kinases, including major impairment of centrosome functions, with abnormal spindle formation characterized by the presence of short microtubules, inhibition of histone H3 phosphorylation, and inability to complete the cytokinesis. The effects of a selective inhibition of either Aurora-A or Aurora-B have been also explored [125, 129, 131]. The selective inhibition of Aurora-B expression, by means of RNA interference, or function, by means of small-molecule compounds (e.g., AZD1152), has been reported to significantly reduce growth and tumorigenicity of ATC-derived cells, both *in vivo* and *in vitro* [125]. In the same way, functional inhibition of Aurora-A by MLN8054 in a panel of ATC-derived cell lines has been shown to block cell proliferation and to induce cell cycle arrest and apoptosis [129]. In xenograft experiments, the drug was capable of reducing tumor volume by 86% [129]. Interestingly, the combined treatment with MLN8054 and bortezomib, targeting the ubiquitin-proteasome system, showed additive effects on ATC-derived cell proliferation and apoptosis, compared with monotherapy [131]. More recently, pazopanib, a multi-target inhibitor of tyrosine kinases including the VEGFR (vascular endothelial growth factor receptor), shown to have impressive therapeutic activity in patients affected by radioactive iodine-refractory DTC, was tested in a phase II clinical trial on ATC patients [132, 133]. Despite several of them treated with pazopanib had a transient disease regression, no response evaluation criteria in solid tumors (RECIST) response was obtained [131]. Moreover, in a preclinical study on a panel of ATC-derived cell lines, pazopanib was found to potentiate the cytotoxic effects of paclitaxel *in vitro* and in xenograft experiments [134]. These pazopanib effects were attributed to an unexpected off-target inhibition of Aurora-A in ATC-derived cell lines. In fact, the same results were obtained when combining paclitaxel and MLN8237, a selective Aurora-A inhibitor. In the same study, the authors also showed that the combined administration of pazopanib and paclitaxel attained a marked and durable regression of lung metastasis in a single ATC patient [134].

In conclusion, the preclinical and clinical data so far available indicate that Aurora kinase inhibitors may have a therapeutic potential for the treatment of the more aggressive thyroid cancers either in monotherapy or, more likely, in combination therapy with antimicrotubule drugs.

Author details

Enke Baldini, Chiara Tuccilli, Salvatore Sorrenti, Domenico Mascagni, Stefano Arcieri, Angelo Filippini and Salvatore Ulisse*

*Address all correspondence to: salvatore.ulisse@uniroma1.it

Department of Surgical Sciences, "Sapienza" University of Rome, Rome, Italy

References

[1] Howlader N, Noone AM, Krapcho M, Garshell J, Miller D, Altekruse SF, Kosary CL, Yu M, Ruhl J, Tatalovich Z, Mariotto A, Lewis DR, Chen HS, Feuer EJ, Cronin KA (eds). SEER Cancer Statistics Review, 1975–2012, Bethesda, MD: National Cancer Institute, http://seer.cancer.gov/csr/1975_2012/.

[2] Grodski S, Brown T, Sidhu S, Gill A, Robinson B, Learoyd D, Sywak M, Reeve T, Delbridge L. Increasing incidence of thyroid cancer is due to increased pathologic detection. Surgery 2008;144:1038–1043.

[3] Trimboli P, Ulisse S, Graziano FM, Marzullo A, Ruggieri M, Calvanese A, Piccirilli F, Cavaliere R, Fumarola A, D'Armiento M. Trend in thyroid carcinoma size, age at diagnosis, and histology in a retrospective study of 500 cases diagnosed over 20 years. Thyroid 2006;16:1151–1155.

[4] Nikiforov YE, Biddinger PW, Thompson LDR. Diagnostic Pathology and Molecular Genetics of the Thyroid. Philadelphia: Volters Kluver & Lippincott Williams & Wilkins; 2009. 382 p.

[5] Nikiforov YE, Nikiforova MN. Molecular genetics and diagnosis of thyroid cancer. Nat Rev Endocrinol 2011;7:569–580.

[6] DeLellis RA, Lloyd R, Heitz PU, Heng C, (eds). World Health Organization Classification of Tumors, Pathology & Genetics – Tumors of Endocrine Organs. Lyon: IARC Press; 2004.

[7] Nikiforov YE. Genetic alterations involved in the transition from well-differentiated to poorly differentiated and anaplastic thyroid carcinomas. Endocr Pathol 2004;15:319–327.

[8] Hunt JL, Tometsko M, LiVolsi VA, Swalsky P, Finkelstein SD, Barnes EL. Molecular evidence of anaplastic transformation in coexisting well-differentiated and anaplastic carcinomas of the thyroid. Am J Surg Pathol 2003;27:1559–1564.

[9] Eloy C, Ferreira L, Salgado C, Soares P, Sobrinho-Simões M. Poorly differentiated and undifferentiated thyroid carcinomas. Turk Patoloji Derg 2015;31:48–59.

[10] Kondo T, Ezzat S, Asa SL. Pathogenetic mechanisms in thyroid follicular-cell neoplasia. Nat Rev Cancer 2006;6:292–306.

[11] Shahedian B, Shi Y, Zou M, Farid NR. Thyroid carcinoma is characterized by genomic instability: evidence from p53 mutations. Mol Gen Metab 2001;72:155–163.

[12] Wressmann VB, Ghossein RA, Patel SG, Harris CP, Schnaser EA, Shaha AR, et al. Genome-wide appraisal of thyroid cancer progression. Am J Pathol 2002;161:1549–1556.

[13] Hanahan D, Weinberg RA. Hallmarks of cancer: the next generation. Cell 2011;144:646–674.

[14] Baldini E, D'Armiento M, Ulisse S. A new aurora in anaplastic thyroid cancer therapy. Int J Endocrinol 2014;2014:816430.

[15] Ito Y, Miyoshi E, Sasaki N, Kakudo K, Yoshida H, Tomoda C, Uruno T, Takamura Y, Miya A, Kobayashi K, Matsuzuka F, Matsuura N, Kuma K, Miyauchi A. Polo-like kinase 1 overexpression is an early event in the progression of papillary carcinoma. Br J Cancer 2004;90:414–418.

[16] The Cancer Genome Atlas Research Network. Integrated genomic characterization of papillary thyroid carcinoma. Cell 2014;159:676–690.

[17] Omur O, Baran Y. An update on molecular biology of thyroid cancer. Crit Rev Oncol Hematol 2014;90:233–252.

[18] Giordano TJ, Au AY, Kuick R, Thomas DG, Rhodes DR, Wilhelm KG Jr, Vinco M, Misek DE, Sanders D, Zhu Z, Ciampi R, Hanash S, Chinnaiyan A, Clifton-Bligh RJ, Robinson BG, Nikiforov YE, Koenig RJ. Delineation, functional validation, and bioinformatic evaluation of gene expression in thyroid follicular carcinomas with the PAX8-PPARG translocation. Clin Cancer Res 2006;12:1983–1993.

[19] Patel KN, Shaha AR. Poorly differentiated and anaplastic thyroid cancer. Cancer Control 2006;13:119–128.

[20] Ito T, Seyama T, Mizuno T, Tsuyama N, Hayashi T, Hayashi Y, Dohi K, Nakamura N, Akiyama M. Unique association of p53 mutations with undifferentiated but not with differentiated carcinomas of the thyroid gland. Cancer Res 1992;52:1369–1371.

[21] Donghi R, Longoni A, Pilotti S, Michieli P, Della Porta G, Pierotti MA. Gene p53 mutations are restricted to poorly differentiated and undifferentiated carcinomas of the thyroid gland. J Clin Invest 1993;91:1753–1760.

[22] Garcia-Rostan G, Camp RL, Herrero A, Carcangiu ML, Rimm DL, Tallini G. Beta-catenin dysregulation in thyroid neoplasms: down-regulation, aberrant nuclear

expression, and CTNNB1 exon 3 mutations are markers for aggressive tumor phenotypes and poor prognosis. Am J Pathol 2001;158:987–996.

[23] Miyake N, Maeta H, Horie S, Kitamura Y, Nanba E, Kobayashi K, Terada T. Absence of mutations in the beta-catenin and adenomatous polyposis coli genes in papillary and follicular thyroid carcinomas. Pathol Int 2001;51:680–685.

[24] Huber MA, Kraut N, Beug H. Molecular requirements for epithelial-mesenchymal transition during tumor progression. Curr Opin Cell Biol 2005;17:548–558.

[25] Vasko V, Espinosa AV, Scouten W, He H, Auer H, Liyanarachchi S, et al. Gene expression and functional evidence of epithelial-to-mesenchymal transition in papillary thyroid carcinoma invasion. Proc Natl Acad Sci USA 2007;104:2803–2808.

[26] Baldini E, Toller M, Graziano FM, Russo FP, Pepe M, Biordi L, Marchioni E, Curcio F, Ulisse S, Ambesi-Impiombato FS, D'Armiento M. Expression of matrix metalloproteinases and their specific inhibitors (TIMPs) in normal and different human thyroid tumor cell lines. Thyroid 2004;14:881–888.

[27] Ulisse S, Baldini E, Toller M, Marchioni E, Giacomelli L, De Antoni E, Ferretti E, Marzullo A, Graziano FM, Trimboli P, Biordi L, Curcio F, Gulino A, Ambesi-Impiombato FS, D'Armiento M. Differential expression of the components of the plasminogen activating system in human thyroid tumour derived cell lines and papillary carcinomas. Eur J Cancer 2006;42:2631–2638.

[28] Ulisse S, Baldini E, Sorrenti S, Barollo S, Gnessi L, Catania A, Pellizzo MR, Nardi F, Mian C, De Antoni E, D'Armiento M, Frati L. High expression of the urokinase plasminogen activator and its cognate 1 receptor associates with advanced stages and reduced disease-free interval in papillary thyroid carcinoma. J Clin Endocrinol Metab 2011;96:504–508.

[29] Ulisse S, Baldini E, Sorrenti S, Barollo S, Prinzi N, Catania A, Nesca A, Gnessi L, Pelizzo MR, Mian C, De Vito C, Calvanese A, Palermo S, Persechino S, De Antoni E, D'Armiento M. In papillary thyroid carcinoma BRAFV600E is associated with increased expression of the urokinase plasminogen activator and its cognate receptor, but not with disease-free interval. Clin Endocrinol 2012;77:780–786.

[30] American Thyroid Association (ATA) Guidelines Taskforce on Thyroid Nodules and Differentiated Thyroid Cancer, Cooper DS, Doherty GM, Haugen BR, Kloos RT, Lee SL, Mandel SJ, Mazzaferri EL, McIver B, Pacini F, Schlumberger M, Sherman SI, Steward DL, Tuttle RM. Revised American Thyroid Association management guidelines for patients with thyroid nodules and differentiated thyroid cancer. Thyroid 2009;19:1167–1214.

[31] Ibrahimpasic T, Ghossein R, Carlson DL, Nixon I, Palmer FL, Shaha AR, Patel SG, Tuttle RM, Shah JP, Ganly I. Outcomes in patients with poorly differentiated thyroid carcinoma. J Clin Endocrinol Metab 2014;99:1245–1252.

[32] Romesser PB, Sherman EJ, Shaha AR, Lian M, Wong RJ, Sabra M, Rao SS, Fagin JA, Tuttle RM, Lee NY. External beam radiotherapy with or without concurrent chemotherapy in advanced or recurrent non-anaplastic non-medullary thyroid cancer. J Surg Oncol 2014;110:375–382.

[33] Antonelli A, Fallahi P, Ferrari SM, Carpi A, Berti P, Materazzi G, Minuto M, Guastalli M, Miccoli P. Dedifferentiated thyroid cancer: a therapeutic challenge. Biomed Pharmacother 2008;62:559–563.

[34] Keutegen XM, Sadowski SM, Kebebew E. Management of anaplastic thyroid cancer. Gland Surg 2015;4:44–51.

[35] Chan CS, Bolstein D. Isolation and characterization of chromosome-gain and increase-in-ploidy mutants in yeast. Genetics 1993;165:677–691.

[36] Glover DM, Leibowitz MH, Mclean DA, Parry H. Mutations in Aurora prevent centrosome separation leading to the formation of monopolar spindle. Cell 1995;81:95–105.

[37] Schumacher JM, Ashcroft N, Donovan PJ, Golden A. A highly conserved centrosomal kinase, AIR1, is required for accurate cell cycle progression and segregation of developmental factors in *Caenorhabditis elegans* embryos. Development 1998:125:4391–4402.

[38] Baldini E, D'Armiento M, Ulisse S. A new aurora in anaplastic thyroid cancer therapy. Int J Endocrinol 2014;2014:816430.

[39] Bischoff JR, Plowman GD. The Aurora/Ipl1 kinase family: regulators of chromosome segregation and cytokinesis. Trend Cell Biol 1999;9:454–459.

[40] Tanaka M, Ueda A, Kanamori H, Ideguchi H, Yang J, Kitajima S, Ishigatsubo Y. Cell-cycle-dependent regulation of human aurora A transcription is mediated by periodic repression of E4TF1. J Biol Chem 2002;277:10719–10726.

[41] Nikulenkov F, Spinnler C, Li H, Tonelli C, Shi Y, Turunen M, Kivioja T, Ignatiev I, Kel A, Taipale J, Selivanova G. Insights into p53 transcriptional function via genome-wide chromatin occupancy and gene expression analysis. Cell Death Differ 2012;19:1992–2002.

[42] D. Fanale, V. Bazan, L. R. Corsini, et al. HIF-1 is involved in the negative regulation of AURKA expression in breast cancer cell lines under hypoxic conditions. Breast Cancer Res Treat 2013;140:505–517.

[43] Lee S, Cinica V, Ramachandra N, Zagzag D, Kalpana GV. Aurora A is a repressed effector target of the chromatin remodeling protein INI1/hSSNF5 required for rhabdoid tumor cell survival. Cancer Res 2011;71:3225–3235.

[44] Latha K, Li M, Chumbalkar V, Gururaj A, Hwang Y, Dakeng S, Sawaya R, Aldape K, Cavenee WK, Bogler O, Furnari FB. Nuclear EGFRvIII-STAT5b complex contributes to

glioblastoma cell survival by direct activation of the Bcl-XL promoter. Int J Cancer 2013;132:509–520.

[45] Murphy DM, Buckley PG, Das S, Watters KM, Bryan K, Stallings RL. Co-localization of the oncogenic transcription factor MYCN and the DNA methyl binding protein MeCP2 at genomic sites in neuroblastoma. PLoS One 2011;6:e21436.

[46] Wakahara K, Ohno T, Kimura M, Masuda T, Nozawa S, Dohjima T, Yamamoto T, Nagano A, Kawai G, Matsuhashi A, Saitoh M, Takigami I, Okano Y, Shimizu K. EWS-Fli1 up-regulates expression of the Aurora A and Aurora B kinases. Mol Cancer Res 2008;6:1937–1945.

[47] Furukawa T, Kanai N, Shiwaku HO, Soga N, Uehara A, Horii A. AURKA is one of the downstream targets of MAPK1/ERK2 in pancreatic cancer. Oncogene 2006;25:4831–4839.

[48] Marumoto T, Zhang D, Saya H. Aurora-A-A guardian of poles. Nat Rev Cancer 2005;5:42–50.

[49] Bolanos-Garcia VM. Aurora kinases. Int J Biochem Cell Biol 2005;37:1572–1577.

[50] Carmena M, Earnshaw WC. The cellular geography of Aurora kinases. Nat Rev Cancer 2003;4:842–854.

[51] Arlot-Bonnemains Y, Klotzbucher A, Giet R, Uzbekov R, Bihan R, Prigent C. Identification of a functional destruction box in the *Xenopus laevis* aurora-A kinase pEG2. FEBS Lett 2001;508:149–152.

[52] Castro A, Arlot-Bonnemains Y, Vigneron S, Labbé JC, Prigent C, Lorca T. APC/Fizzy-related targets Aurora-A kinase for proteolysis. EMBO Rep 2002;3:1–6.

[53] Nikonova AS, Astsaturov I, Serebriiskii IG, Dunbrack Jr RL, Golemis EA. Aurora-A kinase (AURKA) in normal and pathological cell division. Cell Mol Life Sci 2013;70:661–687.

[54] Kimura M, Uchida C, Takano Y, Kitagawa M, Okano Y. Cell cycle-dependent regulation of the human aurora B promoter. 2004;316:930–936.

[55] Shu F, Guo S, Dang Y, Qi M, Zhou G, Guo Z, Zhang Y, Wu C, Zhao S, Yu L. Human Aurora-B binds to a proteosome alpha-subunit HC8 and undergoes degradation in a proteasome-dependent manner Mol Cell Biochem 2003;254:157–162.

[56] Tsou JH, Chang KC, Chang-Liao PY, Yang ST, Lee CT, Chen YP, Lee YC, Lin BW, Lee JC, Shen MR, Chuang CK, Chang WC, Wang JM, Hung LY. Aberrantly expressed AURKC enhances the transformation and tumourigenicity of epithelial cells. J Pathol 2011;225:243–254.

[57] Baldini E, Sorrenti S, D'Armiento E, Prinzi N, Guaitoli E, Favoriti P, Gnessi L, Moretti C, Bianchini M, Alessandrini S, Catania A, De Antoni E, Ulisse S. Aurora kinases: new molecular targets in thyroid cancer therapy. Clin Ter 2012;163:e457–e462.

[58] Joukov V, De Nicolo A, Rodriguez A, Walter JC, Livingstom DM. Centrosomal protein of 192 kDa (Cep192) promotes centrosome-driven spindle assembly by engaging in organelle-specific Aurora A activation. 2010;107:21022–21027.

[59] Berdnik D, Knoblich JA. Drosophila Aurora-A is required for centrosome maturation and actin-dependent asymmetric localization during mitosis. Curr Biol 2002;12:640–647.

[60] Ulisse S, Baldini E, Toller M, Delcros JG, Guého A, Curcio F, De Antoni E, Giacomelli L, Ambesi-Impiombato FS, Bocchini S, D'Armiento M, Arlot-Bonnemains Y. Transforming acidic coiled-coil 3 and Aurora-A interact in human thyrocytes and their expression is deregulated in thyroid cancer tissues. Endocr Relat Cancer 2007;14:831–842.

[61] Kinoshita K, Noetzel TL, Pelletier L, Mechtler K, Drechsel DN, Schwager A, Lee M, Raff JW, Hyman AA. Aurora-A phosphorylation of TACC3/maskin is required for centrosome-dependent microtubule assembly in mitosis. J Cell Biol 2005;170:1047–1055.

[62] Barros TP, Kinoshita K, Hyman AA, Raff JW. Aurora-A activates D-TACC-Msps complexes exclusively at centrosomes to stabilize centrosomal microtubules. J Cell Biol 2005;170:1039–1046.

[63] De Souza CP, Ellem KA, Gabrielli BG. Centrosomal and cytoplasmic Cdc2/cyclin B1 activation precedes nuclear mitotic events. Exp Cell Res 2000;257:11–21.

[64] Seki A, Coppinger JA, Jang CY, Yates JR, Fang. Bora and the kinase Aurora A cooperatively activate the kinase Plk1 and control mitotic entry. Science 2008;320:1655–1658.

[65] Dutertre S, Cazales M, Quaranta M, Froment C, Trabut V, Dozier C, Mirey G, Bouché JP, Theis-Febvre N, Schmitt E, Monsarrat B, Prigent C, Ducommun B. Phosphorylation of CDC25B by Aurora-A at the centrosome contributes to the G2-M transition. J Cell Sci 2004;117:2523–2531.

[66] Van Horn RD, Chu S, Fan L, Yin T, Du J, Beckmann R, Mader M, Zhu G, Toth J, Blanchard K, Ye XS. Cdk1 activity is required for mitotic activation of Aurora A during G2/M transition of human cells. J Biol Chem 2010;285:21849–21857.

[67] Ruchaud S, Carmena M, Earnshaw WC. Chromosomal passengers: conducting cell division. Nat Rev Mol Cell Biol 2007;8:798–812.

[68] Vader G, Medema RH, Lens SM. The chromosomal passenger complex: guiding Aurora-B through mitosis. J Cell Biol 2006;173:833–837.

[69] van der Waal MS, Hengeveld RC, van der Horst A, Lens SM. Cell division control by the chromosomal passenger complex. Exp Cell Res 2012;318:1407–1420.

[70] Sasai K, Katayama H, Stenoien DL, Fujii S, Honda R, Kimura M, Okano Y, Tatsuka M, Suzuki F, Nigg EA, Earnshaw WC, Brinkley WR, Sen S. Aurora-C kinase is a novel

chromosomal passenger protein that can complement Aurora-B kinase function in mitotic cells. Cell Motil Cytoskeleton 2004;59:249–263.

[71] S. D. Slattery, M. A. Mancini, B. R. Brinkley, et al. Aurora-C kinase supports mitotic progression in the absence of Aurora-B. Cell Cycle 2009;8:2984–2994.

[72] Gabillard JC, Ulisse S, Baldini E, Sorrenti S, Cremet JY, Coccaro C, Prigent C, D'Armiento M, Arlot-Bonnemains Y. Aurora-C interacts with and phosphorylates the transforming acidic coiled-coil 1 protein. Biochem Biophys Res Commun 2011;408:647–653.

[73] Hanahan D, Weinberg RA. Hallmarks of cancer: the next generation. Cell 2011;144:646–674.

[74] Gordon DJ, Resio B, Pellman D. Causes and consequences of aneuploidy in cancer. Nat Rev Gen 2012;13:189–203.

[75] Bischoff JR, Anderson L, Zhu Y, Mossie K, Ng L, Souza B, Schryver B, Flanagan P, Clairvoyant F, Ginther C, Chan CS, Novotny M, Slamon DJ, Plowman GD. A homologue of drosophila Aurora kinase is oncogenic and amplified in human colorectal cancers. EMBO J 1998;17:3052–3065.

[76] Ota T, Suto S, Katayama H, Han ZB, Suzuki F, Maeda M, Tanino M, Terada Y, Tatsuka M. Increased mitotic phosphorylation of mitotic histone H3 attributable to AIM-1/ Aurora B overexpression contributes to chromosome number instability. Cancer Res 2002;62:5168–5177.

[77] Khan J, Ezan F, Crémet JY, Fautrel A, Gilot D, Lambert M, Benaud C, Troadec MB, Prigent C. Overexpression of active Aurora-C kinase results in cell transformation and tumour formation. PLoS One 2011;6:e26512.

[78] Tatsuka M, Sato S, Kitajima S, Suto S, Kawai H, Miyauchi M, Ogawa I, Maeda M, Ota T, Takata T. Overexpression of Aurora-A potentiates H-RAS-mediated oncogenic transformation and is implicated in oral carcinogenesis. Oncogene 2005;24:1122–1127.

[79] Kanda A, Kawai H, Suto S, Kitajima S, Sato S, Takata T, Tatsuka M. Aurora-B/Aim-1 kinase activity is involved in Ras-mediated cell transformation. Oncogene 2005;24:7266–7272.

[80] Dar AA, Goff LW, Majid S, Berlin J, El-Rifai W. Aurora kinase inhibitors – rising stars in cancer therapeutics? Mol Cancer Ther 2010;9:268–278.

[81] Lok W, Klein RQ, Saif MW. Aurora kinase inhibitors as anti-cancer therapy. Anticancer Drugs 2010;21:339–350.

[82] Anand S, Penrhyn-Lowe S, Venkitaraman AR. Aurora-A amplification overrides the mitotic spindle assembly checkpoint, inducing resistance to Taxol. Cancer Cell 2003;3:51–62.

[83] Liang X, Wang D, Wang Y, Zhou Z, Zhang J, Li J. Expression of Aurora kinase A and B in chondrosarcoma and its relationship with the prognosis. Diagn Pathol 2012;7:84.

[84] Liu ZG, Yi W, Tao YL, Chan HC, Zeng MS, Xia YF. Aurora-A is an efficient marker for predicting poor prognosis in human nasopharyngeal carcinoma with aggressive local invasion: 208 cases with a 10-year follow-up from a single institution. Oncol Lett 2012;3:1237–1244.

[85] Ali HR, Dawson SJ, Blows FM, Provenzano E, Pharoah PD, Caldas C. Aurora kinase A outperforms Ki67 as a prognostic marker in ER-positive breast cancer. Br J Cancer 2012;106:1798–1806.

[86] Lehman NL, O'Donnell JP, Whiteley LJ, Stapp RT, Lehman TD, Roszka KM, Schultz LR, Williams CJ, Mikkelsen T, Brown SL, Ecsedy JA, Poisson LM. Aurora A is differentially expressed in gliomas, is associated with patient survival in glioblastoma and is a potential chemotherapeutic target in gliomas. Cell Cycle 2012;11:489–502.

[87] Dotan E, Meropol NJ, Zhu F, Zambito F, Bove B, Cai KQ, Godwin AK, Golemis EA, Astsaturov I, Cohen SJ. Relationship of increased aurora kinase A gene copy number, prognosis and response to chemotherapy in patients with metastatic colorectal cancer. Br J Cancer 2012;106:748–755.

[88] Wang J, Yang S, Zhang H, Song Y, Zhang X, Qian H, Han X, Shi Y. Aurora-A as an independent molecular prognostic marker in gastric cancer. Oncol Rep 2011;26:23–32.

[89] Yang F, Guo X, Yang G, Rosen DG, Liu J. AURKA and BRCA2 expression highly correlate with prognosis of endometrioid ovarian carcinoma. Mod Pathol 2011;24:836–845.

[90] Bibby RA, Tang C, Faisal A, Drosopoulos K, Lubbe S, Houlston R, Bayliss R, Linardopoulos S. A cancer-associated aurora A mutant mislocalized and misregulated due to loss of interaction with TPX2. J Biol Chem 2009;284:33177–33184.

[91] Lukasiewicz KB, Lingle WL. Aurora A, centrosome structure, and the centrosome cycle. Environ Mol Mutagen 2009;50:602–619.

[92] D'Assoro AB, Haddad T, Galanis E. Aurora-A kinase as a promising therapeutic target in cancer. Front Oncol 2016;5:295.

[93] D'Assoro AB, Liu T, Quatraro C, Amato A, Opyrchal M, Leontovich A, Ikeda Y, Ohmine S, Lingle W, Suman V, Ecsedy J, Iankov I, Di Leonardo A, Ayers-Inglers J, Degnim A, Billadeau D, McCubrey J, Ingle J, Salisbury JL, Galanis E. The mitotic kinase Aurora – a promotes distant metastases by inducing epithelial-to-mesenchymal transition in ERα(+) breast cancer cells. Oncogene 2014;33:599–610.

[94] Nguyen HG, Makitalo M, Yang D, Chinnappan D, St Hilaire C, Ravid K. Deregulated Aurora-B induced tetraploidy promotes tumorigenesis. FASEB J 2009;23:2741–2748.

[95] Pannone G, Hindi SA, Santoro A, Sanguedolce F, Rubini C, Cincione RI, De Maria S, Tortorella S, Rocchetti R, Cagiano S, Pedicillo C, Serpico R, Lo Muzio L, Bufo P. Aurora

B expression as a prognostic indicator and possible therapeutic target in oral squamous cell carcinoma. Int J Immunopathol Pharmacol 2011;24:79–88.

[96] Lin ZZ, Jeng YM, Hu FC, Pan HW, Tsao HW, Lai PL, Lee PH, Cheng AL, Hsu HC. Significance of Aurora B overexpression in hepatocellular carcinoma. Aurora B Overexpression in HCC. BMC Cancer 2010;10:461.

[97] Kimura M, Matsuda Y, Yoshioka T, Okano Y. Cell cycle-dependent expression and centrosome localization of a third human aurora/Ipl1-related protein kinase, AIK3. J Biol Chem 1999;274:7334–7440.

[98] Ulisse S, Delcros JG, Baldini E, Toller M, Curcio F, Giacomelli L, Prigent C, Ambesi-Impiombato FS, D'Armiento M, Arlot-Bonnemains Y. Expression of Aurora kinases in human thyroid carcinoma cell lines and tissues. Int J Cancer 2006;119:275–282.

[99] Baldini E, Arlot-Bonnemains Y, Mottolese M, Sentinelli S, Antoniani B, Sorrenti S, Salducci M, Comini E, Ulisse S, D'Armiento M. Deregulation of Aurora kinase gene expression in human testicular germ cell tumours. Andrologia 2010;42:260–267.

[100] Baldini E, Arlot-Bonnemains Y, Sorrenti S, Mian C, Pelizzo MR, De Antoni E, Palermo S, Morrone S, Barollo S, Nesca A, Moretti CG, D'Armiento M, Ulisse S. Aurora kinases are expressed in medullary thyroid carcinoma (MTC) and their inhibition suppresses in vitro growth and tumorigenicity of the MTC derived cell line TT. BMC Cancer 2011;11:411.

[101] Manchado E, Guillamot M, Malumbres M. Killing cells by targeting mitosis. Cell Death Differ 2012;19:369–377.

[102] Cheung CH, Coumar MS, Chang JY, Hsieh HP. Aurora kinase inhibitor patents and agents in clinical testing: an update (2009–10). Exp Opin Ther Pat 2011;21:857–884.

[103] Karthigeyan D, Prasad SBB, Shandilya J, Agrawal S, Kundu TK. Biology of Aurora A kinase: implications in cancer manifestation and therapy. Med Res Rev 2011;31:757–93.

[104] Matthews N, Visintin C, Hartzoulakis B, Jarvis A, Selwood DL. Aurora A and B kinases as targets for cancer: will they be selective for tumors? Exp Rev Anticancer Ther 2006;61:109–120.

[105] Kollareddy M, Zheleva D, Dzubak P, Brahmkshatriya PS, Lepsik M, Hajduch M. Aurora kinase inhibitors: progress towards the clinic. Invest New Drugs 2012;30:2411–2432.

[106] Lapenna S, Giordano A. Cell cycle kinases as therapeutic targets for cancer. Nat Rev Drug Discov 2009;8:547–566.

[107] Boss DS, Beijnen JH, Schellens JHM. Clinical experience with Aurora kinase inhibitors: a review. Oncologist 2009;14:780–793.

[108] Kitzen JJEM, de Jonge MJA, Verweij J. Aurora kinase inhibitors. Crit Rev Oncol Hematol, 2010;73:99–110.

[109] Cicenas J. The Aurora kinase inhibitors in cancer research and therapy. J Cancer Res Clin Oncol 2016; DOI 10.1007/s00432-016-2136-1.

[110] Falchook GS, Bastida CC, Kurzrockc R. Aurora kinase inhibitors in oncology clinical trials: current state of the progress. Semin Oncol 2015;42:832–848.

[111] Paller CJ, Wissing MD, Mendonca J, Sharma A, Kim E, Kim HS, Kortenhorst MS, Gerber S, Rosen M, Shaikh F, Zahurak ML, Rudek MA, Hammers H, Rudin CM, Carducci MA, Kachhap SK. Combining the pan-aurora kinase inhibitor AMG 900 with histone deacetylase inhibitors enhances antitumor activity in prostate cancer. Cancer Med 2014;3:1322–1335.

[112] Geuns-Meyer S, Cee VJ, Deak HL, Du B, Hodous BL, Nguyen HN, Olivieri PR, Schenkel LB, Vaida KR, Andrews P, Bak A, Be X, Beltran PJ, Bush TL, Chaves MK, Chung G, Dai Y, Eden P, Hanestad K, Huang L, Lin MH, Tang J, Ziegler B, Radinsky R, Kendall R, Patel VF, Payton M. Discovery of N-(4-(3-(2-aminopyrimidin-4-yl)pyridin-2-yloxy) phenyl)-4-(4-methylthiophen-2-yl)phthalazin-1-amine (AMG 900), a highly selective, orally bioavailable inhibitor of aurora kinases with activity against multidrug-resistant cancer cell lines. J Med Chem 2015;58:5189–5207.

[113] VanderPorten EC, Taverna P, Hogan JN, Ballinger MD, Flanagan WM, Fucini RV. The Aurora kinase inhibitor SNS-314 shows broad therapeutic potential with chemotherapeutics and synergy with microtubule-targeted agents in a colon carcinoma model. Mol Cancer Ther 2009;8:930–939.

[114] Lin YG, Immaneni A, Merritt WM, Mangala LS, Kim SW, Shahzad MM, Tsang YT, Armaiz-Pena GN, Lu C, Kamat AA, Han LY, Spannuth WA, Nick AM, Landen CN Jr, Wong KK, Gray MJ, Coleman RL, Bodurka DC, Brinkley WR, Sood AK. Targeting aurora kinase with MK-0457 inhibits ovarian cancer growth. Clin Cancer Res 2008;14:5437–5446.

[115] Yao R, Zheng J, Zheng W, Gong Y, Liu W, Xing R. VX680 suppresses the growth of HepG2 cells and enhances the chemosensitivity to cisplatin. Oncol Lett 2014;7:121–124.

[116] Wu X, Liu W, Cao Q, Chen C, Chen Z, Xu Z, Li W, Liu F, Yao X. Inhibition of Aurora B by CCT137690 sensitizes colorectal cells to radiotherapy. J Exp Clin Cancer Res 2014;33:13.

[117] Traynor AM, Hewitt M, Liu G, Flaherty KT, Clark J, Freedman SJ, Scott BB, Leighton AM, Watson PA, Zhao B, O'Dwyer PJ, Wilding G. Phase I dose escalation study of MK-0457, a novel Aurora kinase inhibitor, in adult patients with advanced solid tumors. Cancer Chemother Pharmacol 2011;67:305–314.

[118] Pollard JR, Mortimore M. Discovery and development of aurora kinase inhibitors as anticancer agents. J Med Chem. 2009;52:2629–2651.

[119] Giles FJ, Cortes J, Jones D, Bergstrom D, Kantarjian H, Freedman SJ. MK-0457, a novel kinase inhibitor, is active in patients with chronic myeloid leukemia or acute lymphocytic leukemia with the T315I BCR-ABL mutation. Blood 2007;109:500–502.

[120] Giles FJ, Swords RT, Nagler A, Hochhaus A, Ottmann OG, Rizzieri DA, Talpaz M, Clark J, Watson P, Xiao A, Zhao B, Bergstrom D, Le Coutre PD, Freedman SJ, Cortes JE. MK-0457, an Aurora kinase and BCR-ABL inhibitor, is active in patients with BCR-ABL T315I leukemia. Leukemia 2013;27:113–117.

[121] Seymour JF, Kim DW, Rubin E, Haregewoin A, Clark J, Watson P, Hughes T, Dufva I, Jimenez JL, Mahon FX, Rousselot P, Cortes J, Martinelli G, Papayannidis C, Nagler A, Giles FJ. A phase 2 study of MK-0457 in patients with BCR-ABL T315I mutant chronic myelogenous leukemia and Philadelphia chromosome-positive acute lymphoblastic leukemia. Blood Cancer J 2014;4:e238.

[122] Sorrentino R, Libertini S, Pallante PL, Troncone G, Palombini L, Bavetsias V, Spalletti-Cernia D, Laccetti P, Linardopoulos S, Chieffi P, Fusco A, Portella G. Aurora B overexpression associates with the thyroid carcinoma undifferentiated phenotype and is required for thyroid carcinoma cell proliferation. J Clin Endocrinol Metab 2005;90:928–935.

[123] Wiseman SM, Masoudi H, Niblock P, et al. Anaplastic thyroid carcinoma: expression profile of targets for therapy offers new insights for disease treatment. Ann Surg Oncol 2007;14:719–729.

[124] Rodrigues RF, Roque L, Rosa-Santos J, Cid O, Soares J. Chromosomal imbalances associated with anaplastic transformation of follicular thyroid carcinomas. Br J Cancer 2004;90:492–496.

[125] Libertini S, Abagnale A, Passaro C, Botta G, Barbato S, Chieffi P, Portella G. AZD1152 negatively affects the growth of anaplastic thyroid carcinoma cells and enhances the effects of oncolytic virus dl922-947. Endocr Relat Cancer 2011;18:129–141.

[126] Arlot-Bonnemains Y1, Baldini E, Martin B, Delcros JG, Toller M, Curcio F, Ambesi-Impiombato FS, D'Armiento M, Ulisse S. Effects of the Aurora kinase inhibitor VX-680 on anaplastic thyroid cancer-derived cell lines. Endocr Relat Cancer 2008;15:559–568.

[127] E. Baldini, S. Sorrenti, E. D'Armiento, et al., Effects of the Aurora kinases pan-inhibitor SNS-314 mesylate on anaplastic thyroid cancer derived cell lines. Clin Ter 2012;163:e307–313.

[128] Baldini E1, Tuccilli C, Prinzi N, Sorrenti S, Antonelli A, Gnessi L, Catania A, Moretti C, Mocini R, Carbotta G, Morrone S, Persechino S, Redler A, De Antoni E, D' Armiento M, Ulisse S. The dual Aurora kinase inhibitor ZM447439 prevents anaplastic thyroid cancer cell growth and tumorigenicity. J Biol Regul Homeost Agents 2013;27:705–715.

[129] Wunderlich A, Fischer M, Schlosshauer T, et al. Evaluation of Aurora kinase inhibition as a new therapeutic strategy in anaplastic and poorly differentiated follicular thyroid cancer. Cancer Sci 2011;102:762–768.

[130] Baldini E, Tuccilli C, Prinzi N, Sorrenti S, Antonelli A, Fallahi P, Mian C, Barollo S, Catania A, Morrone S, Tartaglia F, Mascagni D, Coccaro C, Pepe M, Filippini A, D'Armiento M, Ulisse S. Selective inhibitors of aurora kinases inhibit proliferation, reduce cell viability and impair cell cycle progression in papillary thyroid carcinoma cells. J Biol Regul Homeost Agents 2015;29:793–803.

[131] Wunderlich A, Roth S, Ramaswamy A. Combined inhibition of cellular pathways as a future option in fatal anaplastic thyroid cancer. Endocrine 2012;42:637–646.

[132] Bible KC, Suman VJ, Molina JR, Smallridge RC, Maples WJ, Menefee ME, Rubin J, Sideras K, Morris JC 3rd, McIver B, Burton JK, Webster KP, Bieber C, Traynor AM, Flynn PJ, Goh BC, Tang H, Ivy SP, Erlichman C; Endocrine Malignancies Disease Oriented Group; Mayo Clinic Cancer Center; Mayo Phase 2 Consortium. Efficacy of pazopanib in progressive, radioiodine-refractory, metastatic differentiated thyroid cancers: results of a phase 2 consortium study. Lancet Oncol 2010;11:962–972.

[133] Bible KC, Suman VJ, Menefee ME, Smallridge RC, Molina JR, Maples WJ, Karlin NJ, Traynor AM, Kumar P, Goh BC, Lim WT, Bossou AR, Isham CR, Webster KP, Kukla AK, Bieber C, Burton JK, Harris P, Erlichman C; Mayo Phase 2 Consortium; Mayo Clinic Endocrine Malignances Disease Oriented Group. A multiinstitutional phase 2 trial of pazopanib monotherapy in advanced anaplastic thyroid cancer. J Clin Endocrinol Metab 2012;97:3179–3184.

[134] Isham CR, Bossou AR, Negron V. Pazopanib enhances paclitaxel-induced mitotic catastrophe in anaplastic thyroid cancer. Sci Transl Med 2013;5:166ra3.

4

Computational Studies and Biosynthesis of Natural Products with Promising Anticancer Properties

Aurélien F.A. Moumbock, Conrad V. Simoben,
Ludger Wessjohann, Wolfgang Sippl,
Stefan Günther and Fidele Ntie-Kang

Abstract

We present an overview of computational approaches for the prediction of metabolic pathways by which plants biosynthesise compounds, with a focus on selected very promising anticancer secondary metabolites from floral sources. We also provide an overview of databases for the retrieval of useful genomic data, discussing the strengths and limitations of selected prediction software and the main computational tools (and methods), which could be employed for the investigation of the uncharted routes towards the biosynthesis of some of the identified anticancer metabolites from plant sources, eventually using specific examples to address some knowledge gaps when using these approaches.

Keywords: anticancer, biosynthesis, computational prediction, natural products, plant metabolism

1. Introduction

An immense number of secondary metabolites (SMs) exist in nature, originating from plants, bacteria, fungi and marine life forms, serving as drugs for the treatment of many life-threatening diseases, including cancer [1–4]. Taxol, vinblastine, vincristine, podophyllotoxin and camptothecin, for example, are typically well-known drugs used in cancer treatment, which are of plant origin. The search for drugs against cancer has often resorted to plants and marine life for lead compounds. To illustrate this, Newmann and Cragg published a recent study in which it was shown that ~49% of drugs used in cancer treatment were either natural products

(NPs) or their derivatives [5]. We would henceforth refer to SMs and NPs interchangeably, since NPs are the products of secondary (or specialised) metabolism, as opposed to primary metabolism, which results in molecules playing a key role in physiological processes of the organism and are thus necessary for the plant's survival. It should be mentioned that SMs are important for the plant's defence against attacks by other organisms. Several efforts have also been made towards the collection of data on naturally occurring plant metabolites showing anticancer properties. As an example, Mangal and co-workers published the naturally occurring plant-based anti-cancer compound activity-target database (NPACT), containing about 1,500 NPs [6]. In addition to the experimentally verified *in vitro* and *in vivo* data for these NPs, the authors also include biological activities (in the form of IC_{50}s, ED_{50}s, EC_{50}s, GI_{50}s, etc.), along with physical, elemental and topological properties of the NPs, the tested cancer types, cell lines, protein targets, commercial suppliers and drug likeness of the NPACT compounds. A similar effort was published the following year, for NPs from African flora, resulting in a dataset of about 400 compounds, named AfroCancer [7]. A further study showed that the NPACT and AfroCancer datasets showed little intersection, thus providing us a combined dataset of about 2,000 NPs [8]. The anticancer properties of some of the most promising AfroCancer compounds have been described in detail in recent reviews [9–12]. Further curation of data from Northern African species has recently resulted in the Northern African Natural Products Database (NANPDB), a web accessible and completely downloadable vast database of NPs, with a significant proportion of anticancer metabolites [13]. The NANPDB effort was founded on the observation that the Northern Africa region is particularly highly endowed with diverse vegetation types, serving as a huge reservoir of bioactive natural products [14–16].

For decades, NPs were identified exclusively by using chemical identification based on bioactivity-guided screening approaches. Recently, it has been postulated that genomics and bioinformatics would transform the approach of natural products discovery, even though genome mining has had only little influence on the advancement of natural product discovery until now [17]. Several algorithms have been developed for the mining of the (meta)genomic data, which continue to be generated. Computational methods and tools for the identification of biosynthetic gene clusters (BGCs, which are physically clustered groups of a few genes in a particular genome that together encode a biosynthetic pathway for the production of a specialised metabolite) in genome sequences and the prediction of chemical structures of their products have been developed [18]. BGCs for SM biosynthetic pathways are important in bacteria and filamentous fungi, with examples being recently discovered in plants [19, 20], although some metabolic processes in plants, for example, the thalianol pathway for triterpene synthesis in *Arabidopsis thaliana* has been suggested to be controlled by operon-like (clusters of unrelated) gene clusters [21]. This, coupled with the rapid progress in sequencing technologies has led to the development of new screening methods, which focus on whole genome sequences of the organisms producing the NPs. Genome mining approaches for NP discovery basically focus on:

- identifying the genes of the organism involved in the biosynthesis of the NPs,
- identifying the metabolic pathways by which the NPs are biosynthesised and
- predicting the products of the identified pathways (**Figure 1A**).

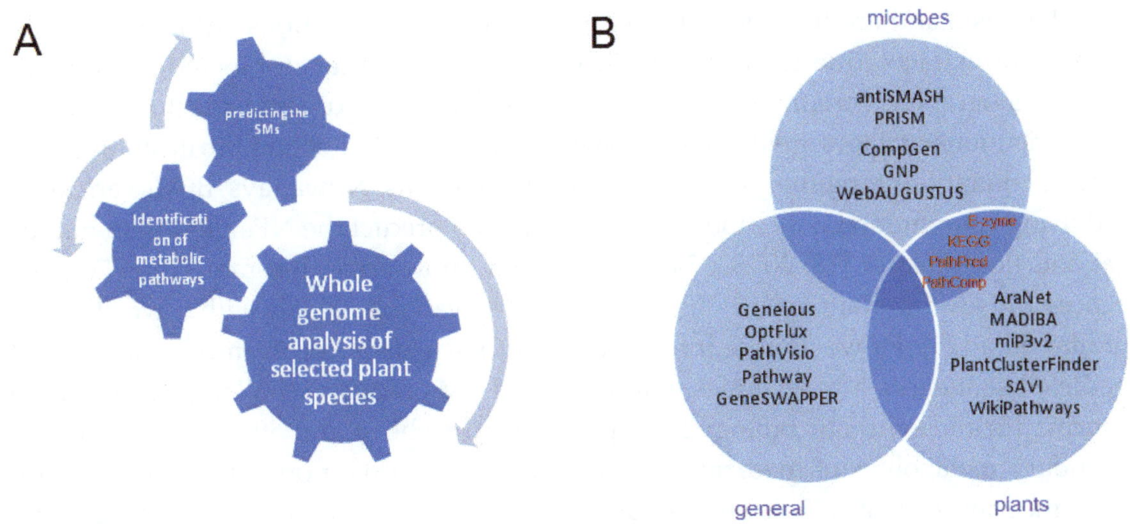

Figure 1. (A) Summary of genome mining approaches for the discovery of SMs and (B) classification of tools by applicability domain.

The four main strategies that are mostly employed to identify such pathways are based on processes involved in the production of plant secondary metabolites, for example, physical clustering, co-expression, evolutionary co-occurrence and epigenomic co-regulation of the genes [22–25]. Such approaches have been successfully applied for the investigation of fungal and microbial metabolites [26–28]. Since the discovery of the first gene cluster for secondary metabolism in *Zea mays*, the corn species [29], BGCs for plant secondary metabolism have become an emerging theme in plant biology [30]. It is even believed that synthetic biology technologies will eventually lead to the effective functional reconstitution of candidate pathways using a variety of genetic systems [25]. A knowledge of BGCs and their manipulation is therefore important in understanding how to activate a number of 'silent' gene clusters observed from the investigation of whole-genome sequencing of organisms. This would make available a wealth of new chemical entities (NCEs), which could be evaluated as drug leads and biologically active compounds [20].

This chapter aims at discussing the metabolic pathways by which plants biosynthesise compounds with anticancer activities, with a focus on selected very promising anticancer SMs from the African flora. We also aim to provide an overview of computational tools, which have been used to predict metabolic pathways and eventually address knowledge gaps when using the former. Additionally, we will present some databases for the retrieval of useful genomic data, discuss the strengths and limitations of selected computational (prediction) tools, which could be employed for the investigation of the uncharted routes towards the biosynthesis of some of the identified anticancer metabolites from plant sources, with specific examples. It is believed that properly addressing knowledge gaps that exist would lay the foundation for proper future investigations.

2. Natural products and plant genomic data

Genome data mining indicates that the vast majority of plant-based NPs have not yet been discovered [24, 25]. In addition, SMs are normally produced only at later growth stages of plant metabolism and are frequently found only at low concentrations within complex mixtures in plant extracts, due to several factors. Some of these factors include physiological variations, geographic variations, environmental conditions and genetic factors [25, 31, 32]. The aforementioned factors are the main drawbacks in the isolation and purification of NPs in meaningful quantities for either research or commercial aims. Nowadays, BGCs can be investigated using computational methodologies and used to predict the NPs present in microbial, fungal and floral matter [18, 20, 33, 34]. It is current knowledge that more than 70 genome sequences for several plant species have been made available, along with a wealth of transcriptome data [25]. However, the interpretation of such data, for example, the translation of predicted sequences into enzymes, pathways and SMs remains challenging. Advances in bioinformatics and synthetic biology have permitted the cheap and efficient overproduction of secondary metabolites of medicinal interest in heterologous (non-native) host organisms by reengineering of BGCs [35]. This is carried out through reengineering of BGCs as well as the activation of silent BGCs to yield unreported natural products of the target chemical space [17, 36], for example, an engineered *Escherichia coli* strain was used as the heterologous host organism for the production of taxadiene (a vital precursor of paclitaxel, an anticancer agent isolated from the bark of *Taxus brevifolia*), a precursor of the anticancer agent taxol [37]. In this way, quite a number of interesting SMs of plant origin (e.g. resveratrol, vanillin, conolidin, etc.) have been objects of pathway engineering in bacteria, yeast and other plants [38]. Thus, chemical libraries of diverse and novel hybrid natural products analogues can now be generated through combinatorial biosynthesis by manipulation of biosynthetic enzymes [39], for example, several analogues of the antibiotic erythromycin were obtained *via* combinatorial biosynthesis [40]. Such bioengineered libraries of 'unnatural' natural products show promises in drug discovery campaigns against multidrug-resistant cancer cells.

3. Some database resources for retrieving secondary metabolism prediction information

A summary of databases for retrieving information on BGCs is provided in **Table 1**. A majority of them focus on microbial BGCs, for example, ClusterMine360, ClustScan, DoBISCUIT, IMG-ABC and the Recombinant ClustScan Database. Details on the utility of the aforementioned databases have been provided in excellent recent reviews [26–28, 53]. Further efforts towards the construction of plant-based BGC and genomic databases include those of the Medicinal Plants Genomics and Metabolomics Resource consortium [47]. This effort has been focused on 14 medicinal plants and includes a BLAST search module, a genome browser, a genome putative search function tool and transcriptome search tools. While the entire database is available for download, similar efforts from the Plant Metabolic Network (PMN) have the advantage of having included several plant metabolic pathway databases, mostly among food crops [49, 50]. The PMN, for example, currently houses one multi-species reference database called PlantCyc and 22 species/taxon-specific databases, providing access to manually curated and/or computationally predicted information about enzymes, pathways, and more for individual species.

Database	Description	Web accessibility	Advantages	Disadvantages	Reference
ClusterMine360	A database of microbial polyketide and non-ribosomal peptide gene clusters.	http://www.clustermine360.ca/	Users can make contributions. Automation leads to high data consistency and quality data.	Focuses only on microbial PKS/NRPS biosynthesis	[41, 42]
ClustScan Database	A database for *in silico* detection of promising new compounds.	http://csdb.bioserv.pbf.hr/csdb/ClustScanWeb.html	Allows easy extraction of DNA and protein sequences of polypeptides, modules, and domains.	Currently includes data for only 57 SMs (PKS), 51 SMs (NRPS) and 62 SMs (PKS-NRPS hybrid) biosynthesis.	[43, 44]
DoBISCUIT	A database of secondary metabolite biosynthetic gene clusters.	http://www.bio.nite.go.jp/pks/	Provides standardised gene/module/domain descriptions related to the gene clusters. Available for download	Contains mostly data relating to bacterial species, mostly of the genus *Streptomyces*.	[45]
GenomeNet	A network of databases and computational services for genome research and related research areas in biomedical sciences.	http://www.genome.jp/	Provides several web accessible tools, e.g. KEGG, E-zyme, etc. See **Table 2**.		
IMG-ABC	A knowledge base for biosynthetic gene clusters for the discovery of novel SMs.	https://img.jgi.doe.gov/cgi-bin/abc-public/main.cgi	Integrates structural and functional genomics with annotated BGCs and associated SMs.	Not available for download. Limited to data on microbes	[46]
Medicinal Plants Genomics Resource	A database for medicinal plants genome sequence data.	http://medicinalplantgenomics.msu.edu/	Available for download	Only genomic data for 14 species are currently available.	[47]
Medicinal Plants Metabolomics Resource	A database for medicinal plants metabolomics data.	http://metnetweb.gdcb.iastate.edu/mpmr_public/	Available for download	Currently limited to metabolite data for 2 medicinal plant species.	[48]

Database	Description	Web accessibility	Advantages	Disadvantages	Reference
Minimum Information about a Biosynthetic Gene cluster (MIBiG)	A community standard for annotations and metadata on biosynthetic gene clusters and their molecular products.	http://mibig.secondarymetabolites.org/index.html	Facilitates the standardised deposition and retrieval of biosynthetic gene cluster data. Useful for the development of comprehensive comparative analysis tools. Available for download		[18]
Plant Metabolic Network (PMN)	Several plant metabolic pathway databases.	http://www.plantcyc.org/	Includes species/taxon-specific data for more than 22 plant species.		[49, 50]
Plant Reactome/"Cyc" Pathways	A pathway database for several crops and model plant species.	http://gramene.org/pathways	Currently includes gene homology-based pathway projections to 62 plant species.		[51]
Recombinant ClustScan Database	A database of gene cluster recombinants and their corresponding chemical structures.	http://csdb.bioserv.pbf.hr/csdb/RCSDB.html	Provides a virtual compound library, which could be a useful resource for computer-aided drug design of pharmaceutically relevant chemical entities.	Currently contains only 47 cluster combinations	[44, 52]
SMBP	Secondary metabolites bioinformatics portal.	http://www.secondarymetabolites.org/	Includes hand-curated links to all major tools and databases commonly used in the field		[53]

Table 1. Summary of currently available database resources for retrieving genomic data for biosynthesis prediction.

It provides a broad network of plant metabolic pathway databases that contain curated information from the literature and computational analyses about the genes, enzymes, compounds, reactions and pathways involved in primary and secondary metabolism in the included plant species. The PlantCyc database also provides access to manually curated or reviewed information about shared and unique metabolic pathways present in over 350 plant species. On the other hand, Plant Reactome is a pathway database for several crops and model plant species, making use of a framework of a eukaryotic cell model. Currently, it uses rice as a reference species and gene homology-based pathway projections have been made to 62 plant species [51].

4. Some computational tools for the analysis of genomic data and specialised metabolism prediction

Some computational tools for biochemical pathway prediction have been summarised in excellent reviews [54]. We have provided a more detailed summary of the main tools that could be useful in analysing plant and microbial genomic data for metabolism prediction in **Table 2**. Some of the tools are designed for the detection and analysis of specialised metabolism in microbes (e.g. antiSMASH, CompGen, GNP, PRISM and WebAUGUSTUS). Others are specially designed for plant metabolism prediction or may only include data for some specific organisms (e.g. AraNet, MADIBA, miP3v2, PlantClusterFinder, SAVI and WikiPathways for plants), while others are more general tools, useful for both microbial and plant metabolism prediction and BGC analysis (e.g. E-zyme, KEGG, PathPred and PathComp) and others are more useful for developers (e.g. Geneious, OptFlux, PathVisio and Pathway GeneSWAPPER), **Figure 1B**. We could also classify the tools according to their respective tasks; prediction and analysis of BGCs (e.g. antiSMASH, MADIBA, Pathway GeneSWAPPER, WebAUGUSTUS), searching, visualisation and prediction of biosynthetic pathways and reaction paths (e.g. BioCyc, CycSim, FMM, GNP, KEGG, MetaCyc, PathComp, PathPred, PathSearch, PathVisio, Pathway GeneSWAPPER, PlantClusterFinder, SAVI, WikiPathways for plants), prediction of SMs (PRISM), metabolic engineering (OptFlux), other functions (miP3v2). Among the tools for specialised metabolism in plants, AraNet is a probabilistic functional gene network (with currently a total of 27,029 protein-encoding genes) of *A. thaliana*. It is based on a modified Bayesian integration of data from multiple organisms, each data type being weighted based on how well it links genes that are known to function together in *A. thaliana*. Each interaction is associated with a log-likelihood score (LLS), which is a measure of the probability of an interaction representing a true functional linkage between two genes [56]. On the other hand, MADIBA facilitates the interpretation of *Plasmodium* and plant (data currently available for *Oryza sativa* and *A. thaliana*) gene clusters [64]. This tool eases the task by automating the post-processing stage during the assignment of biological meaning to gene expression clusters. MADIBA is designed as a relational database and has stored data from gene to pathway for the aforementioned species. Tools within the GUI allow the rapid analyses of each cluster with the view of identifying the Gene Ontology terms, as well as visualising the metabolic pathways where the genes are implicated, their genomic localisations, putative common

Tool	Utility	Web accessibility	Advantage	Disadvantage	Reference
antiSMASH*	A web server and tool for the automatic genomic identification and analysis of biosynthetic gene clusters.	http://antismash.secondarymetabolites.org.	Detects putative gene clusters of unknown types. Identifies similarities of identified clusters to any of 1172 clusters with known end products, etc.	Designed for analysis of BGCs in microbes.	[55]
AraNet	Gene function identification and genetic dissection of plant traits.	http://www.functionalnet.org/aranet/	Had greater precision than literature-based protein interactions (21%) for 55% of tested genes. Is highly predictive for diverse biological pathways.	Applicability is limited to one species - *A. thaliana*.	[56]
BioCyc/CycSim/MetaCyc	Online tools for genome-scale metabolic modelling.	https://biocyc.org/http://www.genoscope.cns.fr/cycsim https://metacyc.org/	Support the design and simulation of knockout experiments, e.g. deletions mutants on specified media, etc.		[57, 58]
CompGen	Carry out *in silico* homologous recombination between gene clusters.	http://csdb.bioserv.pbf.hr/csdb/RCSDB.html		Focuses on gene clusters encoding PKSs in *Streptomyces* sp. and related bacterial genera.	[52]
E-zyme	Assignment of EC numbers.	http://www.genome.jp/tools/e-zyme/	Classifies enzymatic reactions and links the enzyme genes or proteins to reactions in metabolic pathways.		[59]
From Metabolite to metabolite (FMM)	A web server to find biosynthetic routes between two metabolites within the KEGG database.	http://FMM.mbc.nctu.edu.tw/	Both local and global graphical views of the metabolic pathways are designed.		[60]
Geneious	Organisation and analysis of sequence data.	http://www.geneious.com/basic	Includes a public application programming interface (API) available for developers. Freely available for download.		[61]
Genomes-to-Natural Products platform (GNP)	Prediction, combinatorial design and identification of PKs and NRPs from biosynthetic assembly lines.	http://magarveylab.ca/gnp/	Uses LC–MS/MS data of crude extracts to make predictions in a high-throughput manner.	Focuses on bacterial NPs.	[62]

Tool	Utility	Web accessibility	Advantage	Disadvantage	Reference
Gene Regulatory network inference ACcuracy Enhancement (GRACE)	An algorithm to enhance the accuracy of transcriptional gene regulatory networks.	https://dpb.carnegiescience.edu/labs/rhee-lab/software	Focuses on plant species. Available for download.	Only algorithm is available. Lacks a graphical user interface	
KEGG Mapper	A tool to search a biosynthetic pathway.	http://www.kegg.jp/kegg/tool/map_pathway1.html?rn	KEGG is applicable to all organisms and enables interpretation of high-level functions from genomic and molecular data.		[63]
MicroArray Data Interface for Biological Annotation (MADIBA)	A webserver toolkit for biological interpretation of *Plasmodium* and plant gene clusters.	http://www.bi.up.ac.za/MADIBA	It allows rapid gene cluster analyses and the identification of the relevant Gene Ontology terms, visualisation of metabolic pathways, genomic localisations, etc.	Only 2 plant species are currently considered [rice (*Oryza sativa*), and *A. thaliana*].	[64]
miP3v2	Predicts microproteins in a sequenced genome.	https://github.com/npklein/miP3	Sheds light on the prevalence, biological roles, and evolution of microProteins.	Only the algorithm is available. Lacks a graphical user interface	[65]
OptFlux	A software platform for *in silico* metabolic engineering.	http://www.optflux.org/	Open source platform. Integrates visualisation tools. Allows users to load a genome-scale model of a given organism. Wild type and mutants can be simulated. Available for download.		[66]
PathComp	Possible reaction path computation.	http://www.genome.jp/tools/pathcomp/			
PathPred	Prediction of biodegradation and/or biosynthetic pathways.	http://www.genome.jp/tools/pathpred/	Specifically designed for biosynthesis of SMs (in plants) and xenobiotics biodegradation of environmental compounds (by bacteria).		[67]
PathSearch	Search for similar reaction pathways.	http://www.genome.jp/tools/pathsearch/			

Tool	Utility	Web accessibility	Advantage	Disadvantage	Reference
PathVisio	A biological pathway analysis software that allows users to draw, edit and analyse biological pathways.	http://www.pathvisio.org/	Plugins are included, which provide advanced analysis methods, visualisation options or additional import/export functionality. Available for download.		[68, 69]
Pathway GeneSWAPPER	Maps homologous genes from one species onto the PathVisio pathway diagram of another species.	http://jaiswallab.cgrb.oregonstate.edu/software/PGS	Improves the functionalities of PathVisio and WikiPathways for plants.		[70]
PlantClusterFinder	Predicts metabolic gene clusters from plant genomes.	https://dpb.carnegiescience.edu/labs/rhee-lab/software	Focuses on plant species. Available for download.	Only the algorithm is available. Lacks a graphical user interface	
Prediction informatics for secondary metabolomes (PRISM)	Genomes to natural products prediction informatics for secondary metabolomes.	http://magarveylab.ca/prism/	Open-source, user-friendly web available application.	Focuses on microbial SMs.	[71]
RetroPath	A webserver for retrosynthetic pathway design.	http://www.jfaulon.com/bioretrosynth/	Integrates pathway prediction and ranking, prediction of compatibility with host genes, toxicity prediction and metabolic modeling.		[72, 73]
Semi-Automated Validation Infrastructure (SAVI)	Predicts metabolic pathways using pathway metadata (e.g. taxonomic distribution, key reactions, etc.).	https://dpb.carnegiescience.edu/labs/rhee-lab/software	Decides which pathways to keep, remove or validate manually. Available for download.	Only the algorithm is available. Lacks a graphical user interface.	
WebAUGUSTUS	Gene prediction tool.	http://bioinf.uni-greifswald.de/webaugustus	One of the most accurate tools for eukaryotic gene prediction.	Focuses on eukaryotes.	[74]
WikiPathways for plants	A community pathway curation portal.	http://plants.wikipathways.org	Freely available.	Currently limited to rice and *Arabidopsis* sp.	[70, 75, 76]

*Currently provided detection rules for 44 classes and subclasses of SMs.

Table 2. Summary of current computational tools which could be useful for the plant genomic data analysis.

transcriptional regulatory elements in the upstream sequences, and an analysis specific to the organism being studied.

PlantClusterFinder, SAVI and WikiPathways for plants are all purpose tools designed to assist in the prediction of metabolic gene cluster from plant genomes, although WikiPathways for plants has currently included mostly data for rice and *Arabidopsis* sp. SAVI has the added advantage of offering the user the possibility of including pathway metadata (e.g. taxonomic distribution, key reactions, etc.) and offering the possibility to decide which pathway(s) to keep and which to remove or validate manually.

5. Some computational methods for efficient production and the *de novo* engineering of natural products

Two main areas for computational tools can be distinguished: on the one hand the rational modification of genomes for the production of molecules by host organisms, and on the other hand the modification or the *de novo* design of gene clusters for the biosynthesis of novel NPs. For both genetic engineering approaches, the already known genomes of bacteria, fungi and more and more plants provide the basic datasets. A very important computational approach for a rational modification of NP-producing host organisms is the genome-scale metabolic modelling [77, 78].

Automatic assignments of functional annotations of all genes in a genome are ideally proven by manual curation and enriched by current knowledge about the metabolic network of subjected organisms. The curated genomes are then applied to a complete automatic reconstruction of the metabolic pathways of the cell. These metabolic models are normally encoded in the Systems Biology Markup Language (SBML) and are compatible with various software tools, for example, Cytoscape [79], which can be applied for static network analyses. For instance, missing enzymes (gaps) within the network become apparent by substrates that are not taken up or have not been produced by the cell, as well as products that are not consumed by other reactions and are not secreted from cell. The RAST annotation pipeline provides a full automatic server for predicting all gene functions and discovering new pathways in microbial genomes of bacteria [80]. Such models can then be used to predict the turnover rate of each reaction in a Flux Balance Analysis (FBA) [81]. Several tools have been built, which apply FBA to identify enzymes that should be either introduced or knocked-out in the organism to increase production rate in the host organisms. A widely used FBA package is the MATLAB-based COBRA Toolbox [82]. With CycSim [58], BioMet [83] and FAME [84] powerful web-based FBA applications were published that do not require any software installation.

Within the last 10 years, FBA was applied to support numerous genetic engineering approaches, for example, for the determination of minimal media in *Helicobacter pylori* [85], for growth rate predictions in *Bacillus subtilis* [86] or for the development of metabolic engineering strategies in *Pseudomonas putida* [87]. Based on FBA, it was possible to increase vanillin production in baker's yeast by twofold and enhance sesquiterpene production in the same species [88, 89].

The rational modification of a given genome to design novel molecules needs a detailed understanding of the producing gene clusters. Well-studied gene clusters such as polyketide synthases consist of specific domain types that can be identified by trained hidden Markov models that are stored in related databases, for example, PFAM [90]. Gene cluster analysis tools such as antiSMASH [55, 91] or PRISM [71] analyse a given gene cluster to predict the specific domains and to describe the architecture of a gene cluster. However, the prediction of the structure of the resulting natural products is a difficult task because substrate recognition of active sites and the correct ordering of enzymatic reactions has to be predicted. If subjected enzymes are catalysing multiple substrates, the availability of each substrate has to be predicted. Most frequently, the automatic analysis of a cluster is based on the deduction of information from gene clusters similar to the queried one. If well-annotated similar gene clusters do not exist, the prediction of the structure of the biosynthesised NP is challenging. With more and more knowledge about the structure of natural products and the encoding sequences, the relation between the composition of the active sites and substrate binding will be better understood. Existing algorithms are often based on machine-learning approaches and predict the correct substrates for a selected set of enzyme families [92]. For the prediction of NPs synthesised by non-ribosomal peptide synthetases, such a sequence-based prediction method is integrated in the related web-server NRPSpredictor2 [93]. Rational substitution of residues to generate novel molecules still requires a detailed manual analysis of the encoding gene cluster, and new software tools that propose mutations leading to novel molecules might accelerate this approach considerably in future.

6. Selected natural products with promising anticancer properties from African sources

Recent reviews on the anticancer potential of African flora have discussed the anticancer, cytotoxic, antiproferative and antitumour activities of about 500 NPs [9–12]. In this section, we focus on the most promising (recent) results for anticancer SMs from African flora (**Table 3**, **Figure 2**), published after the last reviews. The isolation of two new lignans; 3α-O-(β-*D*-glucopyranosyl) desoxypodophyllotoxin (**1**) and 4-O-(β-*D*-glucopyranosyl) dehydropodophyllotoxin (**2**), alongside other known lignans (**3** and **4**), have been reported from the species, *Cleistanthus boivinianus* (Phyllanthaceae), collected in Madagascar (coordinates 13°06′37″S 049°09′39″E) [94]. These compounds showed potent to moderate antiproliferative activities against the A2780 ovarian cancer cell line, with compound **1** showing potent antiproliferative activity against the HCT-116 human colon carcinoma cell line (IC_{50} = 0.03 μM). The known compounds with promising activities from this species included the lignans; (±)-β-apopicropodophyllin (**3**, PubChem CID: 6452099), (−)-desoxypodophyllotoxin (**4**, PubChem CID: 345501). The same authors also isolated a new butanolide, macrocarpolide A (**5**, PubChem CID: 122372160) and two new secobutanolides; macrocarpolides B (**6**, PubChem CID: 122372161) and C (**7**, PubChem CID: 122372162), together with other known compounds from the ethanol extract of the roots of the Madagascan

Cpd. No.*	Molecule class	Source species (Family)	Cancer cell line	IC_{50} (μM)	Biosynthetic pathway	References
1	lignan	*Cleistanthus boivinianus* (Phyllanthaceae)	HCT-116 human colon carcinoma cell line	0.03	shikimic acid pathway, via phenylalanine	[94]
			A2780 ovarian cancer cell line	0.02		
2	″	″	″	2.10	″	″
3	″	″	″	0.06	″	
4	″	″	″	0.23	″	
5	butanolide	*Ocotea macrocarpa* (Lauraceae)	″	2.57		[95]
6	secobutanolide	″	″	1.98		″
7	″	″	″	1.67		″
8	butanolide	″	″	2.43		″
9	″	″	″	1.65		″
10	polyoxygenated cyclohexene derivative	*Cleistochlamys kirkii* (Annonaceae)	MDA-MB-231 triple-negative human breast cancer cell line	0.03	Shikimic acid pathway	[96]
11	″	″	″	0.29	″	″
12	″	″	″	0.29	″	″
13	″	″	″	0.12	″	″
14	″	″	″	0.45	″	″
15	″	″	″	2.10	″	″
16	″	″	″	0.09	″	″
17	″	″	″	2.70	″	″
18	″	″	″	0.24	″	″

*Compound number.

Table 3. Summary of recently published selected promising anticancer SMs from African flora.

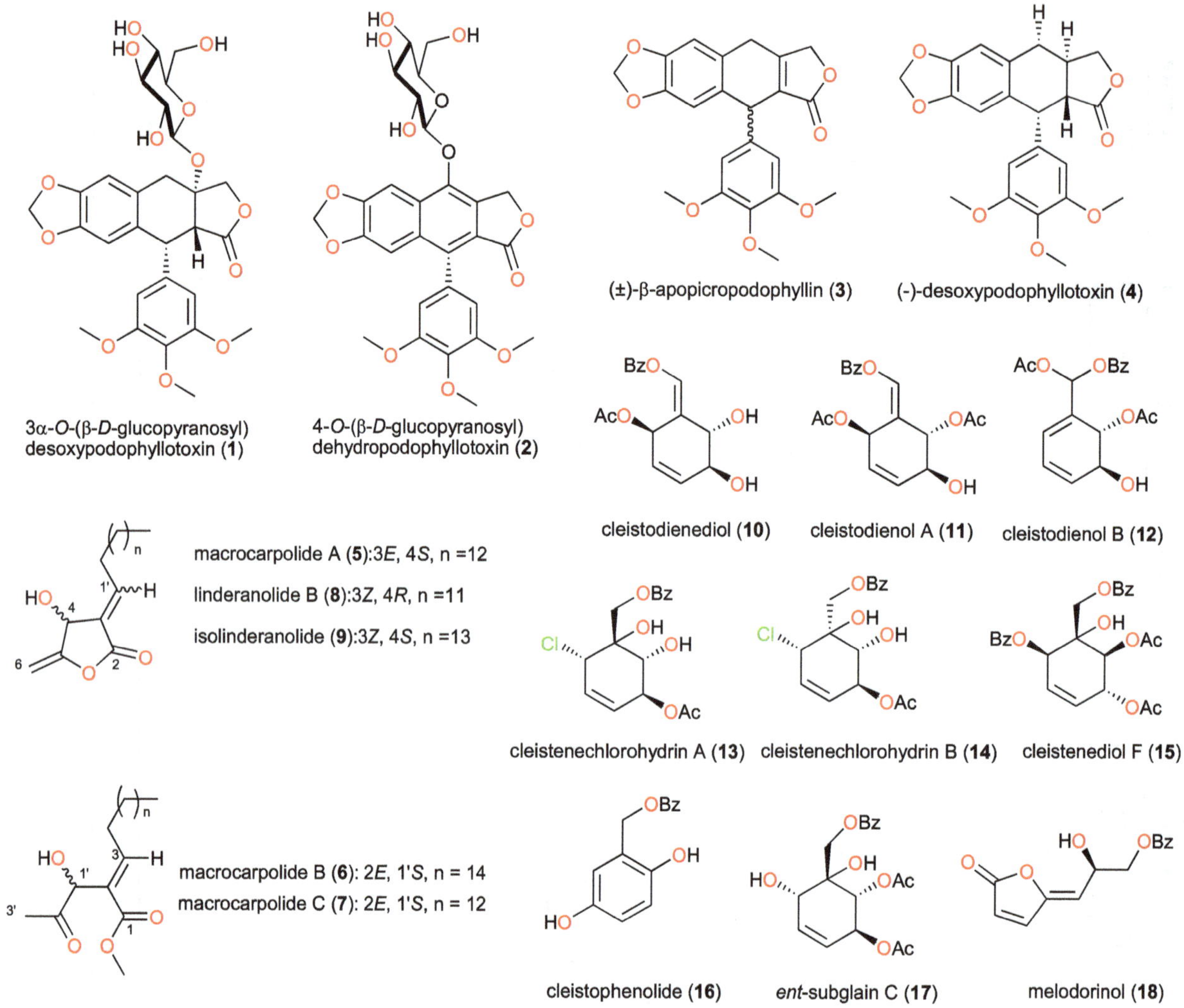

Figure 2. Chemical structures of selected anticancer SMs from African flora.

species *Ocotea macrocarpa* (Lauraceae), which showed antiproliferative activities against the A2780 ovarian cell line [95]. The known isolates included the butanolides; linderanolide B (**8**, PubChem CID: 53308122) and isolinderanolide (**9**, PubChem CID: 44576054). The anticancer activities showed IC_{50} values of 2.57 (**5**), 1.98 (**6**), 1.67 (**7**), 2.43 (**8**) and 1.65 μM (**9**) against A2780 ovarian cancer cell lines. Additionally, the leaves of *Cleistochlamys kirkii* (Annonaceae) from Tanzania have been recently shown to be a rich source of polyoxygenated cyclohexene derivatives with antiplasmodial activities, along with very potent activities against MDA-MB-231 triple-negative human breast cancer cell line [96]. The isolates; cleistodienediol (**10**), cleistodienol A (**11**), cleistodienol B (**12**), cleistenechlorohydrin A (**13**), cleistenechlorohydrin B (**14**), cleistenediol F (**15**), cleistophenolide (**16**), *ent*-subglain C (**17**) and melodorinol (**18**, PubChem CID: 6438687) showed some activities as low as IC_{50} = 0.09 μM against the aforementioned cancer cell lines. To the best of our knowledge, mode of action studies have not yet been conducted for the SMs **1** to **18** and *in vivo* activity data is currently unavailable.

7. Case studies

In this section, we shall discuss specific examples of the investigation of biosynthesis of anticancer plant-based SMs by (computational) analysis of genomic data.

7.1. Biogenesis of several anticancer metabolites by *Ocimum tenuiflorum* (Lamiaceae)

Species from the genus *Ocimum* are well known for their high medicinal values and are therefore used to cure a variety of ailments in Ayurveda, an Indian system of medicine [97, 98]. About 30 SMs have been reported from the genus *Ocimum*, with a variety of biological properties [99]. Only 14 of these SMs belong to the five basic groups of compounds having a complete biosynthetic pathway information in the PMN database [49, 50], thereby leaving us with ~15 medicinally relevant metabolites from *Ocimum* sp. with unknown pathways. This has prompted further investigation on SMs with uncharted biosynthetic pathways. Several bioactive SMs, including the anticancer compounds; apigenin (**19**, PubChem CID: 5280443), rosmarinic acid (**20**, PubChem CID: 5281792), taxol (**21**, PubChem CID: 36314), ursolic acid (**22**, PubChem CID: 64945), oleanolic acid (**23**, PubChem CID: 10494) and the plant steroid sitosterol (**24**, PubChem CID: 222284) have been identified from the herb Krishna Tulsi (*O. tenuiflorum*, Lamiaceae), with the mature leaves retaining the medicinally relevant metabolites [100]. Upadhyay et al. carried out a draft genome analysis of the species and generated paired-end and mate-pair sequence libraries for the whole sequenced genome, together with transcriptomic analysis (RNA-Seq) of two subtypes of *O. tenuiflorum* (Krishna and Rama Tulsi) and reporting the relative expression of genes in the both varieties. The authors further investigated the pathways, which lead to the biosynthesis of the identified SMs, with respect to similar pathways in *A. thaliana* and other model plants (e.g. *Oryza sativa japonica*). Six important genes (including *Q8RWT0* and *F1T282*) were expressed and identified from analysis of genome data. These were validated by q-RT-PCR on the different studied tissues (e.g. roots, mature leaves, etc.) of five closely related species (e.g. *O. gratissimum, O. sacharicum, O. kilmund, Solanum lycopersicum* and *Vitis vinifera*), which showed a high extent of urosolic acid-producing genes in young leaves. The other identified anticancer metabolites included eugenol and ursolic acid. As an example, the authors employed sequence search algorithms to search for the three enzymes of the three-step synthetic pathway of ursolic acid from squalene in the Tulsi genome. Each of these enzymes in Tulsi (squalene epoxidase, α-amyrin synthase and α-amyrin 2,8 monoxygenase) were queried from the PlantCyc database, starting from their protein sequences. The search for analogous enzymes in the model plants *O. sativa japonica* and *A. thaliana*, showed sequence identity covering from 50 to 80% of the query length. The whole genome and sequence analysis of *O. tenuiflorum* suggested that small amino acid changes at the functional sites of genes involved in metabolite synthesis pathways could confer special medicinal (particularly anticancer) properties to this herb.

7.2. Biosynthesis of the anticancer alkaloid noscapine by *Papaver somniferum* (Papaveraceae)

Noscapine (**25**, PubChem CID: 275196) is an antitumour phthalideisoquinoline alkaloid from opium poppy (*Papaver somniferum*, Papaveraceae). Compound **25** is known to bind stoichiometrically to tubulin, alters its conformation, affects microtubule assembly (promotes microtubule polymerisation), hence arresting metaphase and inducing apoptosis in many cell types [101]. It has been demonstrated that the compound has potent antitumour activity against solid murine lymphoid tumours (even when the drug was administered orally). This drug has also shown potency against human breast, ovarian and bladder tumours implanted in nude mice and in dividing human cells [102, 103]. Although the compound is water-soluble and absorbed after oral administration, its chemotherapeutic potential in human cancer could not be fully exploited for drug discovery projects because, like most SMs, this has been limited by the typically small amounts produced in the slow-growing plant species [104]. The quest to improve production levels of the NP is essential for drug discovery. However, such would require a proper understanding biological processes underlying the biosynthesis of this SM, known from isotope-labelling experiments to be derived from scoulerine since the 1960s [105]. Winzer et al. have carried out a transcriptomic analysis, with the aim of elucidating the biosynthetic pathway of this important metabolite for the improvement of its commercial production in both poppy and other systems [106]. The analysis of a high noscapine-producing poppy variety, HN1, showed the exclusive expression of 10 genes encoding five distinct enzyme classes, whereas five functionally characterised genes (*BBE, TNMT, SalR, SalAT* and *T6ODM*) were present in all three of the studied poppy varieties, respectively, rich in morphine, thebaine and noscapine (HM1, HN1 and HT1). The authors analysed the expressed sequence tag (EST) abundance and discovered some previously uncharacterised genes expressed in HN1, which were completely absent from the other (HM1 and HT1) EST libraries. This led to the identification of the corresponding enzymes as three *O*-methyltransferases (*PSMT1, PSMT2, PSMT3*), four cytochrome P450s (*CYP82X1, CYP82X2, CYP82Y1* and *CYP719A21*), an acetyltransferase (*PSAT1*), a carboxylesterase (*PSCXE1*) and a short-chain dehydrogenase/reductase (*PSSDR1*). Further analysis of an F2 mapping population, using HN1 and HM1 as parents, indicated that these genes are tightly linked in HN1. Moreover, bacterial artificial chromosome sequencing confirmed the existence of a complex BGC for plant alkaloids. Based on the knowledge derived from the investigation, the authors could make suggestions for the improved production of noscapine and related bioactive molecules by the molecular breeding of commercial poppy varieties or engineering of new production systems, for example, by virus-induced gene silencing, which resulted in the accumulation of pathway intermediates, thus allowing gene function to be linked to noscapine synthesis [104, 106].

7.3. Biosynthesis of vinblastine and vincristine by *Catharanthus roseus* (Apocynaceae)

Vinblastine (**26**, PubChem CID: 13342) and vincristine (**27**, PubChem CID: 5978) are chemotherapy drugs used to treat a number of cancer types. These are among the >120 known terpenoid indole alkaloids from the medicinal plant *C. roseus,* also known as the Madagascar periwinkle [107]. Since these two very important anticancer compounds have only been produced in very low amounts in *C. roseus,* as opposed to the fairly high levels of several monomeric alkaloids (e.g. ajmalicine and serpentine) [108], attempts to improve the yields of compounds **26** and **27** have led to the genome-wide transcript profiling of elicited *C. roseus* cell cultures, by cDNA-amplified fragment-length polymorphism combined with metabolic profiling [107]. This resulted in the identification of several gene-to-gene and gene-to-metabolite networks obtained by an attempt to establish correlations between the expression profiles of 417 gene tags and the accumulation profiles of 178 metabolite peaks. The results proved that different branches of terpenoid indole alkaloid biosynthesis and various other metabolic pathways are affected by differences in hormonal regulation. Thus, the investigations of Rischer et al. provided the foundations for a proper understanding of secondary metabolism in *C. roseus*, thereby enhancing the applicability of metabolic engineering of Madagascar periwinkle. This study provided the possibility of exploring a select number of genes (e.g. *STR*, *10HGO*, *T16H* and *DAT*) involved in biosynthesis of terpenoid indole alkaloids [107].

8. The way forward

The case studies show that the detailed computational analysis of the transcriptomic and metabolomic data of a plant species could reveal its metabolic capacity and hence help identify candidate genes involved in the biosynthesis of the important SMs it contains. Thus, modifying the plant genes could represent a premise for improving metabolite yield. It should be mentioned that other compounds from some of the aforementioned compound classes (**Table 3**), from both floral and microbial sources, have shown promising anticancer activities [109–113], e.g. isolinderanolide B (**28**, PubChem CID: 53308122) (**Figure 3**), a butanolide from the stems of *Cinnamomum subavenium* (Lauraceae) had shown antiproliferative activity in T24 human bladder cancer cells by blocking cell cycle progression and inducing apoptosis [112]. In addition, subamolide B (**29**, PubChem CID: 16104907), another butanolide from this same species, is known to induce cytotoxicity in human cutaneous squamous cell carcinoma through mitochondrial and CHOP-dependent cell death pathways [113]. Meanwhile, obtusilactone B (**30**, PubChem CID: 101286261), from *Machilus thunbergii* (Lauraceae), is known to target barrier-to-autointegration factor to treat cancer [111].

From the African flora, apart from the Lauraceae, Phyllanthaceae and Annonaceae, known to be rich in anticancer metabolites, the genus *Tacca* of the yam family (Dioscoreaceae) is known for the abundant presence of taccalonolides, which are microtubule stabilisers with clinical potential for cancer treatment [114]. Additionally, the genus *Tamarix* (e.g. *T. aphylla*

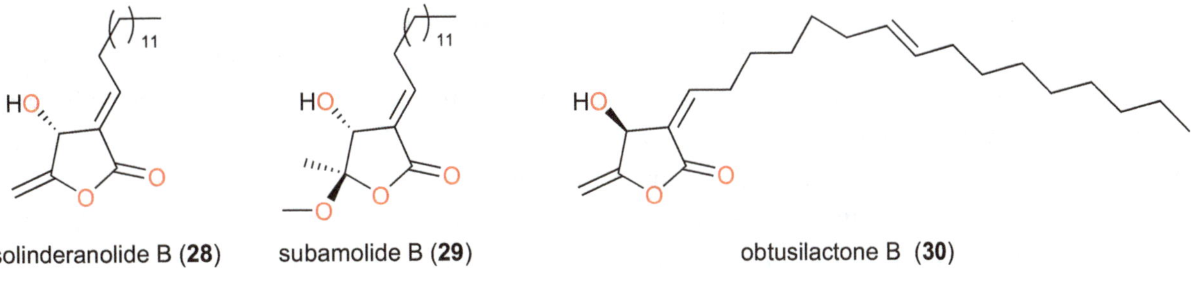

isolinderanolide B (**28**) subamolide B (**29**) obtusilactone B (**30**)

Figure 3. Chemical structures of selected anticancer butanolides from Lauraceae.

and *T. nilotica* from Northern Africa), together with the genus *Reaumuria* (Tamaricaceae) are known for the abundant presence of tannins (gallo-ellagitannin, gallotannins) with remarkable cytotoxic effects. The high salt content of the leaves of *Tamarix* species, rendering them useful locally as a fire barrier, and their adaptability to drought and high salinity are of equal interest. It therefore becomes urgent to investigate the genomics of some of the aforementioned plant species, particularly those from the *Cinnamomum* sp., *Ocotea* sp. and *Machilus* sp. (Lauraceae), *Tacca* sp. (Dioscoreaceae), *Cleistanthus* sp. (Phyllanthaceae), *Cleistochlamys* sp. (Annonaceae), *Tamarix* sp. (Tamaricaceae) and so on, and hence further investigate the genes or BGCs responsible for secondary metabolism with the view of understanding and better exploring the biosynthetic pathways of the anticancer SMs.

9. Conclusions

It has been our intention in this chapter to provide a detailed overview of the important computational tools and resources for the analysis of plant genomic data and for the prediction of biosynthetic pathways in plants. We have taken a few case studies of anticancer SMs to illustrate this. Even though it is unclear how widespread plant genes are clusters, genes that encode the biosynthesis of several small plant SMs are well known, including the vital genes for the production of some highly potent anticancer drugs. With the use of the tools and databases described, along with the drop in the cost of whole genome sequencing in plant species, the future for the discovery of new plant-based anticancer metabolites would involve the identification of one or more genes or BGCs encoding the enzymes in the biosynthetic pathway for the target compound(s), followed by the co-expression analysis, also exploiting the knowledge of the chemical structure of the target compound, for the identification of other enzymes that might be involved in this pathway. As an example, the exploration of the pathway for podophyllotoxin biosynthesis by the use transcriptome mining in *Podophyllum hexandrum* led to the identification biosynthetic genes, 29 of which were combinatorially expressed in the tobacco plant (*Nicotiana benthamiana*), leading to the identification of six pathway enzymes, among which is oxoglutarate-dependent dioxygenase responsible for closing the core cyclohexane ring of the aryltetralin scaffold [115]. An alternative approach could be, if the metabolic pathway and nature of SMs are unknown, then the identified co-expressed genes encoding the enzymes for secondary metabolism could be subjected to untargeted metabolomics for the elucidation of unknown pathways and chemical structures. As an example, a single pathogen-induced P450 enzyme, CYP82C2, with a combination of untargeted metabolomics and co-expression analysis was used to uncover the complete biosynthetic pathway, which leads to the metabolite 4-hydroxyindole-3-carbonyl nitrile, previously unknown to *Arabidopsis* sp. This rare and hitherto unprecedented plant metabolite, with a cyanogenic functionality revealed a hidden capacity of *Arabidopsis* sp. for cyanogenic glucoside biosynthesis. This was confirmed by expressing 4-OH-ICN engineering biosynthetic enzymes in *Saccharomyces cerevisiae* and *Nicotiana benthamiana*, to reconstitute the complete pathway *in vitro* and *in vivo*, thus validating the functions of the enzymes involved in the pathway [116].

Acknowledgements

FNK acknowledges a Georg Forster fellowship from the Alexander von Humboldt Foundation, Germany. CVS is currently a doctoral candidate financed by the German Academic Exchange Services (DAAD), Germany.

Competing interests

The authors declare that they have no competing interests.

Abbreviations

AfroCancer	African Anticancer Natural Products Database
BGC	Biosynthetic gene clusters
EC_{50}	Half maximal effective concentration, that is, the concentration of a drug, antibody or toxicant, which induces a response halfway between the baseline and maximum after a specified exposure time
ED_{50}	The median effective dose, a dose that produces the desired effect in 50% of a population
FBA	Flux Balance Analysis
GI_{50}	The growth inhibition of 50%, drug concentration resulting in a 50% reduction in the net protein increase.
IC_{50}	The drug concentration causing 50% inhibition of the desired activity
IMG-ABC	The Integrated Microbial Genomes Atlas of Biosynthetic gene Clusters
NANPDB	Northern African Natural Products Database
NP	Natural product
NPACT	Naturally Occurring Plant-based Anti-cancer Compound Activity-Target Database
NRP	Nonribosomal peptide
NRPS	Nonribosomal peptide synthase
PK	Polyketide
PKS	Polyketides synthase
PMN	Plant Metabolic Network
PRISM	PRediction Informatics for Secondary Metabolomes
SM	Secondary metabolite

Author details

Aurélien F.A. Moumbock[1], Conrad V. Simoben[2], Ludger Wessjohann[3], Wolfgang Sippl[2], Stefan Günther[4] and Fidele Ntie-Kang[1,2]*

*Address all correspondence to: ntiekfidele@gmail.com

1 Department of Chemistry, University of Buea, Buea, Cameroon

2 Department of Pharmaceutical Chemistry, Martin-Luther University of Halle-Wittenberg, Halle, Germany

3 Leibniz Institute of Plant Biochemistry, Halle, Germany

4 Pharmaceutical Bioinformatics, Albert-Ludwig-University Freiburg, Freiburg, Germany

References

[1] Cragg GM, Newman DJ. Plants as a source of anti-cancer and anti-HIV agents. Ann Appl Biol. 2003;143:127-133. doi:10.1111/j.1744-7348.2003.tb00278.x

[2] Cragg GM, Grothaus PG, Newman DJ. Impact of natural products on developing new anti-cancer agents. Chem Rev. 2009;109:3012-3043. doi:10.1021/cr900019j

[3] Lamari FN, Cordopatis P. Exploring the potential of natural products in cancer treatment. In: Missailidis S, editor. *Anticancer therapeutics*. West Sussex: Wiley-Blackwell; 2008, pp. 3-16.

[4] Pan L, Chai HB, Kinghorn AD. Discovery of new anticancer agents from higher plants. Front Biosci (Schol Ed). 2013;4:142-156.

[5] Newman DJ, Cragg GM. Natural products as sources of new drugs from 1981 to 2014. J Nat Prod. 2016;79:629-661. doi:10.1021/acs.jnatprod.5b01055

[6] Mangal M, Sagar P, Singh H, Raghava GPS, Agarwal SM. NPACT: naturally occurring plant-based anti-cancer compound activity-target database. Nucleic Acids Res. 2013;41:D1124-D1129. doi:10.1093/nar/gks1047

[7] Ntie-Kang F, Nwodo JN, Ibezim A, Simoben CV, Karaman B, et al. Molecular modeling of potential anticancer agents from African medicinal plants. J Chem Inf Model. 2014;54:2433-2450. doi:10.1021/ci5003697

[8] Ntie-Kang F, Simoben CV, Karaman B, Ngwa VF, Judson PN, et al. Pharmacophore modeling and *in silico* toxicity assessment of potential anticancer agents from African medicinal plants. Drug Des Dev Ther. 2016;10:2137-2154. doi:10.2147/DDDT.S108118

[9] Beutler JA, Cragg GM, Iwu M, Newman DJ, Okunji C. Anticancer potential of African plants: the experience of the United States National Cancer Institute and National

Institutes of Health. In: Gurib-Fakim A, editor. Novel plant bioresources: applications in food, medicine and cosmetics, 1st ed. Oxford: John Wiley & Sons Ltd; 2014, pp. 133-149. doi:10.1002/9781118460566.ch10

[10] Nwodo JN, Ibezim A, Simoben CV, Ntie-Kang F. Exploring cancer therapeutics with natural products from African medicinal plants, part II: alkaloids, terpenoids and flavonoids. Anticancer Agents Med Chem. 2016;16:108-127. doi:10.2174/1871520615666150520143827

[11] Simoben CV, Ibezim A, Ntie-Kang F, Nwodo JN, Lifongo LL. Exploring cancer therapeutics with natural products from African medicinal plants, part I: xanthones, quinones, steroids, coumarins, phenolics and other classes of compounds. Anticancer Agents Med Chem. 2015;15:1092-1111. doi:10.2174/1871520615666150113110241

[12] Simoben CV, Ntie-Kang F. African medicinal plants: an untapped reservoir of potential anticancer agents. In: Prasad S, Tyagi AK, editors. Cancer preventive and therapeutic compounds: gift from mother nature. Beijing: Bentham Science Publishers; 2016. p. 78-95.

[13] Ntie-Kang F, Telukunta KK, Döring K, Simoben CV, Moumbock, et al. The Northern African Natural Products Database (NANPDB), 2016. www.african-compounds.org/nanpdb

[14] Ntie-Kang F, Yong JN. The chemistry and biological activities of natural products from Northern African plant families: from Aloaceae to Cupressaceae. RSC Adv. 2014;4:61975-61991. doi:10.1039/C4RA11467A

[15] Yong JN, Ntie-Kang F. The chemistry and biological activities of natural products from Northern African plant families: from Ebenaceae to Solanaceae. RSC Adv. 2015;5:26580-26595. doi:10.1039/C4RA15377D

[16] Ntie-Kang F, Njume LE, Malange YI, Günther S, Sippl W, et al. The chemistry and biological activities of natural products from Northern African plant families: from Taccaceae to Zygophyllaceae. Nat Prod Bioprospect. 2016;6:63-96. doi:10.1007/s13659-016-0091-9

[17] Medema MH, Fischbach M. Computational approaches to natural product discovery. Nat Chem Biol. 2015;11:639-648. doi:10.1038/nchembio.1884

[18] Medema MH, Kottmann R, Yilmaz P, Cummings M, Biggins JB, et al. Minimum information about a biosynthetic gene cluster. Nat Chem Biol. 2015;11:625-631. doi:10.1038/nchembio.1890

[19] Nützmann HW, Osbourn A. Gene clustering in plant specialized metabolism. Curr Opin Biotechnol. 2014;26:91-99. doi:10.1016/j.copbio.2013.10.009

[20] Osbourn A. Secondary metabolic gene clusters: evolutionary toolkits for chemical innovation. Trends Genet. 2010;26:449-457. doi:10.1016/j.tig.2010.07.001

[21] Osbourn AE, Field B. Operons. Cell Mol Life Sci. 2009;66:3755-3775. doi:10.1007/s00018-009-0114-3

[22] Rhee SY, Mutwil M. Towards revealing the functions of all genes in plants. Trends Plant Sci. 2014;19:212-221. doi:10.1016/j.tplants.2013.10.006

[23] Xu M, Rhee SY. Becoming data-savvy in a big-data world. Trends Plant Sci. 2014;19:619-622. doi:10.1016/j.tplants.2014.08.003

[24] Chae L, Lee I, Shin J, Rhee SY. Towards understanding how molecular networks evolve in plants. Curr Opin Plant Biol. 2012;15:177-184. doi:10.1016/j.pbi.2012.01.006

[25] Medema MH, Osbourn A. Computational genomic identification and functional reconstitution of plant natural product biosynthetic pathways. Nat Prod Rep. 2016;33:951-962. doi:10.1039/c6np00035e

[26] Weber T. *In silico* tools for the analysis of antibiotic biosynthetic pathways. Int J Med Microbiol. 2014;304:230-235. doi:10.1016/j.ijmm.2014.02.001

[27] Li YF, Tsai KJ, Harvey CJ, Li JJ, Ary BE, et al. Comprehensive curation and analysis of fungal biosynthetic gene clusters of published natural products. Fungal Genet Biol. 201689:18-28. doi:10.1016/j.fgb.2016.01.012

[28] van der Lee TA, Medema MH. Computational strategies for genome-based natural product discovery and engineering in fungi. Fungal Genet Biol. 2016;89:29-36. doi:10.1016/j.fgb.2016.01.006

[29] Frey M, Chomet P, Glawischnig E, Stettner C, Grun S, et al. Analysis of a chemical plant defense mechanism in grasses. Science. 1997;277:696-699. doi:10.1126/science.277.5326.696

[30] Osbourn A. Gene clusters for secondary metabolic pathways: an emerging theme in plant biology. Plant Physiol. 2010;154:531-535. doi:10.1104/pp.110.161315

[31] Figueiredo AC, Barroso JG, Pedro LG, Scheffer JJC. Factors affecting secondary metabolite production in plants: volatile components and essential oils. Flavour Fragr J. 2008;23:213-226. doi:10.1002/ffj.1875

[32] Leal MC, Hilario A, Munro MHG, Blunt JW, Calado R. Natural products discovery needs improved taxonomic and geographic information. Nat Prod Rep. 2016;33:747-750. doi:10.1039/c5np00130g

[33] Luo Y, Enghiad B, Zhao H. New tools for reconstruction and heterologous expression of natural product biosynthetic gene clusters. Nat Prod Rep. 2016;33:174-182. doi:10.1039/c5np00085h

[34] Carbonell P, Currin A, Jervis AJ, Rattray NJW, Swainston N, et al. Bioinformatics for the synthetic biology of natural products: integrating across the Design-Build-Test cycle. Nat Prod Rep. 2016;33:925-932. doi:10.1039/c6np00018e

[35] Song MC, Kim EJ, Kim E, Rathwell K, Nama SJ, et al. Microbial biosynthesis of medicinally important plant secondary metabolites. Nat Prod Rep. 2014;31:1497-1509. doi:10.1039/c4np00057a

[36] Zhao H, Medema MH. Standardization for natural product synthetic biology. Nat Prod Rep. 2016;33:920-924. doi:10.1039/c6np00030d

[37] Ajikumar PK, Xiao WH, Tyo KE, Wang Y, Simeon F, et al. Isoprenoid pathway optimization for Taxol precursor overproduction in *Escherichia coli*. Science. 2010;330:70-74. doi:10.1126/science.1191652

[38] De Luca V, Salim V, Atsumi SM, Yu F. Mining the biodiversity of plants: a revolution in the making. Science. 2012;336:1658-1661. doi:10.1126/science.1217410

[39] Kim E, Moore BS, Yoon YJ. Reinvigorating natural product combinatorial biosynthesis with synthetic biology. Nat Chem Biol. 2015;11:639-659. doi:10.1038/nchembio.1893

[40] Menzella HG, Reid R, Carney JR, Chandran SS, Reisinger SJ, et al. Combinatorial polyketide biosynthesis by *de novo* design and rearrangement of modular polyketide synthase genes. Nat Biotechnol. 2005;23:1171-1176. doi:10.1038/nbt1128

[41] Conway KR, Boddy CN. ClusterMine360: a database of microbial PKS/NRPS biosynthesis. Nucleic Acids Res. 2013;41:D402-D407. doi:10.1093/nar/gks993

[42] Tremblay N, Hill P, Conway KR, Boddy CN. The use of ClusterMine360 for the analysis of polyketide and nonribosomal peptide biosynthetic pathways. Methods Mol Biol. 2016;1401:233-252. doi:10.1007/978-1-4939-3375-4_15

[43] Starcevic A, Zucko J, Simunkovic J, Long PF, Cullum J, et al. ClustScan: an integrated program package for the semi-automatic annotation of modular biosynthetic gene clusters and *in silico* prediction of novel chemical structures. Nucleic Acids Res. 2008;36:6882-6892. doi:10.1093/nar/gkn685

[44] Diminic J, Zucko J, Ruzic IT, Gacesa R, Hranueli D, et al. Databases of the thiotemplate modular systems (CSDB) and their *in silico* recombinants (r-CSDB). J Ind Microbiol Biotechnol. 2013;40:653-659. doi:10.1007/s10295-013-1252-z

[45] Ichikawa N, Sasagawa M, Yamamoto M, Komaki H, Yoshida Y, et al. DoBISCUIT: a database of secondary metabolite biosynthetic gene clusters. Nucleic Acids Res. 2013;41:D408-D414. doi:10.1093/nar/gks1177

[46] Hadjithomas M, Chen IA, Chu K, Ratner A, Palaniappan K, et al. IMG-ABC: a knowledge base to fuel discovery of biosynthetic gene clusters and novel secondary metabolites. mBio. 2015;6:e00932-15. doi:10.1128/mBio.00932-15

[47] Kellner F, Kim J, Clavijo BJ, Hamilton JP, Childs KL, et al. Genome-guided investigation of plant natural product biosynthesis. Plant J. 2015;82:680-692. doi:10.1111/tpj.12827

[48] Hur M, Campbell AA, Almeida-de-Macedo M, Li L, Ransom N, et al. A global approach to analysis and interpretation of metabolic data for plant natural product discovery. Nat Prod Rep. 2013;30:565-583. doi:10.1039/c3np20111b

[49] Chae L, Kim T, Nilo-Poyanco R, Rhee SY. Genomic signatures of specialized metabolism in plants. Science. 2014;344: 510-513. doi:10.1126/science.1252076

[50] Dreher K. Putting the plant metabolic network pathway databases to work: going offline to gain new capabilities. Methods Mol Biol. 2014;1083:151-171. doi:10.1007/978-1-62703-661-0_10

[51] Naithani S, Preece J, D'Eustachio P, Gupta P, Amarasinghe V, et al. Plant Reactome: a resource for plant pathways and comparative analysis. Nucleic Acids Res. 2017;45:D1029-D1039. doi:10.1093/nar/gkw932

[52] Starcevic A, Wolf K, Diminic J, Zucko J, Ruzic IT, et al. Recombinatorial biosynthesis of polyketides. J Ind Microbiol Biotechnol. 2012;39:503-511. doi:10.1007/s10295-011-1049-x

[53] Weber T, Kim HU. The secondary metabolite bioinformatics portal: computational tools to facilitate synthetic biology of secondary metabolite production. Synth Syst Biotechnol. 2016;1:69-79. doi:10.1016/j.synbio.2015.12.002

[54] Medema MH, van Raaphorst R, Takano E, Breitling R. Computational tools for the synthetic design of biochemical pathways. Nat Rev Microbiol. 2012;10:191-202. doi:10.1038/nrmicro2717

[55] Weber T, Blin K, Duddela S, Krug D, Kim HU, et al. antiSMASH 3.0—a comprehensive resource for the genome mining of biosynthetic gene clusters. Nucleic Acids Res. 2015;43:W237-W243. doi:10.1093/nar/gkv437

[56] Lee I, Ambaru B, Thakkar P, Marcotte EM, Rhee SY. Rational association of genes with traits using a genome-scale gene network for *Arabidopsis thaliana*. Nat Biotechnol. 2010;28:149-156. doi:10.1038/nbt.1603

[57] Caspi R, Billington R, Ferrer L, Foerster H, Fulcher CA, et al. The MetaCyc database of metabolic pathways and enzymes and the BioCyc collection of pathway/genome databases. Nucleic Acids Res. 2016;44:D471-D480. doi:10.1093/nar/gkv1164

[58] Le Fèvre F, Smidtas S, Combe C, Durot M, d'Alché-Buc F, et al. CycSim—an online tool for exploring and experimenting with genome-scale metabolic models. Bioinformatics. 2009;25:1987-1988. doi:10.1093/bioinformatics/btp268

[59] Yamanishi Y, Hattori M, Kotera M, Goto S, Kanehisa M. E-zyme: predicting potential EC numbers from the chemical transformation pattern of substrate-product pairs. Bioinformatics. 2009;25:i179-i186. doi:10.1093/bioinformatics/btp223

[60] Chou CH, Chang WC, Chiu CM, Huang CC, Huang HD. FMM: a web server for metabolic pathway reconstruction and comparative analysis. Nucleic Acids Res. 2009;37:W129-W134. doi:10.1093/nar/gkp264

[61] Kearse M, Moir R, Wilson A, Stones-Havas S, Cheung M, et al. Geneious basic: an integrated and extendable desktop software platform for the organization and analysis of sequence data. Bioinformatics. 2012;28:1647-1649. doi:10.1093/bioinformatics/bts199

[62] Johnston CW, Skinnider MA, Wyatt MA, Li X, Ranieri MRM, et al. An automated Genomes-to-Natural Products platform (GNP) for the discovery of modular natural products. Nat Commun. 2015;6:8421. doi:10.1038/ncomms9421

[63] Kanehisa M. KEGG bioinformatics resource for plant genomics and metabolomics. Methods Mol Biol. 2016;1374:55-70. doi:10.1007/978-1-4939-3167-5_3

[64] Law PJ, Claudel-Renard C, Joubert F, Louw AI, Berger DK. MADIBA: a web server toolkit for biological interpretation of *Plasmodium* and plant gene clusters. BMC Genomics. 2008;9:105. doi:10.1186/1471-2164-9-105

[65] de Klein N, Magnani E, Banf M, Rhee SY. microProtein Prediction Program (miP3): a software for predicting microProteins and their target transcription factors. Int J Genomics. 2015;2015:734147. doi:10.1155/2015/734147

[66] Rocha I, Maia P, Evangelista P, Vilaça P, Soares S, et al. OptFlux: an open-source software platform for *in silico* metabolic engineering. BMC Syst Biol. 2010;4:45. doi:10.1186/1752-0509-4-45

[67] Moriya Y, Shigemizu D, Hattori M, Tokimatsu T, Kotera M, et al. PathPred: an enzyme-catalyzed metabolic pathway prediction server. Nucleic Acids Res. 2010;38:W138-W143. doi:10.1093/nar/gkq318

[68] Kutmon M, van Iersel MP, Bohler A, Kelder T, Nunes N, et al. PathVisio 3: an extendable pathway analysis toolbox. PLoS Comput Biol. 2015;11:e1004085. doi:10.1371/journal.pcbi.1004085

[69] van Iersel MP, Kelder T, Pico AR, Hanspers K, Coort S, et al. Presenting and exploring biological pathways with PathVisio. BMC Bioinformat. 2008;9:399. doi:10.1186/1471-2105-9-399

[70] Hanumappa M, Preece J, Elser J, Nemeth D, Bono G, et al. WikiPathways for plants: a community pathway curation portal and a case study in rice and *Arabidopsis* seed development networks. Rice. 2013;6:14. doi:10.1186/1939-8433-6-14

[71] Skinnider MA, Dejong CA, Rees PN, Johnston CW, Li H, et al. Genomes to natural products PRediction Informatics for Secondary Metabolomes (PRISM). Nucleic Acids Res. 2015;43:9645-9662. doi:10.1093/nar/gkv1012

[72] Carbonell P, Planson AG, Fichera D, Faulon JL. A retrosynthetic biology approach to metabolic pathway design for therapeutic production. BMC Syst Biol. 2011;5:122. doi:10.1186/1752-0509-5-122

[73] Planson AG, Carbonell P, Grigoras I, Faulon JL. A retrosynthetic biology approach to therapeutics: from conception to delivery. Curr Opin Biotechnol. 2012;23:948-956. doi:10.1016/j.copbio.2012.03.009

[74] Hoff KJ, Stanke M. WebAUGUSTUS - a web service for training AUGUSTUS and predicting genes in eukaryotes. Nucleic Acids Res. 2013;41:W123-W128. doi:10.1093/nar/gkt418

[75] Kelder T, van Iersel MP, Hanspers K, Kutmon M, Conklin BR, et al. WikiPathways: building research communities on biological pathways. Nucleic Acids Res. 2012,40:D1301-D1307. doi:10.1093/nar/gkr1074

[76] Kutmon M, Riutta A, Nunes N, Hanspers K, Willighagen EL, et al. WikiPathways: capturing the full diversity of pathway knowledge. Nucleic Acids Res. 2016;44:D488-D494. doi:10.1093/nar/gkv1024

[77] Durot M, Bourguignon PY, Schachter V. Genome-scale models of bacterial metabolism: reconstruction and applications. FEMS Microbiol Rev. 2009;33:164-190. doi:10.1111/j.1574-6976.2008.00146.x

[78] Feist AM, Herrgård MJ, Thiele I, Reed JL, Palsson BØ. Reconstruction of biochemical networks in microorganisms. Nat Rev Microbiol. 2009;7:129-143. doi:10.1038/nrmicro1949

[79] Shannon P, Markiel A, Ozier O, Baliga NS, Wang JT, et al. Cytoscape: a software environment for integrated models of biomolecular interaction networks. Genome Res. 2003;13:2498-2504. doi:10.1101/gr.1239303

[80] Overbeek R, Olson R, Pusch GD, Olsen GJ, Davis JJ, et al. The SEED and the Rapid Annotation of microbial genomes using Subsystems Technology (RAST). Nucleic Acids Res. 2014;42:D206-D214. doi:10.1093/nar/gkt1226

[81] Orth JD, Thiele I, Palsson BØ. What is flux balance analysis? Nat Biotechnol. 2010;28:245-248. doi:10.1038/nbt.1614

[82] Schellenberger J, Que R, Fleming RM, Thiele I, Orth JD, et al. Quantitative prediction of cellular metabolism with constraint-based models: the COBRA Toolbox v2.0. Nat Protoc. 2011;6:1290-1307. doi:10.1038/nprot.2011.308

[83] Garcia-Albornoz M, Thankaswamy-Kosalai S, Nilsson A, Väremo L, Nookaew I, Nielsen J. BioMet Toolbox 2.0: genome-wide analysis of metabolism and omics data. Nucleic Acids Res. 2014;42:W175-W181. doi:10.1093/nar/gku371

[84] Boele J, Olivier BG, Teusink B. FAME, the flux analysis and modeling environment. BMC Syst Biol. 2012;6:8. doi:10.1186/1752-0509-6-8

[85] Schilling CH, Covert MW, Famili I, Church GM, Edwards JS, Palsson BO. Genome-scale metabolic model of *Helicobacter pylori* 26695. J Bacteriol. 2002;184:4582-4593. doi:10.1128/JB.184.16.4582-4593.2002

[86] Oh YK, Palsson BO, Park SM, Schilling CH, Mahadevan R. Genome-scale reconstruction of metabolic network in *Bacillus subtilis* based on high-throughput phenotyping and gene essentiality data. J Biol Chem. 2007;282:28791-28799. doi:10.1074/jbc.M703759200

[87] Puchałka J, Oberhardt MA, Godinho M, Bielecka A, Regenhardt D, et al. Genome-scale reconstruction and analysis of the *Pseudomonas putida* KT2440 metabolic network facilitates applications in biotechnology. PLoS Comput Biol. 2008;4:e1000210. doi:10.1371/journal.pcbi.1000210

[88] Henry CS, Broadbelt LJ, Hatzimanikatis V. Thermodynamics-based metabolic flux analysis. Biophys J. 2007;92:1792-1805. doi:10.1529/biophysj.106.093138

[89] Asadollahi MA, Maury J, Patil KR, Schalk M, Clark A, Nielsen J. Enhancing sesquiterpene production in *Saccharomyces cerevisiae* through *in silico* driven metabolic engineering. Metab Eng. 2009;11:328-334. doi:10.1016/j.ymben.2009.07.001

[90] Finn RD, Coggill P, Eberhardt RY, Eddy SR, Mistry J, et al. The Pfam protein families database: towards a more sustainable future. Nucleic Acids Res. 2016;44:D279-D285. doi:10.1093/nar/gkv1344

[91] Blin K, Medema MH, Kottmann R, Lee SY, Weber T. The antiSMASH database, a comprehensive database of microbial secondary metabolite biosynthetic gene clusters. Nucleic Acids Res. 2017;45:D555-D559. doi:10.1093/nar/gkw960

[92] Röttig M, Rausch C, Kohlbacher O. Combining structure and sequence information allows automated prediction of substrate specificities within enzyme families. PLoS Comput Biol. 2010;6:e1000636. doi:10.1371/journal.pcbi.1000636

[93] Röttig M, Medema MH, Blin K, Weber T, Rausch C, et al. NRPSpredictor2: a web server for predicting NRPS adenylation domain specificity. Nucleic Acids Res. 2011;39:W362-W367. doi:10.1093/nar/gkr323

[94] Liu Y, Young K, Rakotondraibe LH, Brodie PJ, Wiley JD, et al. Antiproliferative compounds from *Cleistanthus boivinianus* from the Madagascar dry forest. J Nat Prod. 2015;78:1543-1547. doi:10.1021/np501020m

[95] Liu Y, Cheng E, Rakotondraibe LH, Brodie PJ, Applequist W, et al. Antiproliferative compounds from *Ocotea macrocarpa* from the Madagascar dry forest. Tetrahedron Lett. 2015;56:3630-3632. doi:10.1016/j.tetlet.2015.01.172

[96] Nyandoro SS, Munissi JJE, Gruhonjic A, Duffy S, Pan F, et al. Polyoxygenated cyclohexenes and other constituents of *Cleistochlamys kirkii* leaves. J Nat Prod. 2016. doi:10.1021/acs.jnatprod.6b00759. PMID: 28001067

[97] Prakash P, Gupta N. Therapeutic uses of *Ocimum sanctum* Linn (Tulsi) with a note on eugenol and its pharmacological actions: a short review. Indian J Physiol Pharmacol. 2005;49:125-131. PMID: 16170979

[98] Willis JC. A dictionary of the flowering plants and ferns. Cambridge: The University Press; 1919

[99] Khare CP. Indian medicinal plants: an illustrated dictionary. Heidelberg: Springer; 2007, p. 443

[100] Upadhyay AK, Chacko AR, Gandhimathi A, Ghosh P, Harini K, et al. Genome sequencing of herb Tulsi (*Ocimum tenuiflorum*) unravels key genes behind its strong medicinal properties. BMC Plant Biol. 2015;15:212. doi:10.1186/s12870-015-0562-x

[101] Ke Y, Ye K, Grossniklaus HE, Archer DR, Joshi HC, et al. Noscapine inhibits tumor growth with little toxicity to normal tissues or inhibition of immune responses. Cancer Immunol Immunother. 2000;49:217-225. PMID: 10941904

[102] Ye K, Ke Y, Keshava N, Shanks J, Kapp JA, et al. Opium alkaloid noscapine is an anti-tumor agent that arrests metaphase and induces apoptosis in dividing cells. Proc Natl Acad Sci USA. 1998;95:1601-1606. PMID: 9465062

[103] Zhou J, Gupta K, Yao J, Ye K, Panda D, et al. Paclitaxel-resistant human ovarian cancer cells undergo c-Jun NH_2-terminal kinase-mediated apoptosis in response to noscapine. J Biol Chem. 2002;277:39777-39785. doi:10.1074/jbc.M203927200

[104] DellaPenna D, O'Connor SE. Plant gene clusters and opiates. Science. 2012;336:1648-1649. doi:10.1126/science.1225473

[105] Battersby AR, Hirst M, McCaldin DJ, Southgate R, Staunton J. Alkaloid biosynthesis. XII. The biosynthesis of narcotine. J Chem Soc Perkin 1. 1968;17:2163-2172. PMID: 5691486

[106] Winzer T, Gazda V, He Z, Kaminski F, Kern M, et al. A *Papaver somniferum* 10-gene cluster for synthesis of the anticancer alkaloid noscapine. Science. 336:1704-1708. doi:10.1126/science.1220757

[107] Rischer H, Oresic M, Seppänen-Laakso T, Katajamaa M, Lammertyn F, et al. Gene-to-metabolite networks for terpenoid indole alkaloid biosynthesis in *Catharanthus roseus* cells. Proc Natl Acad Sci USA. 2006;103:5614-5619. doi:10.1073/pnas.0601027103

[108] Noble RL. The discovery of the vinca alkaloids-chemotherapeutic agents against cancer. Biochem Cell Biol. 1990;68:1344-1351. doi:10.1139/o90-197

[109] Dong HP, Wu HM, Chen SJ, Chen CY. The effect of butanolides from *Cinnamomum tenuifolium* on platelet aggregation. Molecules. 2013;18:11836-11841. doi:10.3390/molecules181011836

[110] Hoshino S, Wakimoto T, Onaka H, Abe I. Chojalactones A-C, cytotoxic butanolides isolated from *Streptomyces* sp. cultivated with mycolic acid containing bacterium. Org Lett. 2015;17:1501-1504. doi:10.1021/acs.orglett.5b00385

[111] Kim W, Lyu HN, Kwon HS, Kim YS, Lee KH, et al. Obtusilactone B from *Machilus thunbergii* targets barrier-to-autointegration factor to treat cancer. Mol Pharmacol. 2013;83:367-376. doi:10.1124/mol.112.082578

[112] Shen KH, Lin ES, Kuo PL, Chen CY, Hsu YL. Isolinderanolide B, a butanolide extracted from the stems of *Cinnamomum subavenium*, inhibits proliferation of T24 human bladder cancer cells by blocking cell cycle progression and inducing apoptosis. Integr Cancer Ther. 2011;10:350-358. doi:10.1177/1534735410391662

[113] Yang SY, Wang HM, Wu TW, Chen YJ, Shieh JJ, et al. Subamolide B isolated from medicinal plant *Cinnamomum subavenium* induces cytotoxicity in human cutaneous squamous cell carcinoma cells through mitochondrial and CHOP-dependent cell death pathways. Evid Based Complement Alternat Med. 2013,2013:630415. doi:10.1155/2013/630415

[114] Risinger AL, Mooberry SL. Taccalonolides: novel microtubule stabilizers with clinical potential. Cancer Lett. 2010;291:14-19. doi:10.1016/j.canlet.2009.09.020

[115] Lau W, Sattely ES. Six enzymes from mayapple that complete the biosynthetic pathway to the etoposide aglycone. Science. 2015;349:1224-1228. doi:10.1126/science.aac7202

[116] Rajniak J, Barco B, Clay NK, Sattely ES. A new cyanogenic metabolite in *Arabidopsis* required for inducible pathogen defence. Nature. 2015;525:376-379. doi:10.1038/nature14907

5

Natural Products for Treatment of Chronic Myeloid Leukemia

Kalubai Vari Khajapeer and Rajasekaran Baskaran

Abstract

Chronic myeloid leukemia (CML) is a hematological malignancy that arises due to reciprocal translocation of 3′ sequences from c-Abelson (*abl*) protooncogene on chromosome 9 with 5′ sequence of truncated break point cluster region (*bcr*) to chromosome 22. The fusion gene product BCR-ABL, a functional oncoprotein p210, is a constitutively activated tyrosine kinase that activates several cell proliferative signaling pathways. BCR-ABL-specific tyrosine kinase inhibitors (TKIs) such as imatinib, nilotinib and ponatinib potently inhibit CML progression. However, drug resistance owing to BCR-ABL mutations and overexpression is still an issue. Natural products are chemical compounds or substances produced by living organisms. They are becoming an important research area for cancer drug discovery due to their low toxicity and cost-effectiveness. Several lines of evidence show that many NPs such as alkaloids, flavonoids, terpenoids, polyketides, lignans and saponins inhibit CML cell proliferation and induce apoptosis. NPs not only differentiate CML cells into monocyte/erythroid lineage but also can reverse the multi-drug resistance (MDR) in CML cells. In this chapter, we review the anti-CML activity of various NPs.

Keywords: chronic myeloid leukemia (CML), BCR-ABL, TKIs, natural products (NPs), multi-drug resistance (MDR)

1. Chronic myeloid leukemia

Chronic myeloid leukemia (CML) is a hematoproliferative neoplasm that is marked by uncontrolled myeloid cell divisions in the bone marrow [1]. CML arises due to a reciprocal translocation between chromosome 9 and chromosome 22 [(9;22) (q34;q11)], eventually culminating in the genesis of the *bcr-abl* oncogene. Approximately 90% of CML patients have shortened chromosome called "Philadelphia chromosome" (Ph) [2].

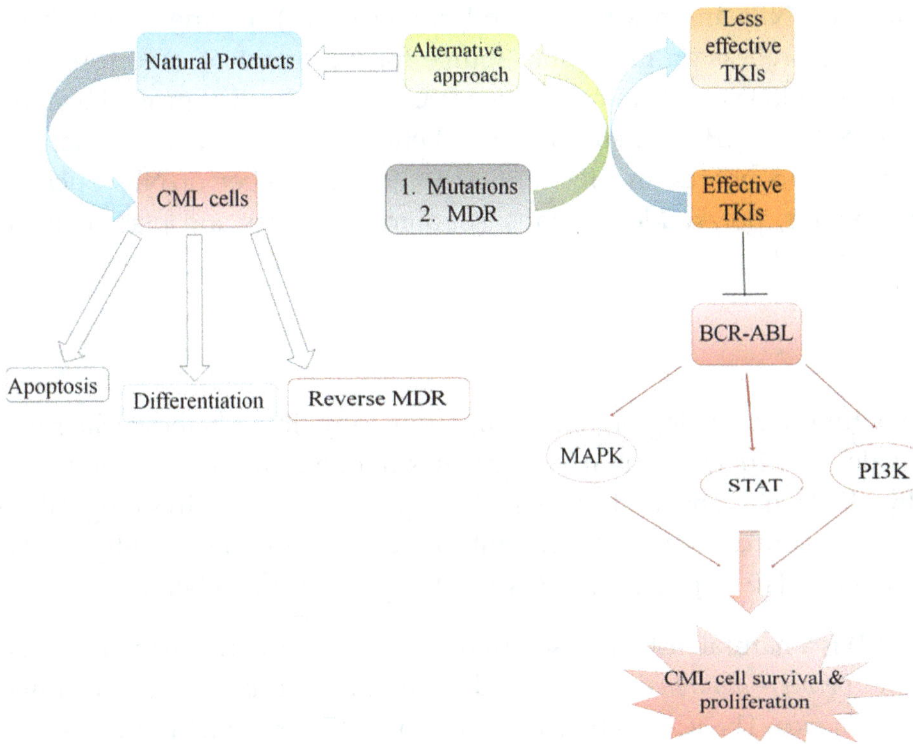

Figure 1. Schematic representation of NPs and TKIs on BCR-ABL inhibition and downregulation of downstream signaling pathways (NP—natural products, TKI—tyrosine kinase inhibitor, CML—chronic myeloid leukemia, MDR—multi-drug resistance).

The *bcr-abl* oncogene encodes a constitutively activated tyrosine kinase, BCR-ABL. The catalytically activated kinase, in turn, activates multiple cell proliferatory signaling pathways such as RAS, a small GTPase, mitogen activated protein kinase (MAPK), signal transducers and activator of transcription (STAT), and phosphoinositide-3-kinase (PI3K) pathways [3].

Targeting Abl kinase is clearly a proven successful strategy to combat CML. First generation tyrosine kinase inhibitor (TKI), imatinib, also known as Gleevac or STI571 inhibited BCR-ABL and suppressed CML progression [4]. Second generation TKIs such as nilotinib, dasatinib & bosutinib and third generation TKIs (Ponatinib) that are more potent to inhibit BCR-ABL kinase are currently used to treat CML [5, 6]. All these TKIs were approved by the US Food and Drug Administration (FDA). TKIs have changed the clinical course of CML. However, mutations in *bcr-abl* and multi-drug resistance (MDR) due to efflux of the drug as a result of overexpression of p-glycoprotein (p-gp) make TKIs less effective. Primary or secondary resistance to TKIs therapy still exists; however, there is a constant need for alternative therapeutic strategy (**Figure 1**) [7].

2. Natural products

Natural products (NPs) represent a large family of diverse secondary metabolites with profound biological activities. NPs are produced in several organisms like bacteria, fungi, plants and marine animals. NPs are inexpensive and have less (or) no side effects; hence, NPs are currently being explored as an invaluable source for treatment of cancerous and infectious diseases. As of 2013, 1453 new chemical entities (NCEs) have been approved by the US FDA, of which 40% are NPs or NP-inspired (semi-synthetic NP derivatives, synthetic compounds based on NP pharmacophores, or NP mimics) [8, 9]. A number of NPs Such as alkaloids, flavonoids, terpenoids, polyketides, lignans, saponins, peptides and plant extracts exhibited potent anti-CML activity.

2.1. Alkaloids

Alkaloids are naturally occurring organic compounds containing heterocyclic ring with nitrogen atom. Alkaloids, widely distributed in plant kingdom, are bitter secondary metabolites synthesized by plants, microbes and animals. They possess several physiological activities like anti-malarial, anti-asthmatic, anti-cancer, anti-bacterial, antiviral, anti-hyperglycemic and vasodilatory activities [10–13]. Their anti-CML activity is described below.

Berbamine (BBM) is a natural bisbenzylisoquinoline product, isolated from traditional Chinese herbal medicine *Berberis amurensis,* was tested on imatinib resistant K562 cell line (K562/IR) both *in vitro* and *in vivo*. The IC_{50} value was found to be 17.1 and 11.1 μM at 24 and 48 h. BBM downregulated Bcl-2, Bcl-xL, mdr-1 mRNA, p-gp levels and enhanced Bax & cytochrome C (cyt.C) release. BALB/c or nu/nu mice were injected with K562-r subcutaneously and the tumor-bearing mice, when treated with BBM [60 mg/kg body weight (BW)] intravenously effectively suppressed the xenotransplated tumors in these mice [14]. BBM also induced apoptosis in CML cells *via* downregulating survivin protein levels [15]. At 8 μg/ml dose of BBM, NFκB nuclear, IKK-α, IKB-α [16], BCR-ABL, p-BCR-ABL level were decreased [17]. Furthermore, BBM-induced differentiation of CML cells into RBC, granulocyte and megakaryocytes [18]. Interestingly, BBM is a heat shock protein 90 (Hsp90) inhibitor [19]. BBM inhibited MDR K562/adriamycin (ADR) [20] and K562/A02 cell lines consequently inducing apoptosis by reducing mdr-1 gene expression and reversing MDR effect [21]. 4-chlorobenzoyl berbamine (BBD9), an analogue of BBM was also tested against K562/IR. BBD9 with IC_{50} 0.5 μg/ml was found to be more effective than BBM (IC_{50} 8 μg/ml), BBD9-lowered BCR-ABL, IKK a, nuclear NF-κB. Furthermore, it increased the cleaved caspases 3,9, Poly(ADP-Ribose) polymerase (PARP) and LC3-phosphatidylethanolamine conjugate (LC3 II) expression levels. In nude mice model bearing K562 tumors, BBD9 was effective in reducing the tumor weight, promoting tumor regression [22]. E6, a derivative of BBM, was tested against MDR K562/doxorubicin (DOX) with 1, 3, 10 and 30 μM concentrations, and it significantly reduced the IC_{50} of DOX from 79.19 μM to 35.18, 21.86, 6.31 and 1.97 μM. Co-treatment of E6 with DOX arrested K562 cells at G2/M phase [23].

Camptothecin, isolated from *Camptotheca acuminate,* is documented to display anti-CML activity. Homocampthothecin (hCPT), a synthetic analogue of camptothecin, showed potent activity at IC_{50} value of 11 nM suggesting its potential use compared to parent compound camptothecin (IC_{50} 57 nM) [24]. BN80927, an analogue of camptothecin, effectively inhibited K562 cell proliferation with IC_{50} of 8.4 nM [25]. NSC606985, an analogue of camptothecin, inhibited CML cell growth in a dose-dependent manner. The IC_{50} was found to be 6.25 nM

[26]. Combination of imatinib and camptothecin increased Bax, cleavage of PARP-1, DNA-dependent protein kinase (DNA–PK) in CML cells [27].

Capsaicin, an active component of capsicum genus, is a homovanillic acid derivative experimentally is shown to exhibit anti-mutagenic activity [28]. Capsaicin treatment of K562 cells decreased microRNA (miRNA) expression such as miR-520a-5p, a putative target of STAT3. Hence, capsaicin induced apoptosis *via* reducing mRNA involved in JNK/STAT pathway [29]. Capsaicin also stimulated GATA-1 promoter in CML cells which is an essential transcriptional factor for the development of erythroid cells [30].

Homoharringtonine (HHT), isolated from *Cephalotaxus harringtona,* has been documented to inhibit CML cell proliferation in a dose-dependent manner. The IC_{50} was found to be 43.89 ng/ml. HHT arrested K562 cells at G0/G1 phase and, in addition, downregulated Bcl-2, NF-κB, p-JAK2, p-STAT5, p-Akt, p-BCR-ABL levels [31, 32].

Sanguinarine, a benzophenanthridine alkaloid, isolated from blood root plant *Sanguinaria canadensis,* belonging to the Papaveraceae family inhibited CML cell growth in a dose-dependent manner. At 1.5 μg/ml, sanguinarine induced apoptosis in CML cells. At higher concentration (12.5 μg/ml), sanguinarine caused blister formation in CML cells [33].

Staurosporine, an alkaloid isolated from the bacterium *Streptomyces staurosporeus,* not only inhibited CML cell growth but also induced differentiation of myeloid cell lineage to megakaryocytic lineage resulting in polypoidy formation. Staurosporine treatment resulted in upregulation and activation of JAK/STAT3, p-STAT3 nuclear translocation and downregulation of c-myc [34, 35]. Staurosporine also induced differentiation of CML cells into erythroid cells *via* increased CD61 and CD42b levels [36]. 7-Hydroxy staurosporine (UCN-01), a potent PKC inhibitor is effective in inhibiting CML cell proliferation at a concentration of 3 μM for 24 h [37, 38].

Tetrandrine is a bis-benzylisoquinoline alkaloid that is isolated from Chinese herb *Stephania tetrandra*. Combination of tetrandine and imatinib showed syngerisitic effect significantly inhibited CML cell growth. The combination treatment arrested CML cells at G1/S phase, enhanced caspase 3 mRNA, protein levels and decreased Bcl-2 mRNA, protein levels [39]. Combination of nilotinib and tetrandrine also effectively decreased the IC_{50} of daunorubicin (DNR) on K562/A02 to 3.12 ± 0.13 μg/ml. This combinational effect not only increased Bax mRNA and protein levels but also decreased the survivin mRNA and protein levels [40]. Tetrandrine citrate, a novel tetrandrine salt which is highly soluble in water, Inhibited the growth of K562/IR, primary leukemic cells and primitive CD34 (+) leukemic cells with IC_{50} ranging from 1.2 to 2.97 μg/ml. Tetrandrine citrate lowered BCR-ABL mRNA and β-catenin protein levels. Nude mice bearing CML tumors when orally administered with tetrandrine citrate (100 mg/kg BW), reduced the tumor growth [41]. Combination of 5-bromotetrandrine (analogue of tetrandrine) and DNR decreased p-JNK 11,2 and MDR/p-gp levels in ADR resistant K562 cells [42].

Alkaloids from plant and microbial source inhibited CML cell proliferation in micromole (μM)/ microgram (μg) concentration (**Table 1**) (**Figure 2**) [43–66]. Alkaloids are well documented to

Alkaloid	Source of isolation	IC_{50} value on K562 cells	Mechanism of action	References
Berbamine (bisbenzylisoquinoline alkaloid)	*Berberis amurensis*	8 μg/ml	↓Bcl-2, Bcl-xL, NFκB (nuclear), IKK-α, IKB-α, BCR-ABL, p-BCR-ABL, Hsp90	[14–17]
Camptothecin (quinoline alkaloid)	*Camptotheca acuminate*	57 nM	↑Bax, cleavage of PARP-1, DNA—PK adducts	[24]
Homoharringtonine	*Cephalotaxus harringtona*	43.89 ng/ml	↓Bcl-2, NF-κB, p-JAK2, p-STAT5, p-Akt, p-BCR-ABL and ⊥G_0/G_1 phase	[31, 32]
Sanguinarine (benzophenanthridine alkaloid)	*Sanguinaria canadensis*	–	At 1.5 μg/ml induced apoptosis	[33]
Tetrandrine (bis-benzylisoquinoline alkaloid)	*Stephania tetrandra*	–	↑Caspase 3 mRNA, protein and ↓Bcl-2 mRNA, protein	[39, 40]
Ancistrotectorine E (napthylisoqunoline alkaloid)	70% EtOH extract of *Ancistrocladus tectorius*	4.18 μM	–	[43]
1,2,3-Trimethoxy-5-oxonoraporphine and ouregidion (aporphine alkaloids)	Crude HEX, EtOAc and AQE extracts of *Pseuduvaria rugosa* (Blume) Merr	*63 and 64%	–	[44]
Cathachunine	*Catharanthus roseus* (L.) G. Don	9.3 ± 1.8 μM	–	[45]
Cepharanthine	*Stephania* sp.	–	↓p-gp	[46]
Crebanine	*Stephania venosa*	13 μg/ml	↓Cyclin A, D & ↑Caspases 3,9,8 & PARP and ⊥G_0/G_1 phase	[48]
Curine	*Chondrodendron platyphyllum*	17.8 ± 5.2 μM	–	[49]
Cyanogramide	*Actinoalloteichus cyanogriseus* WHI-2216-6	–	At 5 μM, reversed MDR in K562/ADR	[50]
9-Deacetoxyfumigaclavine C	*Aspergillus fumigatus*	3.1 μM	–	[51]
Evodiamine (quinazolinocarboline alkaloid)	*Evodia rutaecarpa*	34.43 μM	–	[53]
Naamidine J (imidazole containing alkaloid)	*Pericharax heteroraphis*	11.3 μM	–	[54]
Salvicine (diterpenoid alkaloid)	*Salvia prioniti*	7.82 ± 2.81 μM	⊥G_1 phase	[56]
Solamargine (glycoalkaloid)	*Solanum species*	5.2 μM	↑Caspases and ↓Bcl-2	[57, 58]
α-Tomatine (glycoalkaloid)	*Solanum lycopersicum*	1.51 μM	Loss of MMP. ↑Bak, Mcl-1s, AIF and ↓survivin	[59]
Tylophora alkaloids (tylophorine, tylophorinine, tylophorindine)	*Tylophora indica*	–	Nuclear condensation, ↑Caspases activation, release of cyt.C	[60]
		44 and 53 μM	–	[61]

Alkaloid	Source of isolation	IC_{50} value on K562 cells	Mechanism of action	References
5-Chlorosclerotiamide and 10-episclerotiamide (prenylated indole alkaloids)	*Aspergillus westerdijkiae* DFFSCS013			
Eupolauramine and sampangine (azaphenanthrene alkaloids)	*Anaxagorea dolichocarpa* Sprague and sandwith	18.97 and 10.95 μg/ml	–	[62]
Arthpyrones A, B and C (4-hydroxy-2-pyridone alkaloids)	*Arthrinium arundinis* ZSDS1-F3	0.24—45 μM	-	[63]
Auranomides A, B and C	*Penicillium aurantiogriseum*	*20.48, 76.36 and 5.78%	–	[64]
Malonganenones 1–3 (tetraprenylated alkaloids)	*Euplexauria robusta*	0.35—10.82 μM	–	[65]
Virosecurinine	*Securinega suffruticosa*	32.984 μM	↑PTEN & ↓mTOR, SHIP-2 BCR-ABL, and ⊥G_1/S phase	[66]

↑ – upregulation, ↓ – downregulation, ⊥ – cell cycle arrest & * – Inhibition rate (IR) at 100 μg/ml.

Table 1. Anti-CML activity of alkaloids.

potently reduce tumor growth in *in vivo* models (**Table 2**). Besides, some alkaloids such as capasaicin, staurosporine induces differentiation of CML cells (**Table 3**).

2.2. Flavonoids

Flavonoids belong to polyphenolic compounds which are prevalent in plants. They contain two phenyl rings A, B and a heterocyclic ring C (commonly referred as C6-C3-C6 skeleton) and are classified into many major classes like flavones, flavonols, flavanones, flavanonols and isoflavonoids (**Figure 3**). They exhibit antioxidant, anti-inflammatory, anti-bacterial, antiviral and anti-cancer activities and play a significant role in human health [67–74].

Oroxylin A, an O-methylated flavone, found in the medicinal plant *Scutellaria baicalensis*, was tested against MDR K562/ADR cells. Oroxylin A specifically enhanced the sensitivity of K562/ADR to ADR by selectively inducing apoptosis. The treatment downregulated CXCR4 expression and inhibited PI3K/Akt/NF-κB pathways [75]. NOD/SCID mice-bearing K562 xenograft, treated with oroxylin A (30 mg/kg BW) alone or in combination with imatinib enhanced the sensitivity of imatinib to K562 cells through suppression of STAT3 pathway, decreasing p-gp levels thus reversing MDR in CML cells [76].

Quercetin (Q), a major flavonol, found in the kingdom Plantae, exhibits many biological effects including Antioxidant, anti-inflammatory, anti-cancer and anti-diabetic activities [77]. While evaluating the anti-proliferative effect of pytoestrogens, it was found that Q specifically inhibits K562 and MDR K562/A cell growth [78]. When K562 cells were treated with Q at a

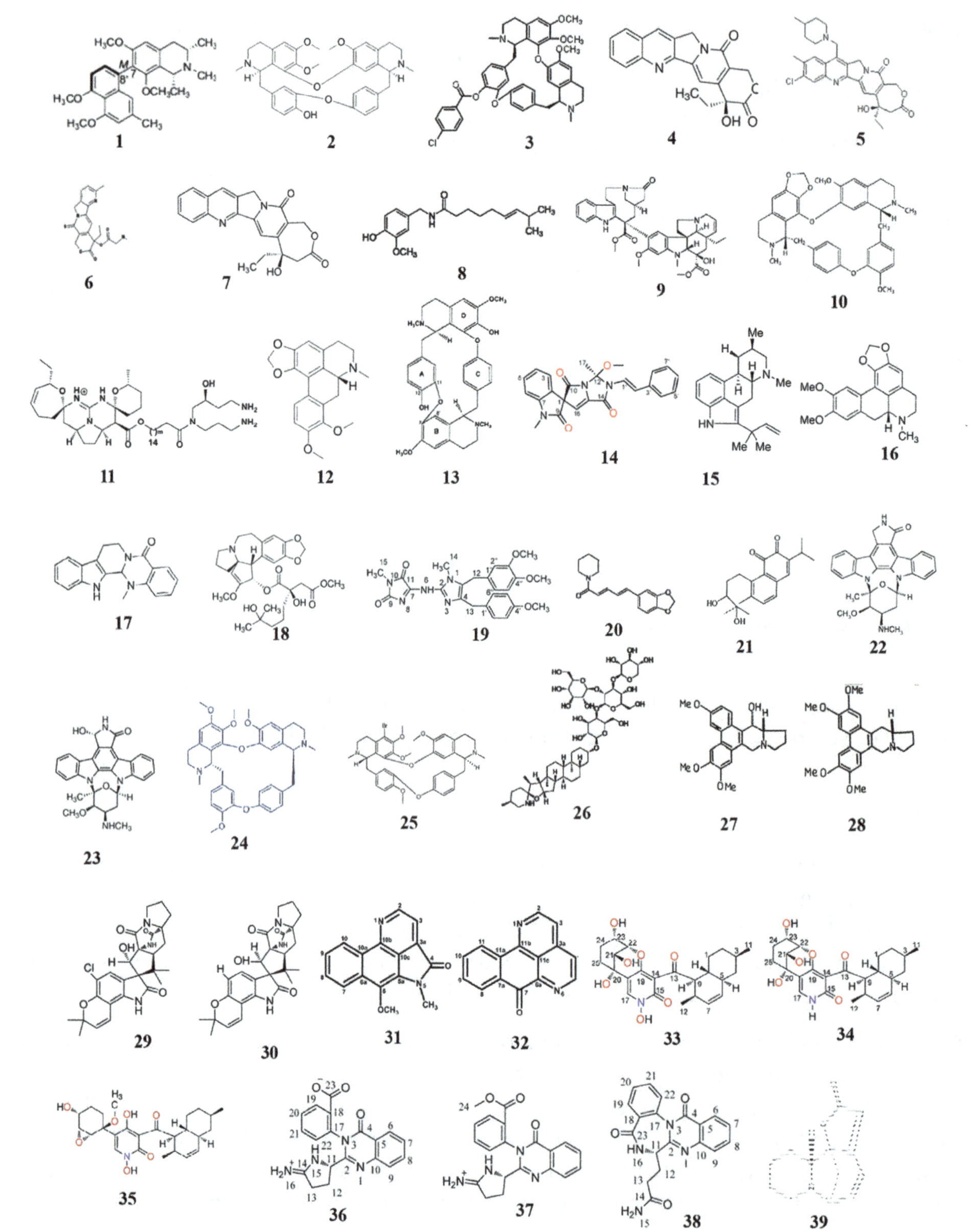

Figure 2. List of anti-CML alkaloids as 1—Ancistrotectorine E, 2—Berbamine, 3—BBD9, 4—Camptothecin, 5—BN80927, 6—NSC606985, 7—Homocamptothecin, 8—Capsaicin, 9—Cathachunine, 10—Cephranathine, 11—Crambescidin 800, 12—Crebanine, 13—Curine, 14—Cyanogramide, 15—9-deacetoxyfumigaclavine C, 16—d-Dicentrine, 17—Evodiamine, 18—Homoharringtonine, 19—Naamidine J, 20—Piperine, 21—Salvicine, 22—Staurosporine, 23—UCN-01, 24—Tetrandrine, 25—5-bromotetrandrine, 26—α-tomatine, 27—tylophorine, 28—tylophorinine, 29—5-chlorosclerotiamide, 30—10-episclerotiamide, 31—Eupolauramine, 32—Sampangine, 33, 34, 35—Arthpyrones A, B and C, 36–38—Auranomides A, B and C and 39—Virosecurinine.

Name of NP	Type of NP	Mice strain	Type of CML cells used to induce tumors	Dosage	Mode of administration	Mechanism of action	References
BBM	Alkaloid	Balb/c	K562-r	60 mg/ kg BW	Intravenously	↓*mdr*-1 mRNA, p-gp protein	[14]
BBD9	Analogue of BBM	nu−/−	K562/IR	15 and 30 mg/ kg BW	–	↓p-BCR-ABL, IKKa, NF-κBp65	[22]
Tetrandrine citrate	Alkaloid	nu−/−	K562/IR	100 mg/ kg BW	Orally	↓BCR-ABL, β-catenin	[41]
d-Dicentrine	Alkaloid	SCID	K562	100 mg/ kg BW	Intraperitoneal	↓tumor size	[52]
Oroxylin A	Flavonoid	SCID	K562	80 mg/ kg BW	Intravenously	↓STAT3 pathway	[76]
Nobiletin	Flavonoid	Nude mice	K562	12.5, 25, 50 mg/ kg BW	–	↓VEGF	[99]
dEpoF	Polyketide	Nude mice	K562	6 mg/kg	Intravenously	Complete tumor regression	[147]
HSS	Protein extract from *Tegillarca granosa*	–	K562/ADM	–	–	↓mdr1, BCR-ABL and sorcin	[177]
Gambogic acid	*Garcinia hanburyi*	Balb/c	KBM5-T315I	3 mg/kg/ 2 days	Intraperitoneal	↓Bcr-Abl, Akt, Erk1/2, and STAT5	[229]
TAF273	Fraction of *Eurycoma longifolia MeOH extract*	Balb/c	K562	50 mg/ kg	Intraperitoneal	↑apoptosis and ↓blood vessel formation	[258]
NPB001–05	Piper betle extract	–	T315I	500 mg/ kg	Orally	↓PI3K/AKT, MAPK pathways	[275]

Table 2. In vivo results of anti-CML NPs.

concentration of 9.2 mg/ml for 72 h, it induced apoptosis and reduced the BCR-ABL levels in CML cells [79]. Combination of Q and ADR was tested on MDR K562/ADR cells. Combined treatment enhanced activation of caspases 3,8 and loss of mitochondrial membrane potential (MMP). Furthermore, it lowered Bcl-2, Bcl-xl and enhanced the p-c-Jun-N terminal kinase and p-p38 mitogen-activated protein kinase (p-p38-MAPK). Q also significantly decreased the p-gp levels [80] and sensitized MDR K562/ADM to DNR and reversed MDR in CML cells [81]. Q inhibited K562 and MDR K562/A in the range of 5–160 μM. Q treatment of K562/ADR cells (5 μM) enhanced accumulation of ADR and, in addition, decreased the expression of MDR-causing proteins like ABC, solute carrier (SLC). Moreover, it reduced Bcl-2, TNF expression reversing MDR in CML cells [82]. Moreover, Q arrested CML cells at G2/M phase [83]. IC_{50} of Q on K562 and K562/ADR was found to be 11 ± 2 μM and 5 ± 0.4 μM [84]. It also inhibited the

Name of NP	NP class	Differentiation of CML cells into	Mechanism of action	References
Capsaicin	Alkaloid	Erythroid cells	↑GATA-1 promoter	[28–30]
Staurosporine	Alkaloid	Megakaryocytes	↑CD61, CD42b and ↓c-myc	[34–36]
Crambescidin 800	Alkaloid	Erythroblasts, induction of hemoglobin production	⊥S-phase	[47]
Piperine	Alkaloid	Macrophages/monocytes (20/40 μM)	–	[55]
Apigenin	Flavonoid	Erythroid lineage	↑ α and ϒ hemoglobin mRNA expression	[87]
Galangin	Flavonoid	Monocytes	↑CD61	[90]
Genistein	Flavonoid	Erythroid lineage	–	[92]
EtOH extract of *Olea europaea*	Plant extract	Monocyte lineage	↑CD14	[243]
EtOH extract of *Stellera chamaejasme*	Plant extract	Granulocytes	↑CD11b	[250]
Huangqi (Astragalus membranaceus)	Traditional Chinese medicine	Erythroid lineage	↑β-globin gene expression	[272]

Table 3. List of some NPs and its differentiation capacity.

Hsp70 levels in CML cells [85]. Q induced apoptosis *via* inhibiting the telomerase enzyme by enhancing human telomerase reverse transcriptase (hTERT) enzymes in CML cells [86].

In sum, flavonoids not only inhibit the growth of CML cells (**Table 4**) but also induce their differentiation into erythroid or monocyte lineage (**Table 3**). Flavonoid fractions of plant extracts also inhibit CML cell proliferation and induced apoptosis [87–109].

2.3. Terpenoids

Terpenoids are naturally occurring products representing the largest secondary metabolites. Approximately 60% of NPs are terpenoids. They are basically made up of five carbon isoprene units (IU). Depending upon the number of isoprene units present, terpenoids has been classified into hemiterpenoids (1 IU), monoterpenoids (2 IU), sesquiterpenoids (3 IU), diterpenoids (4 IU), sesterterpenoids (5 IU), triterpenoids (6 IU), tetraterpenoids (8 IU) and polyterpenoid (n IU). They have been documented to possess antioxidant, anti-inflammatory, anti-helminitic and anti-cancer activities [110–115].

Sesquiterpenoids, diterpenoids, sesterterpenoids and triterpenoidshas been shown to potently inhibit CML cell proliferation and induce apoptosis (**Figure 3**) (**Table 5**) [116–144]. Other diterpenoids such as scapaundulin C (from *Scapania undulate* (L.) Dum.,) [120], parvifoline Z, parvifoline AA (from *Isodon parvifolius*) [121], labdane-type diterpenes (from *Chloranthus henryi* Hemsl.) [124] and sesterterpenoid compounds 3, 11 and 12 (from *Sarcotragus* sp.) [133] and triterpenoid compounds 1, 2, 5, 7 and 9 (from *Ganoderma hainanense)* [135], (24R/S)-24-hydroxy-

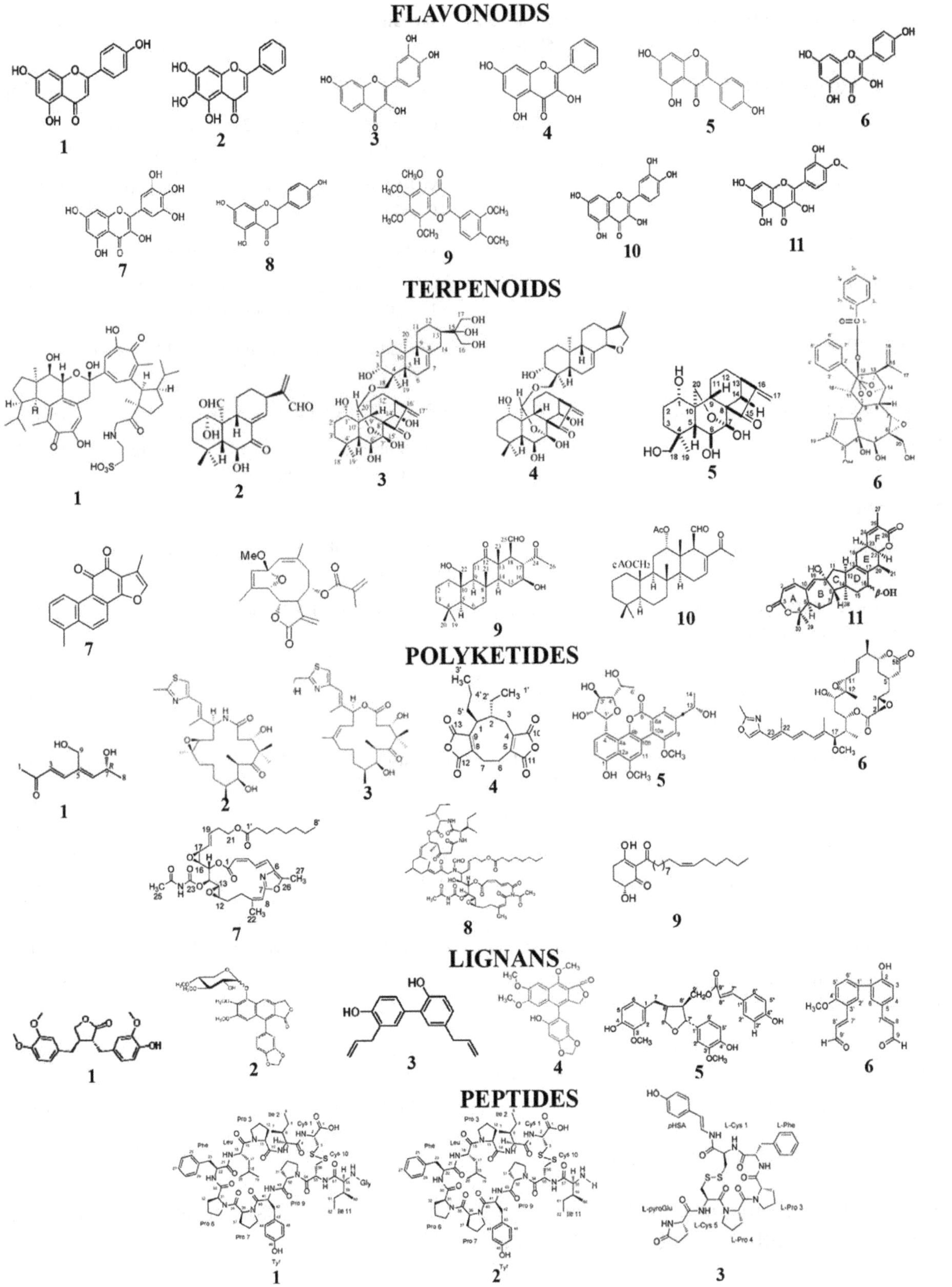

Figure 3. Anti-CML activity of some NPs which include - flavonoids: 1—Apigenin, 2—Baicalein, 3—Fistein, 4—Galangin, 5—Genistein, 6—Kaempferol, 7—Myricetin, 8—Naringenin, 9—Nobiletin, 10—Oroxylin A and 11—Tamarixetin. Terpenoids: 1—Gukulenin A, 2-4—Hebeiabinin A, D & E, 5—Parvifolines C, 6—3-hydrogenwadaphnin, 7—Tanshinone I, 8—EM23, 9, 10—Felixins F & G, 11—Kadlongilactone D. Polyketides: 1—Epiaspinonediol, 2—aza-EpoB, 3—dEpoF, 4—Heveadride, 5—Gilvocarin HE, 6—Rhizoxin, 7—Salarin C, 8—Tausalarin C, 9—Trineurone E. Lignans: 1—Arctigenin, 2—Cleistanthin A, 3—Honokiol, 4—6-hydroxyjusticidin C, 5—(+) -lariciresinol 9'-p-coumarate, 6—4-methoxy magndialdehyde. Peptides: 1, 2—chujamide A, B, 3—gombamide A.

Flavonoids/flavonoid fraction	IC_{50} value on K562 cells	Mechanism of action	References
Oroxylin A (o-methylated flavone)	–	↓CXCR4, PI3K/Akt/NF-κB pathways	[75, 76]
Quercetin (flavonol)	11 ± 2 μM	Loss of MMP. ↑caspases 3,8 & ↓Bcl-2, Bcl-xl, Hsp70, telomerase and ⊥G_2/M phase	[77–86]
Apigenin (flavone)	–	↓Mcl-1, Bcl-2 & ↑caspases activation and ⊥G_2/M phase	[87, 91]
Baicalein (flavone)	–	↑ caspase 3, Fas gene and ⊥ S phase	[88]
Fistein (flavonol)	–	Induced apoptosis and Altered JAK/STAT, KIT pathways and ⊥S & G_2/M phases	[89, 97]
Galangin (flavonol)	–	↓pRb, cdk4, cdk1, cycline B & Bcl-2 levels and ⊥G_0/G_1 phase	[90]
Kaempferol (flavonol)	–	↑ Bax, SIRT3, caspases 3, 9 and ↓ Bcl-2	[93]
Myricetin (flavonol)	–	Myricetin pre-treatment enhanced Natural killer cells to kill K562	[96, 97]
Naringenin (flavanone)	–	↑ p21/WAF1 and ⊥G_0/G_1 phase	[98]
Tamarixetin (o-methylated flavonol)	–	↑ cyclin B1, Bub1, p21, caspases and ↓tublin polymerization	[100]
3,5-Dihydroxy-6,7,3′,4′-tetramethoxyflavone (DHTMF) (polymethoxyflavone)	7.85 μg/ml	↑caspases 3, 9 & PARP cleavage	[101]
2″,3″-Diidroochnaflavone (*Luxemburgia nobilis*)	89 μM	–	[102]
Isochamaejasmin (biflavonoid) (*Stellera chamaejasme* L)	24.51 ± 1.62 μM	↑caspases 3, 9 and PARP cleavage	[103]
Protoapigenone (total flavonoid fraction of *Macrothelypteris torresiana*)	0.9 μg/ml	–	[104]
Total flavonoids from *Lysimachia clethroides* Duby (ZE4)	–	↓Bcl-2 and ↑Fas, TRAIL & DR5	[105]
Total flavonoids of *Astragali Radix*	98.63 mg/L	↓ cyclin D1 mRNA levels and ⊥G_0/G_1 phase	[106]
Total oligomer flavonoids of *Rhamnus alaternus*	196 μg/ml	–	[107]
Flavonoid-enriched *Rhamnus alaternus* root and leaf extracts	165 and 210.73 μg/ml	–	[108]
Epigallocatechin-3-gallate (*Camellia sinensis*)	50 μM	↓CyclinD1, CDC25A and ↑TGF-β2	[109]

Table 4. Anti-CML activity of flavonoids.

3α 10α-epoxy-9-eip-cucurbita-25-ene (1a, b) (from *Fructus Viticis* Negundo) [136] are also shown to efficiently inhibit CML cell proliferation.

2.4. Polyketides

Polyketides represent a large group of natural products that are produced by microorganisms and plants. These are secondary metabolites, derived by the repetitive condensation of acetate

Terpenoid class	Name of terpenoid	Source of isolation	IC_{50} value on K562 cells	Mechanism of action	References
Sesquiterpenoids	EM23	*Elephantopus mollis*	10.8 μM	↑ caspases, PARP cleavage and ↓ NFκB. Loss of MMP	[116]
Diterpenoids	Caesalminaxin D and H	*Caesalpinia minax*	9.9 ± 1.7 and 9.2 ± 0.9 μM	–	[117]
	Gukulenin A and diterpenoid pseudodimers (2–5)	*Phorbas gukhulensis*	*0.26 ± 0.03, 0.12 ± 0.01, 0.44 ± 0.01, 0.32 ± 0.05 and 0.04 ± 0.09 μM	–	[118]
	Diterpene compounds 11, 12, 13, 14 and 15	petroleum ether soluble fraction of the aerial parts of *Tirpitzia ovoidea* ethanol extract	86.4, 66.3, 91, 45.1 and 58.6 μM	–	[119]
	7β,11β,14β-Trihydroxy-ent-kaur-20-al-6,15-dioxo-16-ene	*Isodon xerophilus*	0.04 μM	–	[122]
	Hebeiabinin A, D and E	*Isodon rubescens* var. rubescens	53.21, 5.05 and 0.91 μM	–	[123]
	Parvifolines C	*Isodon parvifolius*	13.8 μM	–	[125]
	3-Hydrogenwadaphnin	*Dendrostellera lessertii*	15 nM con. caused 45% apoptosis	–	[126]
	Enanderianins K—P, Rabdocoetsin B and D	*Isodon enanderianus*	0.13–0.87 μg/ml	–	[127]
	Ludongnin J	*Isodon rubescens* var. lushiensis	0.18 μg/ml	–	[128]
	Tanshinone I	*Salvia miltiorrhiza* Bunge.	38 ± 5.2 μM	↑ Bax, caspase 3 and ↓Survivin	[129]
	ent-Kaurane diterpenoids 11, 16, 17 and 20	*Isodon nervosus*	2.39, 4.11, 1.05 and 1.55 μM		[130]
	5-Episinuleptolideacetate	*Sinularia species*	4.09 μg/ml	↓c-ABL, Akt, NFκB	[144]
Sesterterpenoids	Felixins F and G	*Ircinia felix*	1.27 and 19.9 μM	–	[131]
	Compounds 8, 9	*Smenospongia* sp.	*0.11 and 0.97μ/ml	–	[132]
	Two linear furanosesterterpenes	*Smenospongia* sp.	3 and 31.6 μg/ml	–	[134]
Triterpenoids	3β,21β,24-Trihydroxyserrat-14-en-24-(4′-hydroxybenzoate)	*Palhinhaea cernua*	56.1 μg/ml	–	[137]
	L-Arabinopyranosyloleanolic acid	*Garcinia hanburyi* resin	4.15 μM	–	[138]

Terpenoid class	Name of terpenoid	Source of isolation	IC_{50} value on K562 cells	Mechanism of action	References
	Nortriterpenoids	*Schisandra propinqua* var. propinqua	>100 μM	–	[139]
	Kadlongilactone D	*Kadsura longipedunculata*	1.92 μM	–	[140]
	Six triterpenes	fractions of *Aceriphyllum rossii* methanolic extract	12.2—28.7 μM	–	[141]
	Argetatin B	*Parthenium argentatum*	Cytotoxic at 5—25 μM con.	–	[142]
	Celastrol (quinone methide triterpene)	*Tripterygium wilfordii Hook F*	–	↓pSTAT5, p-CRKL, pERK1/2, p-Akt, p-BCR-ABL, Bcl-xL, Mcl-1, survivin, Hsp90	[143]

*LC_{50}, lethal concentation.

Table 5. Anti-CML activity of terpenoids.

units or other short carboxylic acids catalyzed by multi-functional enzymes called polyketide synthases (PKSs) which is similar to fatty acid synthases [145]. Many polyketides suppress CML cell proliferation and induce apoptosis (**Figure 3**) (**Table 6**) [146–155].

2.5. Lignans

Lignans, natural compounds that are exclusively found in plants, are derived from amino acid phenyl alanine. They possess anti-oxidant and anti-cancer activities [156]. Various lignans effectively inhibit CML cell proliferation and induced apoptosis (**Figure 3**) (**Table 6**) [157–163].

2.6. Saponins

Saponins are a diverse group of secondary metabolites widely distributed in the plant kingdom. They produce soap-like foam when shaken in aqueous solutions. Their structure comprise of triterpene or steroid aglycone and one or more sugar chains. They exhibit anti-cancer and anti-cholesterol activities [164, 165]. Various saponins inhibited CML cell proliferation (**Table 6**) [166–174].

2.7. Peptides

Two peptides, chujamides A (1) and B (2), isolated from the marine sponge *Suberites waedoensis* inhibited K562 cell growth with LC_{50} values of 37 and 55.6 μM [175]. Another peptide, gombamide A (1), isolated from the marine sponge *Clathria gombawuiensis* inhibited CML cell proliferation with LC_{50} of 6.9 μM [176]. Haishengsu (HSS), a protein extract from

Type of NP	Name of compound	Source of isolation	IC_{50} value on K562	Mechanism of action	References
Polyketides	Epiaspinonediol	*Aspergillus* sp. 16–02–1	44.3 μg/mL	–	[146]
	Geldanamycin	*Streptomyces Hygroscopicus*	–	↓c-Raf, Akt, BCR-ABL	[148]
	Heveadride	*Ascomycota Dichotomyces cejpii*	82.7 ± 11.3 μM	↑ TNFα	[149]
	Gilvocarin HE	Streptomyces sp. QD01–2	45 μM	–	[150]
	Radicicol	*Diheterospora chlamydosporia* and *Monosporium bonorden*	–	↓p-Raf1, p-BCR-ABL	[151]
	Rhizoxin	*Burkholderia rhizoxina*	$5{\times}10^{-7}$ μg/ml	–	[152]
	Salarin C	*Fascaplysinopis* sp.	0.1 μM	↑ caspase 3 and 9 cleavage	[153]
	Tausalarin C	*Fascaplysinopis* sp.	1 μM	–	[154]
	Trineurone E	*Peperomia trineura*	26 μM	–	[155]
Lignans	Arctigenin	Asteraceae family	–	↑Bax and ↓ Bcl-2	[157]
	Cleistanthin A	*Cleistanthus collinus* (Rox B)	0.4 μM	–	[158]
	5,5′-Dimethoxylariciresinol-4′-O-β-D-glucoside (DMAG)	Mahonia	–	↓IC_{50} of DOX from 34.93 to 12.51 μM	[159]
	Honokiol	*Magnolia officinalis* Rend. Et wils.	28.4 μM	–	[160]
	6-Hydroxyjusticidin C	*Justica procumbens*	43.9 ± 2.9 μM	↑ROS levels, casapase 3	[161]
	(+)-Lariciresinol 9′-p-coumarate	*Larix olgensis* var. koreana.	2.9 μg/ml	–	[162]
	4-Methoxy magndialdehyde	*Magnolia officinalis*	3.9 μg/ml	–	[163]
Saponins	Astrgorgiosides A, B, C (19-norand aromatized B ring bearing steroid aglycone)	*Astrogor dumbea*	26.8—45.6 μM	–	[168]
	Wattoside G, H, and I (steroidal saponins)	*Tupistra wattii* Hook.F.	35.67, 76.16 and 76.96 μM	–	[169]
	Tenacissoside C (steroidal saponins)	*Marsdenia tenacissima*	31.4 μM	↓ cyclin D, Bcl-2, Bcl-xL and ↑caspases 3, 9, Bax and Bak	[170]
	Compounds 14 and 15 (C21-steroidal pregnane sapogenins)	*Cynanchum wilfordii* roots	6.72 μM	–	[171]
	Total saponin content	*Aralia Taibaiensis*	–	Loss of MMP. ↑ Bax and ↓ Bcl-2	[172]

Type of NP	Name of compound	Source of isolation	IC_{50} value on K562	Mechanism of action	References
	Saponin rich fraction (GSE)	*Gleditsia sinensis* Lam. fruit extract	18 ± 1.6 μg/ml	↑ Bax and ↓ Bcl-2, PCNA	[173]
	23-Hydroxybetulinic acid	Total saponin content of *Pulsatilla chinensis* (Bunge) Regel	–	↑ Bax, caspase 3 cleavage and ↓ Bcl-2, survivin	[174]
Peptides	Chujamides A and B	*Suberites waedoensis*	*37 and 55.6 μM	–	[175]
	Gombamide A	*Clathria gombawuiensis*	*6.9 μM	–	[176]

*LC_{50}—lethal concentation.

Table 6. Anti-CML activities of polyketides, lignans, saponins and peptides.

Tegillarca granosa, when administered in mice-bearing MDR K562/ADM cell tumors inhibited tumor growth and downregulated *mdr1* gene, BCR-ABL and sorcin [177]. HSS was also tested against MDR K562/ADR cells, and it induced apoptosis at 20 mg/l [178]. HSS also inhibited K562 cells at G0/G1 and S phase and lowered Bcl-2 and enhanced Bax levels (**Figure 2**) (**Table 6**) [179].

2.8. Others natural products

Other natural products such as acetylenic metabolites, betanin, bufadienolide, mamea a/ba, cryptotanshinone, bavachalcone, polyanthumin, cubebin, denbinobin, digallic acid, perforanoid A, β- and α-mangostin, parthenolide, perezone, polyphyllin D, squamocin, toxicarioside H, tripolide, woodfordin I and rhodexin A inhibited CML cell proliferation (**Table 7**) [180–230]. Moreover, many plant crude extracts enriched with NPs inhibited the CML cell proliferation and induced apoptosis (**Table 8**) [231–280].

2.9. Natural products in clinical trials

Of the several natural products, Homoharringtonine (alkaloid) (NCT00114959) is currently under phase II study sponsored by Chem Genex pharmaceuticals to reverse the Gleevac resistance in CML patients [281]. 17-AAG (analogue of glendamycin–polyketide) (NCT00100997) is currently under phase I clinical trial sponsored by Jonsson Comprehensive Cancer Center collaborated with National Cancer Institute (NCI). Efforts are underway to determine the side effects and optimal dose of 17-AAG for treating patients with CML in chronic phase who did not respond to imatinib-mesylate [282]. Paclitaxel (diterpenoid) (NCT00003230) is currently under Phase I/II trials to study the effectiveness in treating patients with refractory or recurrent acute leukemia or CML. This work is sponsored by Swiss Group for Clinical Cancer Research [283].

Name of NP	Source of isolation	IC_{50} value on K562 cells	Mechanism of action	References
Acetylenic metabolites	*Stelletta* sp.	43.5, 51.3 and 62.5 μg/ml	–	[180]
Betanin (betacyanin pigment)	*Opuntia ficus-indica*	40 μM	↑ PARP cleavage, release of Cyt C and ↓ BCl-2. Loss of MMP	[182]
Bufalin 3β-acrylic ester (Bufadienolide)	"Ch'an Su"	6.83 nM	–	[183]
3-Formylcarbazole, methylcarbazole-3-carboxylate and 2-methoxy-1-(3-methyl-buten-1-yl)-9H-carbazole-3-carbaldehyde	*Clausena lansium* (Lour.) Skeels	20.48 ± 1.78, 26.5 ± 2.12 and 23.49 ± 1.85 μg/ml	–	[184]
Toxicarioside F and G	*Latex of Antaris toxicaria (Pers.) Lasch*	–	–	[185]
Pangelin and oxypeucedanin hydrate acetonide	*Angelica dahurica*	8.6–14.6 μg/ml	–	[186]
Mamea A/BA	*Calophyllum brasiliense*	0.04–0.59 μM	–	[187, 188]
Cryptotanshinone (lipid soluble active compound)	*Salvia miltiorrhiza*	–	induced apoptosis ↑ PARP cleavage and ↓BCR-ABL, STAT3, mTOR & eIF4E	[189, 190]
Bavachalcone (Chalcones)	–	2.7 μM	–	[191]
Polyanthumin (novel chalcone trimmer) and sulfuretin	*Memecylon polyanthum H.L. Li.*	45.4 and 30.5 μg/ml	–	[192]
(−)-Cubebin	*Piper cubeba*	8.66 ± 0.43 μM	–	[193]
Denbinobin	5-Hydroxy-3,7-dimethoxy-1,4-phenanthraquinone	1.84 μM	↓ BCR-ABL, CrkL and⊥G2/M phase	[194]
Digallic acid	*Pistascia lentiscus*	–	Induced DNA fragmentation and pro-apoptotic effect in CML cells	[195]
1,4,5-Trihydroxy-7-methoxy-9H-fluoren-9-one, dendroflorin and denchrysan (fluorenones)	*Dendrobium chrysotoxum*	32.18, 26.65 and 52.28 μg/ml	–	[196]
C27-Steroidal glycoside	*Liriope graminifolia* (Linn.) Baker	18.6 μg/ml	–	[198]
9α-Acetoxyartecanin, apressin, inducumenone and centaureidin	*Achillea clavennae*	9.84 ± 2.52, 4.44 ± 0.76, 52.53 ± 8.43 and 5.37 ± 0.8 μM	–	[199]
Perforanoid A (limonoid)	–	4.24 μM	–	[200]
Linoleic acid	Methanol extracts of proso and Japanese millet	68 μM	–	[201]
β- and α-Mangostin	*Garcinia malaccensis*		–	[202, 203]

Name of NP	Source of isolation	IC_{50} value on K562 cells	Mechanism of action	References
		0.40 μM and 0.48 μM		
Nudifloside and linearoside (iridoid)	EtOH extract of the aerial parts of *Callicarpa nudiflora* Hook	20.7 and 36 μg/ml	–	[204]
Parthenolide	–	17.1, 8.67 and 9.42 for 24, 48 and 72 h	Induced apoptosis	[205]
Perezone	*Perezia* spp.	–	Cytotoxic to CML cells at 25, 50 and 100 μM and induced apoptosis	[206]
Compound 6a (phenalenone metabolite)	*Coniothyrium cereal*	8.5 μM	–	[207]
Polyphyllin D	*Paris polyphyllin*	–	↑ p21, Bax, caspase 3 & Cyt. C release and ↓ cyclin B1, cdk1, Bcl-2. Loss of MMP and ⊥ G_2/M phase	[208]
Polysaccharide (PSP001)	*Punica granatum*	52.8 ± 0.9 μg/ml	–	[209]
Riccardin F and Pakyonol (macrocyclic bisbenzyls)	*Plagiochasm intermedium*	0–6 μg/ml	–	[210]
Highly methoxylated bibenzyls	*Frullania inouei*	11.3–49.6 μM	–	[211]
Sarcovagine and β-sitosterol 5- 8	*Sarcococca saligna*	2.5–5 μM	–	[212]
Squamocin (annonaceous acetogenins)	–	–	↑ cdk inhibitors, p21, p27 & ↓ cdk1, cdk25c and ⊥G_2/M phase	[213]
Klyflaccisteroid J	*Klyxum flaccidum*	12.7 μM	–	[214]
Suvanine (N,N-dimethyl-1,3-dimethylherbipoline salt) and suvanine-lactam derivatives (4–8)	*Coscinoderma* sp. sponge	* 2.2, 1.9, 3.9, 4.6, 3.9 and 3.6 μM	–	[215]
ar-Turmerone	*Curcuma longa* L	20–50 μg/ml	Induced DNA fragmentation and apoptosis	[216]
Terpene metabolites (1–3)	*Clathria gombawuiensis*	*4.7, 3.9 and 2.1 μM	–	[217]
Toxicarioside H (nor-cardenolide)	*Antiaris toxicaria* (Pers.) Lesch	0.037 μg/ml	–	[218]
Tripolide	Chinese herbal extract	–	↓ Nrf2 and HIF-1α mRNA and protein expression	[219]
10-(Chrysophanol-7′-yl)-10-hydroxychrysophanol-9-anthrone and ramosin	Fractions of EtOH extract of *Asphodelus microcarpus* Salzm. et Vivi	0.15 ± 0.02 and 0.65 ± 0.01 μM	–	[220]

Name of NP	Source of isolation	IC_{50} value on K562 cells	Mechanism of action	References
Withametelins I, J, K, L and N	MeOH extract of *Datura metel* flowers	0.05, 2.5, 0.12, 0.55 and 0.46 μM	–	[221]
Woodfordin I (macrocyclic ellagitannin dimer)	–	–	↓ Bcl-2, Bcl-xL, Bax, c-Abl & BCR-ABL and Loss of MMP	[222]
Gaudichaudic acid, isogambogenic acid and deoxygaudichaudione A (xanthones)	*Garcinia hanburyi* resin	0.41 ± 0.03, 2.1 ± 0.14 and 1.74 ± 0.22 μg/ml	–	[223]
Xindongnins C–D, A, B, melissoidesin G, dawoensin A and glabcensin V	*Isodon rubescens var. rubescens*	0.3–7.3 μg/ml	–	[224]
Hyperbeanols B and D	MeOH extract of *Hypericum beanie*	16.9 and 20.7 μM	–	[225]
Rhodexin A	*Rhodea japonica*	19 nM	⊥G_2/M phase induced apoptosis	[226]
Curcumin	*Curcumina longa*	20 μg/ml	↓BCR-ABL, Hsp90, WT1	[227, 228]
Gambogic acid	*Garcinia hanburyi*	0.62 μM	↓p-BCR-ABL, pSTAT5, p-CRKL, pERK1/2, p-Akt	[229, 230]

*LC_{50}–lethal concentation.

Table 7. Anti-CML activity of other natural products.

Plant extract	IC_{50} value on K562 cells	Mechanism of action	References
Acetone extract of *Peucedanum nebrodense* (Guss.) Strohl.,	14–10.27 μg/ml	–	[231]
AQE extract of *Cornus officinalis* Sieb. et Zuce	100 μg/ml	–	[232]
AQE extracts of the husk fiber of the typical A and common varieties of *Cocos nucifera* (Palmae)	At 500 μg/ml the cell viability of CML cells was found to be 60.1 ± 8.5 and 47.5 ± 11.9%	–	[233]
AQE extract of *Rhodiola imbricate*	–	↓CML cell proliferation at 100 and 200 μg/ml for 72 hrs. induced ROS & apoptosis and ⊥G_2/M phase	[234]
Abnobaviscum F® (standardized AQE extract of European mistletoe from the host tree *Fraxinus)*	–	↑ caspase 9, JNK-1,2, p38 MAPK and ↓ Bcl-1, Erk-1/2 & PKB phosphorylation	[235]
Chloroform extract of *Polyalthia rumphii* stem	40–60μ/ml	–	[236]
Chloroform extract of *Tecomella undulata* bark	30 μg/ml	↑ FAS, FADD, & caspase 8, 3/7. Induced DNA fragmentation & apoptosis	[237]
DCM) extract of *Psidium guajava* L.	32 μg/ml	–	[238]

Plant extract	IC_{50} value on K562 cells	Mechanism of action	References
DCM extract *Artemisia turanica Krasch*	69 μg/ml	↑ caspases, PARP cleavage. Induced DNA damage and apoptosis	[239]
HEX and DCM extract of *Mesua beccariana*	*20 ± 1.5 and 43.75 ± 0.78 μg/ml	–	[240]
HEX and DCM extract of *Mesua ferrea*	*17.5 ± 1.02 and 22.91 ± 1.25 μg/ ml	–	[240]
HEX extract of *Mesua congestiflora*	40.63 ± 1.45 μg/ml	–	[240]
DCM fraction of *Melissa officinalis*	At 50 μg/ml concentration, it induced 65.04 ± 0.93% apoptotic rate	↑ Fas, Bax mRNA levels and Bax/Bcl-2 ratio	[241]
DCM fraction of the crude EtOH extract of *Echinops grijissi* Hance roots	30 μg/ml	–	[242]
EtOH extract of *Pereskia sacharosa*	130 ± 0.03 μg/ml	↑ caspases, cyt. C release, p21 & p53 and ↓Akt and Bcl-2	[244]
EtOH extract of propolis (NP produced by stingless bee *Melipona orbignyi*)	At 250 and 500 μg/ml promoted cell death of CML cells by 15 ± 1 and 63 ± 2%	–	[245]
EtOH extract of *Isodon japonicas*	2.7 μg/ml	–	[246]
EtOH root extract of *Allamanda schottii*	At 800 μg/ml showed cytotoxicity	–	[247]
EtOH stem and leaf extract of *Physalis peruviana*	0.02 and 0.03 g/ml	–	[248]
Alcoholic extract of *Dendrostellera lessertii*	28 μl and 5×10^{-9}M	–	[249]
EtOH extract of *Rosmarinus officinalis* L	1/400 dilution	–	[251]
EtOH extract of *Goldfussia psilostachys*	0.5 μg/ml	↑ CML cells in G_2/M phase	[252]
Fraction from EtoAc of *Caesalpinia spinosa*	44.5 ± 4.05 μg/ml	induced chromatin condensation. Loss of MMP & ↑ caspase 3	[253]
EtoAc extract of *Helichrysum plicatum* flowers	25.9 μg/ml	–	[254]
MeOH extract of *Linum persicum*	0.1 μg/ml	–	[255]
MeOH extracts of *Echinophora cinerea* and *Cirsium bracteosum*	Less than 20 μg/ml	–	[256]
MeOH extract of *Galium mite*	39.8 μg/ml	–	[256]
MeOH extract *of Cyperus rotundus*	175 ± 1.2 μg/ml	Induced DNA damage	[257]
TAF273, F3 and F4 fractions of MeOH extract of *Eurycoma longifolia* Jack	19, 55 and 62 μg/ml	–	[258]
MeOH extract of *Rhaphidophora korthalsii*	–	Enhanced Natural killer cells to kill K562, ↑IFN-ϒ, TNF-α	[259]

Plant extract	IC_{50} value on K562 cells	Mechanism of action	References
MeOH extract of *Rhinella jimi* Stevaux (Anura: Bufonidae) skin	*235 μg/ml	–	[260]
MeOH extract of *Hypericum perforatum L.*flower extract	–	Induced apoptosis	[261]
HEX, DCM, EtoAc, butanol and MeOH extracts of *Helichrysum zivojinii* Černjavski and Soška	11.78 ± 0.94, 23.82 ± 6.54, 27.52 ± 4.96, 50.37 ± 3.28 and 74.88 ± 7.57 μg/ml (for 72 h)	–	[262]
Acetate: MeOH (95:5), acetate, chloroform and HEX fractions of *Erythroxylum caatingae* plowman	13.1 ± 0.63, 9.86 ± 0.56, 11.21 ± 0.46, 33.58 ± 1.33 μg/ml	–	[263]
DCM extract of *Arctium lappa* root	^17 μg/ml	–	[264]
Alisma orientalis (Sam) Juzep extract	–	Reverse of MDR	[265]
Polyphenolic extract of *Ichnocarpus fructescens* leaves	–	At 5, 10, 20 μg/ml con. ↓K562 cell proliferation	[266]
EtOH extract of *Orbignya speciosa*	33.9 ± 4.3 μg/ml	–	[267]
Coptis chinensis and Epimedium sagittatum extracts	29 and74 μg/ml	–	[268]
Sangre de Drago is red viscous latex extract of *Croton lechleri*	2.5 ± 0.3 μg/ml	–	[269]
Dionysia termeana extract	20 μg/ml	–	[270]
Ganoderma lucidum extract	*50 μg/ml	–	[271]
Crude MeOH extracts of *Luehea candicans* Mart. et Zucc. branches and leaves	#8.1–5.4 μg/ml	–	[273]
Nerium oleander extract	–	↓p-gp	[274]
Ponicidin (*Rabdosia rubescens* extract)	–	↓ Bcl-2 and ↑ Bax, caspase 3 & PARP cleavage	[276]
Scutellaria litwinowii Bornm. and Sint. ex Bornm.	–	↑ caspase 3,8, PARP cleavage, Bax/ Bcl-2 ratio	[278]
Swietenia mahagoni leaf extract	–	↑ caspases 3,9, Cyt. C release and ⊥G_2-M phase	[279]
Viscin, (lipophilic extract from *Viscum album* L)	252 ± 37 μg/ml	–	[280]

AQE, aqueous, DCM, dichloromethane, HEX, hexane, EtOH, ethanol, EtoAc, ethyl acetate, MeOH, methanol, ^TGI, tumor growth inhibition,*ED50, –effective concentration; # GI^{50}, growth inhibition.

Table 8. Anti-CML activity of plant extracts.

3. Conclusion

CML is a hematological malignancy that arises due to chromosomal translocation resulting in the presence of Ph chromosome. Initially, TKIs were designed to compete with the ATP binding site of BCR-ABL. TKIs effectively inhibited wild-type BCR-ABL; however, mutations in BCR-ABL and overexpression of drug efflux proteins following treatment decreased their potency.

Since, there is a need for alternative strategy to develop new BCR-ABL inhibitors; NPs (obtaining from living organisms) offers an alternate, effective and inexpensive design for CML therapy. Moreover, they have less (or) no side effects. Studies conducted so far have revealed that many NPs inhibit CML cell proliferation and, in addition, induce cell death through apoptosis. NPs alone or in combination with other TKIs are able to reverse the MDR, thereby increasing the sensitivity of TKIs towards CML. Moreover, many NPs are able to differentiate CML cells into erythroid, monocyte or macrophage lineage. *In vivo* results have clearly shown that NPs potently suppress tumor growth. In sum, NPs serve as an inexhaustible source which renders an attractive alternate strategy to combat CML.

Conflict of interests

The authors declare that they do not have any competing interests.

Abbreviations

CML	chronic myeloid leukemia
Ph	Philadelphia chromosome
MAPK	mitogen activated protein kinase
STAT	signal transducers and activator of transcription
PI3K	phosphoinositide 3-kinase
TKIs	tyrosine kinase inhibitor
FDA	Food and Drug Administration
MDR	multi drug resistance
p-gp	p-glycoprotein
NPs	natural products
NCEs	new chemical entities
BBM	berbamine
K562/IR	imatinib resistant K562 cell line
cyt. C	cytochrome C
BW	body weight
ADR	adriamycin
Hsp90	heat shock protein 90
BBD9	4-chlorobenzoyl berbamine
PARP	Poly(ADP-Ribose) polymerase
LC3 II	LC3-phosphatidylethanolamine conjugate
DOX	doxorubicin

hCPT	homocampthothecin
DNA-PK	DNA-dependent protein kinase
miRNA	microRNA
HHT	homoharringtonine
UCN-01	7-hydroxy staurosporine
μM	micromole
μg	microgram
Q	quercetin
DNR	daunorubicin
MMP	mitochondrial membrane potential
p-p38-MAPK	p-p38 mitogen-activated protein kinase
SLC	solute carrier
hTERT	human telomerase reverse transcriptase
IU	isoprene units
PKSs	polyketide synthases
DMAG	5,5′-dimethoxylariciresinol-4′-O-β-D-glucoside
HJC	6-hydroxyjusticidin C
HSS	Haishengsu

Author details

Kalubai Vari Khajapeer and Rajasekaran Baskaran*

*Address all correspondence to: baskaran.rajasekaran@gmail.com

Department of Biochemistry and Molecular Biology, School of Life Sciences, Pondicherry University, Pondicherry, India

References

[1] Shahrabi S, Azizidoost S, Shahjahani M, Rahim F, Ahmadzadeh A, Saki N. New insights in cellular and molecular aspects of BM niche in chronic myelogenous leukemia. Tumour Biol. 2014;35(11):10627–33. doi:10.1007/s13277-014-2610-9. PubMed PMID: 25234716.

[2] Deininger MW, Goldman JM, Melo JV. The molecular biology of chronic myeloid leukemia. Blood. 2000;96(10):3343–56. PubMed PMID: 11071626.

[3] Sattler M, Griffin JD. Molecular mechanisms of transformation by the BCR-ABL oncogene. Semin Hematol. 2003;40(2 Suppl 2):4–10. doi:10.1053/shem.2003.50034. PubMed PMID: 12783368.

[4] Sacha T. Imatinib in chronic myeloid leukemia: an overview. Mediterr J Hematol Infect Dis. 2014;6(1):e2014007. doi:10.4084/MJHID.2014.007. PubMed PMID: 24455116; PubMed Central PMCID: PMCPMC3894842.

[5] Akard LP. Second-generation BCR-ABL kinase inhibitors in CML. N Engl J Med. 2010;363 (17):1672–3; author reply 3–5. PubMed PMID: 20973144.

[6] Shamroe CL, Comeau JM. Ponatinib: a new tyrosine kinase inhibitor for the treatment of chronic myeloid leukemia and Philadelphia chromosome-positive acute lymphoblastic leukemia. Ann Pharmacother. 2013;47(11):1540–6. doi:10.1177/1060028013501144. Pub Med PMID: 24265264.

[7] Ali MA. Chronic myeloid leukemia in the era of tyrosine kinase inhibitors: an evolving paradigm of molecularly targeted therapy. Mol Diagn Ther. 2016;20(4):315–33. doi:10.1007/s40291-016-0208-1. PubMed PMID: 27220498.

[8] Kinch MS, Haynesworth A, Kinch SL, Hoyer D. An overview of FDA-approved new molecular entities: 1827–2013. Drug Discov Today. 2014;19(8):1033–9. doi:10.1016/j.drudis.2014.03.018. PubMed PMID: 24680947.

[9] Demain AL. Importance of microbial natural products and the need to revitalize their discovery. J Ind Microbiol Biotechnol. 2014;41(2):185–201. doi:10.1007/s10295-013-1325-z. PubMed PMID: 23990168.

[10] Cushnie TP, Cushnie B, Lamb AJ. Alkaloids: an overview of their antibacterial, antibiotic-enhancing and antivirulence activities. Int J Antimicrob Agents. 2014;44(5):377–86. doi:10.1016/j.ijantimicag.2014.06.001. PubMed PMID: 25130096.

[11] Kittakoop P, Mahidol C, Ruchirawat S. Alkaloids as important scaffolds in therapeutic drugs for the treatments of cancer, tuberculosis, and smoking cessation. Curr Top Med Chem. 2014;14(2):239–52. PubMed PMID: 24359196.

[12] Qiu S, Sun H, Zhang AH, Xu HY, Yan GL, Han Y, et al. Natural alkaloids: basic aspects, biological roles, and future perspectives. Chin J Nat Med. 2014;12(6):401–6. doi:10.1016/S1875-5364(14)60063-7. PubMed PMID: 24969519.

[13] Russo P, Frustaci A, Del Bufalo A, Fini M, Cesario A. Multitarget drugs of plants origin acting on Alzheimer's disease. Curr Med Chem. 2013;20(13):1686–93. PubMed PMID: 23410167.

[14] Wei YL, Xu L, Liang Y, Xu XH, Zhao XY. Berbamine exhibits potent antitumor effects on imatinib-resistant CML cells in vitro and in vivo. Acta Pharmacol Sin. 2009;30(4):451–7. doi:10.1038/aps.2009.19. PubMed PMID: 19270722; PubMed Central PMCID: PMCPMC 4002272.

[15] Pazhang Y, Ahmadian S, Mahmoudian M, Shafiezadeh M. Berberine-induced apoptosis via decreasing the survivin protein in K562 cell line. Med Oncol. 2011;28(4):1577–83. doi:10.1007/s12032-010-9586-0. PubMed PMID: 20517657.

[16] Wei YL, Xu L, Zhao XY. Mechanism related to inhibition of leukemia K562 cells by berbamine. Zhejiang Da Xue Xue Bao Yi Xue Ban. 2009;38(4):387–91. PubMed PMID: 19693977.

[17] Wei YL, Liang Y, Xu L, Zhao XY. The anhway. Anat Rec (Hoboken).tiproliferation effect of berbamine on k562 resistant cells by inhibiting NF-kappaB pat 2009;292(7):945–50. doi:10.1002/ar.20924. PubMed PMID: 19548306.

[18] Jin L, Liao HJ, Zhang MY, Liu QY, Wang YF. Effect of berberine on the differentiation and apoptosis of K562 cell line. Zhong Yao Cai. 2009;32(3):384–8. PubMed PMID: 19565717.

[19] Sun JR, Zhang XH, He ZW, Gu Y, Yu YZ, Fang YM, et al. The mechanism of apoptosis of chronic myeloid leukemia cells induced by the novel p210 bcr/abl inhibitor berbamine. Zhonghua Yi Xue Za Zhi. 2006;86(32):2246–51. PubMed PMID: 17064567.

[20] Dong QH, Zheng S, Xu RZ, Lu Q, He L. Study on effect of berbamine on multidrug resistance leukemia K562/Adr cells. Zhongguo Zhong Xi Yi Jie He Za Zhi. 2004;24(9):820–2. PubMed PMID: 15495829.

[21] Han YQ, Yuan JY, Shi YJ, Zhu Y, Wu SL. Reversal effect of berbamine on multidrug resistance of K562/A02 cells and its mechanism. Zhongguo Shi Yan Xue Ye Xue Za Zhi. 2003;11(6):604–8. PubMed PMID: 14706144.

[22] Zhang YF, Xu GB, Gan YC, Xu XH, Xu RZ. Inhibitory effect of 4-chlorobenzoyl berbamine on imatinib-resistant K562 cells in vitro and in vivo. Nan Fang Yi Ke Da Xue Xue Bao. 2011;31(12):1997–2001. PubMed PMID: 22200699.

[23] Zhu HJ, Wang JS, Guo QL, Jiang Y, Liu GQ. Reversal of P-glycoprotein mediated multidrug resistance in K562 cell line by a novel synthetic calmodulin inhibitor, E6. Biol Pharm Bull. 2005;28(10):1974–8. PubMed PMID: 16204958.

[24] Lesueur-Ginot L, Demarquay D, Kiss R, Kasprzyk PG, Dassonneville L, Bailly C, et al. Homocamptothecin, an E-ring modified camptothecin with enhanced lactone stability, retains topoisomerase I-targeted activity and antitumor properties. Cancer Res. 1999;59 (12):2939–43. PubMed PMID: 10383158.

[25] Demarquay D, Huchet M, Coulomb H, Lesueur-Ginot L, Lavergne O, Camara J, et al. BN80927: a novel homocamptothecin that inhibits proliferation of human tumor cells in vitro and in vivo. Cancer Res. 2004;64(14):4942–9. doi:10.1158/0008-5472.CAN-03-3872. PubMed PMID: 15256467.

[26] Song MG, Gao SM, Du KM, Xu M, Yu Y, Zhou YH, et al. Nanomolar concentration of NSC606985, a camptothecin analog, induces leukemic-cell apoptosis through protein kinase Cdelta-dependent mechanisms. Blood. 2005;105(9):3714–21. doi:10.1182/blood-2004-10-4011. PubMed PMID: 15671440.

[27] Ju DS, Kim MJ, Bae JH, Song HS, Chung BS, Lee MK, et al. Camptothecin acts synergistically with imatinib and overcomes imatinib resistance through Bcr-Abl independence in human K562 cells. Cancer Lett. 2007;252(1):75–85. doi:10.1016/j.canlet.2006.12.013. PubMed PMID: 17223257.

[28] Surh YJ, Lee E, Lee JM. Chemoprotective properties of some pungent ingredients present in red pepper and ginger. Mutat Res. 1998;402(1–2):259–67. PubMed PMID: 9675305.

[29] Kaymaz BT, Cetintas VB, Aktan C, Kosova B. MicroRNA-520a-5p displays a therapeutic effect upon chronic myelogenous leukemia cells by targeting STAT3 and enhances the anticarcinogenic role of capsaicin. Tumour Biol. 2014;35(9):8733–42. doi:10.1007/s13277-014-2138-z. PubMed PMID: 24870597.

[30] Lee SA, Ryu YS, Choi HI, Han IS. Capsaicin promotes the development of burst-forming units–erythroid (BFU-E) from mouse bone marrow cells. Exp Mol Med. 2007;39(3):278–83. doi:10.1038/emm.2007.31. PubMed PMID: 17603282.

[31] Ye LL, Cao WK, Shi YY, Deng ZK, Tao SD, Ji P, et al. Effect of homoharringtonine on expression of NF-kappaB and BCL-2 proteins in K562 cells. Zhongguo Shi Yan Xue Ye Xue Za Zhi. 2013;21(1):78–81. doi:10.7534/j.issn.1009-2137.2013.01.017. PubMed PMID: 23484696.

[32] Tong H, Ren Y, Zhang F, Jin J. Homoharringtonine affects the JAK2-STAT5 signal pathway through alteration of protein tyrosine kinase phosphorylation in acute myeloid leukemia cells. Eur J Haematol. 2008;81(4):259–66. doi:10.1111/j.1600-0609.2008.01116.x. PubMed PMID: 18616510.

[33] Hallock S, Tang SC, Buja LM, Trump BF, Liepins A, Weerasinghe P. Aurintricarboxylic acid inhibits protein synthesis independent, sanguinarine-induced apoptosis and oncosis. Toxicol Pathol. 2007;35(2):300–9. doi:10.1080/01926230701194211. PubMed PMID: 17366325.

[34] Lerga A, Crespo P, Berciano M, Delgado MD, Canelles M, Cales C, et al. Regulation of c-Myc and Max in megakaryocytic and monocytic-macrophagic differentiation of K562 cells induced by protein kinase C modifiers: c-Myc is down-regulated but does not inhibit differentiation. Cell Growth Differ. 1999;10(9):639–54. PubMed PMID: 10511314.

[35] Peng HY, Liao HF. Staurosporine induces megakaryocytic differentiation through the upregulation of JAK/Stat3 signaling pathway. Ann Hematol. 2011;90(9):1017–29. doi:10.1007/s00277-011-1186-3. PubMed PMID: 21331591.

[36] Ogino T, Kobuchi H, Fujita H, Matsukawa A, Utsumi K. Erythroid and megakaryocytic differentiation of K562 erythroleukemic cells by monochloramine. Free Radic Res. 2014;48(3):292–302. doi:10.3109/10715762.2013.865840. PubMed PMID: 242372 53.

[37] Shao RG, Shimizu T, Pommier Y. 7-Hydroxystaurosporine (UCN-01) induces apoptosis in human colon carcinoma and leukemia cells independently of p53. Exp Cell Res. 1997;234 (2):388–97. doi:10.1006/excr.1997.3650. PubMed PMID: 9260909.

[38] Busby EC, Leistritz DF, Abraham RT, Karnitz LM, Sarkaria JN. The radiosensitizing agent 7-hydroxystaurosporine (UCN-01) inhibits the DNA damage checkpoint kinase hChk1. Cancer Res. 2000;60(8):2108–12. PubMed PMID: 10786669.

[39] Shi DX, Ma LM, Lu YJ, Bai B. Apoptosis-inducing effect of tetrandrine and imatinib on K562/G01 cells and its related mechanism. Zhongguo Shi Yan Xue Ye Xue Za Zhi. 2014;22 (3):723–8. doi:10.7534/j.issn.1009-2137.2014.03.028. PubMed PMID: 24989284.

[40] Cui TY, Chen BA, Ding JH, Gao C, Cheng J, Bao W, et al. Inducing apoptosis and reversal effect of nilotinib in combination with tetrandrine on multidrug resistance of K562/A02 cell line. Zhongguo Shi Yan Xue Ye Xue Za Zhi. 2011;19(1):28–33. PubMed PMID: 21362216.

[41] Xu XH, Gan YC, Xu GB, Chen T, Zhou H, Tang JF, et al. Tetrandrine citrate eliminates imatinib-resistant chronic myeloid leukemia cells in vitro and in vivo by inhibiting Bcr-Abl/beta-catenin axis. J Zhejiang Univ Sci B. 2012;13(11):867–74. doi:10.1631/jzus.B1200021. PubMed PMID: 23125079; PubMed Central PMCID: PMCPMC3494025.

[42] Zhang W, Chen BA, Jin JF, He YJ, Niu YQ. Involvement of c-Jun N-terminal kinase in reversal of multidrug resistance of human leukemia cells in hypoxia by 5-bromotetrandrine. Leuk Lymphoma. 2013;54(11):2506–16. doi:10.3109/10428194.2013.776681. PubMed PMID: 23418897.

[43] Jiang C, Li ZL, Gong P, Kang SL, Liu MS, Pei YH, et al. Five novel naphthylisoquinoline alkaloids with growth inhibitory activities against human leukemia cells HL-60, K562 and U937 from stems and leaves of *Ancistrocladus tectorius*. Fitoterapia. 2013;91:305–12. doi:10.1016/j.fitote.2013.09.010. PubMed PMID: 24076380.

[44] Uadkla O, Yodkeeree S, Buayairaksa M, Meepowpan P, Nuntasaen N, Limtrakul P, et al. Antiproliferative effect of alkaloids via cell cycle arrest from *Pseuduvaria rugosa*. Pharm Biol. 2013;51(3):400–4. doi:10.3109/13880209.2012.734314. PubMed PMID: 23406361.

[45] Wang XD, Li CY, Jiang MM, Li D, Wen P, Song X, et al. Induction of apoptosis in human leukemia cells through an intrinsic pathway by cathachunine, a unique alkaloid isolated from *Catharanthus roseus*. Phytomedicine. 2016;23(6):641–53. doi:10.1016/j.phymed.2016.03.003. PubMed PMID: 27161405.

[46] Ikeda R, Che XF, Yamaguchi T, Ushiyama M, Zheng CL, Okumura H, et al. Cepharanthine potently enhances the sensitivity of anticancer agents in K562 cells. Cancer Sci. 2005;96(6):372–6. doi:10.1111/j.1349-7006.2005.00057.x. PubMed PMID: 15958061.

[47] Aoki S, Kong D, Matsui K, Kobayashi M. Erythroid differentiation in K562 chronic myelogenous cells induced by crambescidin 800, a pentacyclic guanidine alkaloid. Anticancer Res. 2004;24(4):2325–30. PubMed PMID: 15330179.

[48] Wongsirisin P, Yodkeeree S, Pompimon W, Limtrakul P. Induction of G1 arrest and apoptosis in human cancer cells by crebanine, an alkaloid from *Stephania venosa*. Chem Pharm Bull (Tokyo). 2012;60(10):1283–9. PubMed PMID: 22863844.

[49] Dantas BB, Faheina-Martins GV, Coulidiati TH, Bomfim CC, da Silva Dias C, Barbosa-Filho JM, et al. Effects of curine in HL-60 leukemic cells: cell cycle arrest and apoptosis induction. J Nat Med. 2015;69(2):218–23. doi:10.1007/s11418-014-0881-5. PubMed PMID: 25616501.

[50] Fu P, Kong F, Li X, Wang Y, Zhu W. Cyanogramide with a new spiro[indolinone-pyrroloimidazole] skeleton from *Actinoalloteichus cyanogriseus*. Org Lett. 2014;16(14):3708–11. doi:10.1021/ol501523d. PubMed PMID: 24968070.

[51] Ge HM, Yu ZG, Zhang J, Wu JH, Tan RX. Bioactive alkaloids from endophytic *Aspergillus fumigatus*. J Nat Prod. 2009;72(4):753–5. doi:10.1021/np800700e. PubMed PMID: 19256529.

[52] Huang RL, Chen CC, Huang YL, Ou JC, Hu CP, Chen CF, et al. Anti-tumor effects of d-dicentrine from the root of *Lindera megaphylla*. Planta Med. 1998;64(3):212–5. doi:10.1055/s-2006-957411. PubMed PMID: 9581516.

[53] Pan X, Hartley JM, Hartley JA, White KN, Wang Z, Bligh SW. Evodiamine, a dual catalytic inhibitor of type I and II topoisomerases, exhibits enhanced inhibition against camptothecin resistant cells. Phytomedicine. 2012;19(7):618–24. doi:10.1016/j.phymed.2012.02.003. PubMed PMID: 22402246.

[54] Gong KK, Tang XL, Liu YS, Li PL, Li GQ. Imidazole alkaloids from the South China Sea Sponge *Pericharax heteroraphis* and their cytotoxic and antiviral activities. Molecules. 2016;21(2):150. doi:10.3390/molecules21020150. PubMed PMID: 26821008.

[55] Song QF, Qu YC, Zheng HB, Zhang GH, Lin HG, Yang JL. Differentiation of erythroleukemia K562 cells induced by piperine. Ai Zheng. 2008;27(6):571–4. PubMed PMID: 18570727.

[56] Qing C, Zhang JS, Ding J. In vitro cytotoxicity of salvicine, a novel diterpenoid quinone. Zhongguo Yao Li Xue Bao. 1999;20(4):297–302. PubMed PMID: 10452112.

[57] Wei G, Wang J, Du Y. Total synthesis of solamargine. Bioorg Med Chem Lett. 2011;21 (10):2930–3. doi:10.1016/j.bmcl.2011.03.064. PubMed PMID: 21482107.

[58] Sun L, Zhao Y, Li X, Yuan H, Cheng A, Lou H. A lysosomal-mitochondrial death pathway is induced by solamargine in human K562 leukemia cells. Toxicol In Vitro. 2010;24 (6):1504–11. doi:10.1016/j.tiv.2010.07.013. PubMed PMID: 20647040.

[59] Chao MW, Chen CH, Chang YL, Teng CM, Pan SL. alpha-Tomatine-mediated anti-cancer activity in vitro and in vivo through cell cycle- and caspase-independent pathways. PLoS One. 2012;7(9):e44093. doi:10.1371/journal.pone.0044093. PubMed PMID: 22970166; PubMed Central PMCID: PMCPMC3435411.

[60] Ganguly T, Khar A. Induction of apoptosis in a human erythroleukemic cell line K562 by tylophora alkaloids involves release of cytochrome c and activation of caspase 3. Phytomedicine. 2002;9(4):288–95. doi:10.1078/0944-7113-00146. PubMed PMID: 12120809.

[61] Peng J, Zhang XY, Tu ZC, Xu XY, Qi SH. Alkaloids from the deep-sea-derived fungus *Aspergillus westerdijkiae* DFFSCS013. J Nat Prod. 2013;76(5):983–7. doi:10.1021/np400132m. PubMed PMID: 23701598.

[62] Lucio AS, Almeida JR, Barbosa-Filho JM, Pita JC, Branco MV, Diniz Mde F, et al. Azaphenanthrene alkaloids with antitumoral activity from *Anaxagorea dolichocarpa* Sprague & Sandwith (Annonaceae). Molecules. 2011;16(8):7125–31. doi:10.3390/molecules16087125. PubMed PMID: 21860364.

[63] Wang J, Wei X, Qin X, Lin X, Zhou X, Liao S, et al. Arthpyrones A-C, pyridone alkaloids from a sponge-derived fungus *Arthrinium arundinis* ZSDS1-F3. Org Lett. 2015;17(3):656–9. doi:10.1021/ol503646c. PubMed PMID: 25606827.

[64] Song F, Ren B, Yu K, Chen C, Guo H, Yang N, et al. Quinazolin-4-one coupled with pyrrolidin-2–iminium alkaloids from marine-derived fungus *Penicillium aurantiogriseum*. Mar Drugs. 2012;10(6):1297–306. doi:10.3390/md10061297. PubMed PMID: 22822373; PubMed Central PMCID: PMCPMC3397440.

[65] Zhang JR, Li PL, Tang XL, Qi X, Li GQ. Cytotoxic tetraprenylated alkaloids from the South China Sea gorgonian *Euplexaura robusta*. Chem Biodivers. 2012;9(10):2218–24. doi:10.1002/cbdv.201100374. PubMed PMID: 23081922.

[66] Zhang G, Li M, Han S, Chen D, Wang Y, Ye W, et al. Induction of human chronic myeloid leukemia K562 cell apoptosis by virosecurinine and its molecular mechanism. Mol Med Rep. 2014;10(5):2365–71. doi:10.3892/mmr.2014.2531. PubMed PMID: 25189629; PubMed Central PMCID: PMCPMC4214351.

[67] Cushnie TP, Lamb AJ. Recent advances in understanding the antibacterial properties of flavonoids. Int J Antimicrob Agents. 2011;38(2):99–107. doi:10.1016/j.ijantimicag.2011.02.014. PubMed PMID: 21514796.

[68] Gonzalez CA, Sala N, Rokkas T. Gastric cancer: epidemiologic aspects. Helicobacter. 2013;18 Suppl 1:34–8. doi:10.1111/hel.12082. PubMed PMID: 24011243.

[69] Lotito SB, Frei B. Consumption of flavonoid-rich foods and increased plasma antioxidant capacity in humans: cause, consequence, or epiphenomenon? Free Radic Biol Med. 2006;41(12):1727–46. doi:10.1016/j.freeradbiomed.2006.04.033. PubMed PMID: 17157175.

[70] Martinez-Micaelo N, Gonzalez-Abuin N, Ardevol A, Pinent M, Blay MT. Procyanidins and inflammation: molecular targets and health implications. Biofactors. 2012;38(4):257–65. doi:10.1002/biof.1019. PubMed PMID: 22505223.

[71] Romagnolo DF, Selmin OI. Flavonoids and cancer prevention: a review of the evidence. J Nutr Gerontol Geriatr. 2012;31(3):206–38. doi:10.1080/21551197.2012.702534. PubMed PMID: 22888839.

[72] Taylor PW, Hamilton-Miller JM, Stapleton PD. Antimicrobial properties of green tea catechins. Food Sci Technol Bull. 2005;2:71–81. PubMed PMID: 19844590; PubMed Central PMCID: PMCPMC2763290.

[73] Williams RJ, Spencer JP, Rice-Evans C. Flavonoids: antioxidants or signalling molecules? Free Radic Biol Med. 2004;36(7):838–49. doi:10.1016/j.freeradbiomed.2004.01.001. PubMed PMID: 15019969.

[74] Woo HD, Kim J. Dietary flavonoid intake and smoking-related cancer risk: a meta-analysis. PLoS One. 2013;8(9):e75604. doi:10.1371/journal.pone.0075604. PubMed PMID: 24069431; PubMed Central PMCID: PMCPMC3777962.

[75] Wang Y, Miao H, Li W, Yao J, Sun Y, Li Z, et al. CXCL12/CXCR4 axis confers adriamycin resistance to human chronic myelogenous leukemia and oroxylin A improves the sensitivity of K562/ADM cells. Biochem Pharmacol. 2014;90(3):212–25. doi:10.1016/j.bcp.2014.05.007. PubMed PMID: 24858801.

[76] Li X, Miao H, Zhang Y, Li W, Li Z, Zhou Y, et al. Bone marrow microenvironment confers imatinib resistance to chronic myelogenous leukemia and oroxylin A reverses the resistance by suppressing Stat3 pathway. Arch Toxicol. 2015;89(1):121–36. doi:10.1007/s00204-014-1226-6. PubMed PMID: 24671465.

[77] Kawabata K, Mukai R, Ishisaka A. Quercetin and related polyphenols: new insights and implications for their bioactivity and bioavailability. Food Funct. 2015;6(5):1399–417. doi:10.1039/c4fo01178c. PubMed PMID: 25761771.

[78] Shen J, Zhang WJ, Tai YC, Wong CH, Xie Z, Chen CS. Synergistic antileukemic effect of phytoestrogens and chemotherapeutic drugs on leukemic cell lines in vitro. Zhongguo Shi Yan Xue Ye Xue Za Zhi. 2008;16(2):276–81. PubMed PMID: 18426648.

[79] Deora AB, Miranda MB, Rao SG. Down-modulation of P210bcr/abl induces apoptosis/differentiation in K562 leukemic blast cells. Tumori. 1997;83(4):756–61. PubMed PMID: 9349317.

[80] Chen FY, Cao LF, Wan HX, Zhang MY, Cai JY, Shen LJ, et al. Quercetin enhances adriamycin cytotoxicity through induction of apoptosis and regulation of mitogen-activated protein kinase/extracellular signal-regulated kinase/c-Jun N-terminal kinase signaling in multidrug-resistant leukemia K562 cells. Mol Med Rep. 2015;11(1):341–8. doi:10.3892/mmr.2014.2734. PubMed PMID: 25339540.

[81] Cai X, Chen FY, Han JY, Gu CH, Zhong H, Ouyang RR. Restorative effect of quercetin on subcellular distribution of daunorubicin in multidrug resistant leukemia cell lines K562/ADM and HL-60/ADM. Ai Zheng. 2004;23(12):1611–5. PubMed PMID: 15601547.

[82] Han YQ, Cao LJ, Hao HJ, Shi YJ. Effects of quercetin on multidrug resistance and expression of related genes in human erythroleukemic K562/a cells. Zhongguo Shi Yan Xue Ye Xue Za Zhi. 2011;19(4):884–9. PubMed PMID: 21867607.

[83] Philchenkov AA, Zavelevich MP, Mikhailenko VM, Kuyava LM. Apoptosis and content of mobile lipid domains in human leukemia K-562 cells induced to differentiate by quercetin or dimethyl sulfoxide. Ukr Biokhim Zh (1999). 2010;82(2):104–10. PubMed PMID: 20684251.

[84] Kothan S, Dechsupa S, Leger G, Moretti JL, Vergote J, Mankhetkorn S. Spontaneous mitochondrial membrane potential change during apoptotic induction by quercetin in K562 and K562/adr cells. Can J Physiol Pharmacol. 2004;82(12):1084–90. doi:10.1139/y04-113. PubMed PMID: 15644950.

[85] Elia G, Santoro MG. Regulation of heat shock protein synthesis by quercetin in human erythroleukaemia cells. Biochem J. 1994;300 (Pt 1):201–9. PubMed PMID: 8198534; PubMed Central PMCID: PMCPMC1138143.

[86] Avci CB, Yilmaz S, Dogan ZO, Saydam G, Dodurga Y, Ekiz HA, et al. Quercetin-induced apoptosis involves increased hTERT enzyme activity of leukemic cells. Hematology. 2011;16(5):303–7. doi:10.1179/102453311X13085644680104. PubMed PMID: 21902895.

[87] Isoda H, Motojima H, Onaga S, Samet I, Villareal MO, Han J. Analysis of the erythroid differentiation effect of flavonoid apigenin on K562 human chronic leukemia cells. Chem Biol Interact. 2014;220:269–77. doi:10.1016/j.cbi.2014.07.006. PubMed PMID: 25058688.

[88] Dong QH, Zheng S, Xu RZ, Lu QH. Baicalein selectively induce apoptosis in human leukemia K562 cells. Yao Xue Xue Bao. 2003;38(11):817–20. PubMed PMID: 14991992.

[89] Adan A, Baran Y. Fisetin and hesperetin induced apoptosis and cell cycle arrest in chronic myeloid leukemia cells accompanied by modulation of cellular signaling. Tumour Biol. 2016;37(5):5781–95. doi:10.1007/s13277-015-4118-3. PubMed PMID: 26408178.

[90] Tolomeo M, Grimaudo S, Di Cristina A, Pipitone RM, Dusonchet L, Meli M, et al. Galangin increases the cytotoxic activity of imatinib mesylate in imatinib-sensitive and imatinib-resistant Bcr-Abl expressing leukemia cells. Cancer Lett. 2008;265(2):289–97. doi:10.1016/j.canlet.2008.02.025. PubMed PMID: 18374481.

[91] Budhraja A, Gao N, Zhang Z, Son YO, Cheng S, Wang X, et al. Apigenin induces apoptosis in human leukemia cells and exhibits anti-leukemic activity in vivo. Mol Cancer Ther. 2012;11(1):132–42. doi:10.1158/1535-7163.MCT-11-0343. PubMed PMID: 22084167; PubMed Central PMCID: PMCPMC4430727.

[92] Honma Y, Okabe-Kado J, Kasukabe T, Hozumi M, Umezawa K. Inhibition of abl oncogene tyrosine kinase induces erythroid differentiation of human myelogenous leukemia K562 cells. Jpn J Cancer Res. 1990;81(11):1132–6. PubMed PMID: 2125038.

[93] Marfe G, Tafani M, Indelicato M, Sinibaldi-Salimei P, Reali V, Pucci B, et al. Kaempferol induces apoptosis in two different cell lines via Akt inactivation, Bax and SIRT3 activation, and mitochondrial dysfunction. J Cell Biochem. 2009;106(4):643–50. doi:10.1002/jcb.22044. PubMed PMID: 19160423.

[94] Ikegawa T, Ohtani H, Koyabu N, Juichi M, Iwase Y, Ito C, et al. Inhibition of P-glycoprotein by flavonoid derivatives in adriamycin-resistant human myelogenous leukemia (K562/ADM) cells. Cancer Lett. 2002;177(1):89–93. PubMed PMID: 11809535.

[95] Ross JA, Kasum CM. Dietary flavonoids: bioavailability, metabolic effects, and safety. Annu Rev Nutr. 2002;22:19–34. doi:10.1146/annurev.nutr.22.111401.144957. PubMed PMID: 12055336.

[96] Lindqvist C, Bobrowska-Hagerstrand M, Mrowczynska L, Engblom C, Hagerstrand H. Potentiation of natural killer cell activity with myricetin. Anticancer Res. 2014;34(8):3975–9. PubMed PMID: 25075019.

[97] Lopez-Lazaro M, Willmore E, Austin CA. The dietary flavonoids myricetin and fisetin act as dual inhibitors of DNA topoisomerases I and II in cells. Mutat Res. 2010;696(1):41–7. doi:10.1016/j.mrgentox.2009.12.010. PubMed PMID: 20025993.

[98] Li RF, Feng YQ, Chen JH, Ge LT, Xiao SY, Zuo XL. Naringenin suppresses K562 human leukemia cell proliferation and ameliorates Adriamycin-induced oxidative damage in polymorphonuclear leukocytes. Exp Ther Med. 2015;9(3):697–706. doi:10.3892/etm.2015.2185. PubMed PMID: 25667616; PubMed Central PMCID: PMCPMC4316947.

[99] Wang Y, Su M, Yin J, Zhang H. Effect of nobiletin on K562 cells xenograft in nude mice. Zhongguo Zhong Yao Za Zhi. 2009;34(11):1410–4. PubMed PMID: 19771874.

[100] Nicolini F, Burmistrova O, Marrero MT, Torres F, Hernandez C, Quintana J, et al. Induction of G2/M phase arrest and apoptosis by the flavonoid tamarixetin on human leukemia cells. Mol Carcinog. 2014;53(12):939–50. doi:10.1002/mc.22055. PubMed PMID: 23765509.

[101] Cao C, Liu B, Zeng C, Lu Y, Chen S, Yang L, et al. A polymethoxyflavone from *Laggera pterodonta* induces apoptosis in imatinib-resistant K562R cells via activation of the intrinsic apoptosis pathway. Cancer Cell Int. 2014;14(1):137. doi:10.1186/s12935-014-0137-1. PubMed PMID: 25530716; PubMed Central PMCID: PMCPMC4272561.

[102] Oliveira MC, de Carvalho MG, Grynberg NF, Brioso PS. A biflavonoid from *Luxemburgia nobilis* as inhibitor of DNA topoisomerases. Planta Med. 2005;71(6):561–3. doi:10.1055/s-2005-864159. PubMed PMID: 15971129.

[103] Zhang SD, Shan L, Li W, Li HL, Zhang WD. Isochamaejasmin induces apoptosis in leukemia cells through inhibiting Bcl-2 family proteins. Chin J Nat Med. 2015;13 (9):660–6. doi:10.1016/S1875-5364(15)30063-7. PubMed PMID: 26412425.

[104] Huang XH, Xiong PC, Xiong CM, Cai YL, Wei AH, Wang JP, et al. In vitro and in vivo antitumor activity of *Macrothelypteris torresiana* and its acute/subacute oral toxicity. Phytomedicine. 2010;17(12):930–4. doi:10.1016/j.phymed.2010.03.006. PubMed PMID: 20381325.

[105] Liu YL, Tang LH, Liang ZQ, You BG, Yang SL. Growth inhibitory and apoptosis inducing by effects of total flavonoids from *Lysimachia clethroides* Duby in human chronic myeloid leukemia K562 cells. J Ethnopharmacol. 2010;131(1):1–9. doi:10.1016/j.jep.2010.04.008. PubMed PMID: 20420897.

[106] Zhang D, Wang D, Yu Y. Effects and mechanisms of total flavonoids of astragali radix and calycosin on inhibiting human erythroleukemia cell line K562. Zhongguo Zhong Yao Za Zhi. 2011;36(24):3502–5. PubMed PMID: 22368866.

[107] Ammar RB, Neffati A, Skandrani I, Sghaier MB, Bhouri W, Ghedira K, et al. Anti-lipid peroxidation and induction of apoptosis in the erythroleukaemic cell line K562 by extracts from (Tunisian) *Rhamnus alaternus* L. (Rhamnaceae). Nat Prod Res. 2011;25 (11):1047–58. doi:10.1080/14786419.2010.490783. PubMed PMID: 21726127.

[108] Ammar RB, Kilani S, Bouhlel I, Ezzi L, Skandrani I, Boubaker J, et al. Antiproliferative, antioxidant, and antimutagenic activities of flavonoid-enriched extracts from (Tunisian) *Rhamnus alaternus* L.: combination with the phytochemical composition. Drug Chem Toxicol. 2008;31(1):61–80. doi:10.1080/01480540701688725. PubMed PMID: 18161508.

[109] Goker B, Caliskan C, Onur Caglar H, Kayabasi C, Balci T, Erbaykent Tepedelen B, et al. Synergistic effect of ponatinib and epigallocatechin-3-gallate induces apoptosis in chronic myeloid leukemia cells through altering expressions of cell cycle regulatory genes. J BUON. 2014;19(4):992–8. PubMed PMID: 25536607.

[110] Aziz M, Karboune S. Natural antimicrobial/antioxidant agents in meat and poultry products as well as fruits and vegetables: a review. Crit Rev Food Sci Nutr. 2016. doi:10.1080/10408398.2016.1194256. PubMed PMID: 27437876.

[111] da Silveira e Sa Rde C, Andrade LN, de Sousa DP. Sesquiterpenes from essential oils and anti–inflammatory activity. Nat Prod Commun. 2015;10(10):1767–74. PubMed PMID: 26669122.

[112] Evidente A, Kornienko A, Lefranc F, Cimmino A, Dasari R, Evidente M, et al. Sesterterpenoids with anticancer activity. Curr Med Chem. 2015;22(30):3502–22. PubMed PMID: 26295461; PubMed Central PMCID: PMCPMC4955362.

[113] Grassmann J. Terpenoids as plant antioxidants. Vitam Horm. 2005;72:505–35. doi:10.1016/S0083-6729(05)72015-X. PubMed PMID: 16492481.

[114] Mukherjee N, Mukherjee S, Saini P, Roy P, Babu SP. Phenolics and terpenoids; the promising new search for anthelmintics: a critical review. Mini Rev Med Chem. 2015. PubMed PMID: 26586122.

[115] Tholl D. Biosynthesis and biological functions of terpenoids in plants. Adv Biochem Eng Biotechnol. 2015;148:63–106. doi:10.1007/10_2014_295. PubMed PMID: 25583224.

[116] Li H, Li M, Wang G, Shao F, Chen W, Xia C, et al. EM23, a natural sesquiterpene lactone from *Elephantopus mollis*, induces apoptosis in human myeloid leukemia cells through thioredoxin- and reactive oxygen species-mediated signaling pathways. Front Pharmacol. 2016;7:77. doi:10.3389/fphar.2016.00077. PubMed PMID: 27064563; PubMed Central PMCID: PMCPMC4809879.

[117] Zheng Y, Zhang SW, Cong HJ, Huang YJ, Xuan LJ. Caesalminaxins A-L, cassane diterpenoids from the seeds of *Caesalpinia minax*. J Nat Prod. 2013;76(12):2210–8. doi:10.1021/np400545v. PubMed PMID: 24303808.

[118] Jeon JE, Liao L, Kim H, Sim CJ, Oh DC, Oh KB, et al. Cytotoxic diterpenoid pseudodimers from the Korean sponge *Phorbas gukhulensis*. J Nat Prod. 2013;76 (9):1679–85. doi:10.1021/np400389c. PubMed PMID: 24025124.

[119] Su D, Yang XY, Feng X, Shang MY, Cai SQ. The diterpenes ovoideal A-G from *Tirpitzia ovoidea*. Molecules. 2014;19(11):18966–79. doi:10.3390/molecules191118966. PubMed PMID: 25412043.

[120] Kang YQ, Zhou JC, Fan PH, Wang SQ, Lou HX. Scapaundulin C, a novel labdane diterpenoid isolated from Chinese liverwort *Scapania undulate*, inhibits acetylcholinesterase activity. Chin J Nat Med. 2015;13(12):933–6. doi:10.1016/S1875-5364(15)30100-X. PubMed PMID: 26721712.

[121] Li LM, Li GY, Li SH, Weng ZY, Xiao WL, Han QB, et al. Cytotoxic ent-kauranoids from *Isodon parvifolius*. Chem Biodivers. 2006;3(9):1031–8. doi:10.1002/cbdv.200690101. PubMed PMID: 17193336.

[122] Li LM, Weng ZY, Huang SX, Pu JX, Li SH, Huang H, et al. Cytotoxic ent-kauranoids from the medicinal plant *Isodon xerophilus*. J Nat Prod. 2007;70(8):1295–301. doi:10.1021/np070205m. PubMed PMID: 17665952.

[123] Huang SX, Pu JX, Xiao WL, Li LM, Weng ZY, Zhou Y, et al. ent-Abietane diterpenoids from Isodon rubescens var. rubescens. Phytochemistry. 2007;68(5):616–22. doi:10.1016/j.phytochem.2006.11.007. PubMed PMID: 17173940.

[124] Wu B, He S, Wu XD, Pan YJ. Bioactive terpenes from the roots of *Chloranthus henryi*. Planta Med. 2006;72(14):1334–8. doi:10.1055/s-2006-947256. PubMed PMID: 17022005.

[125] Li LM, Li GY, Huang SX, Li SH, Zhou Y, Xiao WL, et al. 7alpha,20-epoxy-ent-kauranoids from *Isodon parvifolius*. J Nat Prod. 2006;69(4):645–9. doi:10.1021/np0600200. PubMed PMID: 16643043.

[126] Moosavi MA, Yazdanparast R, Sanati MH. The cytotoxic and anti-proliferative effects of 3-hydrogenkwadaphnin in K562 and jurkat cells is reduced by guanosine. J Biochem Mol Biol. 2005;38(4):391–8. PubMed PMID: 16053705.

[127] Xiang W, Na Z, Li SH, Li ML, Li RT, Tian QE, et al. Cytotoxic diterpenoids from *Isodon enanderianus*. Planta Med. 2003;69(11):1031–5. doi:10.1055/s-2003-45151. PubMed PMID: 14735442.

[128] Han QB, Zhao AH, Zhang JX, Lu Y, Zhang LL, Zheng QT, et al. Cytotoxic constituents of Isodon rubescens var. lushiensis. J Nat Prod. 2003;66(10):1391–4. doi:10.1021/np030165w. PubMed PMID: 14575445.

[129] Liu JJ, Liu WD, Yang HZ, Zhang Y, Fang ZG, Liu PQ, et al. Inactivation of PI3k/Akt signaling pathway and activation of caspase-3 are involved in tanshinone I-induced apoptosis in myeloid leukemia cells in vitro. Ann Hematol. 2010;89(11):1089–97. doi:10.1007/s00277-010-0996-z. PubMed PMID: 20512574.

[130] Li LM, Li GY, Ding LS, Yang LB, Zhao Y, Pu JX, et al. ent-Kaurane Diterpenoids from Isodon nervosus. J Nat Prod. 2008;71(4):684–8. doi:10.1021/np800027a. PubMed PMID: 18345641.

[131] Lai YY, Chen LC, Wu CF, Lu MC, Wen ZH, Wu TY, et al. New cytotoxic 24-homoscalarane sesterterpenoids from the sponge *Ircinia felix*. Int J Mol Sci. 2015;16(9):21950–8. doi:10.3390/ijms160921950. PubMed PMID: 26378524; PubMed Central PMCID: PMCPMC4613290.

[132] Song J, Jeong W, Wang N, Lee HS, Sim CJ, Oh KB, et al. Scalarane sesterterpenes from the sponge *Smenospongia* sp. J Nat Prod. 2008;71(11):1866–71. doi:10.1021/np8003694. PubMed PMID: 18973387.

[133] Wang N, Song J, Jang KH, Lee HS, Li X, Oh KB, et al. Sesterterpenoids from the sponge *Sarcotragus* sp. J Nat Prod. 2008;71(4):551–7. doi:10.1021/np0780147. PubMed PMID: 18341287.

[134] Rho JR, Lee HS, Shin HJ, Ahn JW, Kim JY, Sim CJ, et al. New sesterterpenes from the sponge *Smenospongia* sp. J Nat Prod. 2004;67(10):1748–51. doi:10.1021/np040103l. PubMed PMID: 15497955.

[135] Ma QY, Luo Y, Huang SZ, Guo ZK, Dai HF, Zhao YX. Lanostane triterpenoids with cytotoxic activities from the fruiting bodies of *Ganoderma hainanense*. J Asian Nat Prod Res. 2013;15(11):1214–9. doi:10.1080/10286020.2013.820712. PubMed PMID: 2390 9866.

[136] Huang D, Qing S, Zeng G, Wang Y, Guo H, Tan J, et al. Lipophilic components from Fructus Viticis Negundo and their anti-tumor activities. Fitoterapia. 2013;86:144–8. doi:10.1016/j.fitote.2013.02.009. PubMed PMID: 23454672.

[137] Yan J, Zhou ZY, Zhang M, Wang J, Dai HF, Tan JW. New serratene triterpenoids from *Palhinhaea cernua* and their cytotoxic activity. Planta Med. 2012;78(12):1387–91. doi:10.1055/s-0032-1314999. PubMed PMID: 22753038.

[138] Wang LL, Li ZL, Song DD, Sun L, Pei YH, Jing YK, et al. Two novel triterpenoids with antiproliferative and apoptotic activities in human leukemia cells isolated from the resin of *Garcinia hanburyi*. Planta Med. 2008;74(14):1735–40. doi:10.1055/s-2008-1081355. PubMed PMID: 18781544.

[139] Lei C, Huang SX, Chen JJ, Yang LB, Xiao WL, Chang Y, et al. Propindilactones E-J, schiartane nortriterpenoids from *Schisandra propinqua* var. propinqua. J Nat Prod. 2008;71(7):1228–32. doi:10.1021/np8001699. PubMed PMID: 18578539.

[140] Pu JX, Huang SX, Ren J, Xiao WL, Li LM, Li RT, et al. Isolation and structure elucidation of kadlongilactones C-F from *Kadsura longipedunculata* by NMR spectroscopy and DFT computational methods. J Nat Prod. 2007;70(11):1706–11. doi:10.1021/np070247a. PubMed PMID: 17970593.

[141] Lee I, Yoo JK, Na M, Min BS, Lee J, Yun BS, et al. Cytotoxicity of triterpenes isolated from *Aceriphyllum rossii*. Chem Pharm Bull (Tokyo). 2007;55(9):1376–8. PubMed PMID: 17827765.

[142] Parra-Delgado H, Garcia-Pillado F, Sordo M, Ramirez-Apan T, Martinez-Vazquez M, Ostrosky-Wegman P. Evaluation of the cytotoxicity, cytostaticity and genotoxicity of argentatins A and B from *Parthenium argentatum* (Gray). Life Sci. 2005;77(22):2855–65. doi:10.1016/j.lfs.2005.05.024. PubMed PMID: 15979099.

[143] Lu Z, Jin Y, Qiu L, Lai Y, Pan J. Celastrol, a novel HSP90 inhibitor, depletes Bcr-Abl and induces apoptosis in imatinib-resistant chronic myelogenous leukemia cells harboring T315I mutation. Cancer Lett. 2010;290(2):182–91. doi:10.1016/j.canlet.2009.09.006. PubMed PMID: 19819619.

[144] Huang KJ, Chen YC, El-Shazly M, Du YC, Su JH, Tsao CW, et al. 5-Episinuleptolide acetate, a norcembranoidal diterpene from the formosan soft coral *Sinularia* sp., induces leukemia cell apoptosis through Hsp90 inhibition. Molecules. 2013;18(3):2924–33. doi:10.3390/molecules18032924. PubMed PMID: 23459302.

[145] Huffman J, Gerber R, Du L. Recent advancements in the biosynthetic mechanisms for polyketide-derived mycotoxins. Biopolymers. 2010;93(9):764–76. doi:10.1002/bip.21483. PubMed PMID: 20578001; PubMed Central PMCID: PMCPMC2894268.

[146] Chen XW, Li CW, Cui CB, Hua W, Zhu TJ, Gu QQ. Nine new and five known polyketides derived from a deep sea-sourced *Aspergillus* sp. 16–02–1. Mar Drugs. 2014;12(6):3116–37. doi:10.3390/md12063116. PubMed PMID: 24871461; PubMed Central PMCID: PMCPMC4071568.

[147] Stachel SJ, Lee CB, Spassova M, Chappell MD, Bornmann WG, Danishefsky SJ, et al. On the interactivity of complex synthesis and tumor pharmacology in the drug discovery process: total synthesis and comparative in vivo evaluations of the 15-aza epothilones. J Org Chem. 2001;66(12):4369–78. PubMed PMID: 11397179.

[148] Nimmanapalli R, O'Bryan E, Bhalla K. Geldanamycin and its analogue 17-allylamino-17-demethoxygeldanamycin lowers Bcr-Abl levels and induces apoptosis and differentiation of Bcr-Abl-positive human leukemic blasts. Cancer Res. 2001;61(5):1799–804. PubMed PMID: 11280726.

[149] Harms H, Orlikova B, Ji S, Nesaei-Mosaferan D, Konig GM, Diederich M. Epipolythiodiketopiperazines from the marine derived Fungus *Dichotomomyces cejpii* with NF-kappaB inhibitory potential. Mar Drugs. 2015;13(8):4949–66. doi:10.3390/md13084949. PubMed PMID: 26258781; PubMed Central PMCID: PMCPMC4557009.

[150] Hou J, Liu P, Qu H, Fu P, Wang Y, Wang Z, et al. Gilvocarcin HE: a new polyketide glycoside from *Streptomyces* sp. J Antibiot (Tokyo). 2012;65(10):523–6. doi:10.1038/ja.2012.61. PubMed PMID: 22854339.

[151] Morceau F, Buck I, Dicato M, Diederich M. Radicicol-mediated inhibition of Bcr-Abl in K562 cells induced p38-MAPK dependent erythroid differentiation and PU.1 down-regulation. Biofactors. 2008;34(4):313–29. doi:10.3233/BIO-2009-1085. PubMed PMID: 19850986.

[152] Scherlach K, Partida-Martinez LP, Dahse HM, Hertweck C. Antimitotic rhizoxin derivatives from a cultured bacterial endosymbiont of the rice pathogenic fungus *Rhizopus microsporus*. J Am Chem Soc. 2006;128(35):11529–36. doi:10.1021/ja062953o. PubMed PMID: 16939276.

[153] Ben-Califa N, Bishara A, Kashman Y, Neumann D. Salarin C, a member of the salarin superfamily of marine compounds, is a potent inducer of apoptosis. Invest New Drugs. 2012;30(1):98–104. doi:10.1007/s10637-010-9521-4. PubMed PMID: 20734109.

[154] Bishara A, Rudi A, Goldberg I, Aknin M, Neumann D, Ben-Califa N, et al. Tausalarin C: a new bioactive marine sponge-derived nitrogenous bismacrolide. Org Lett. 2009;11(16):3538–41. doi:10.1021/ol9011019. PubMed PMID: 19627102.

[155] Ferreira EA, Reigada JB, Correia MV, Young MC, Guimaraes EF, Franchi GC, Jr., et al. Antifungal and cytotoxic 2-acylcyclohexane-1,3-diones from *Peperomia alata* and *P. trineura*. J Nat Prod. 2014;77(6):1377–82. doi:10.1021/np500130x. PubMed PMID: 24905499.

[156] Adlercreutz H. Lignans and human health. Crit Rev Clin Lab Sci. 2007;44(5–6):483–525. doi:10.1080/10408360701612942. PubMed PMID: 17943494.

[157] Wang L, Zhao F, Liu K. Induction of apoptosis of the human leukemia cells by arctigenin and its mechanism of action. Yao Xue Xue Bao. 2008;43(5):542–7. PubMed PMID: 18717345.

[158] Pradheepkumar CP, Panneerselvam N, Shanmugam G. Cleistanthin A causes DNA strand breaks and induces apoptosis in cultured cells. Mutat Res. 2000;464(2):185–93. PubMed PMID: 10648905.

[159] Wang TX, Shi XY, Cong Y, Wang SG, Wang YY, Zhang ZQ. Reversal of multidrug resistance by 5,5′-dimethoxylariciresinol-4-O-beta-D-glucoside in doxorubicin-resistant human leukemia K562/DOX. Indian J Pharmacol. 2013;45(6):597–602. doi:10.4103/0253-7613.121371. PubMed PMID: 24347768; PubMed Central PMCID: PMCPMC3847250.

[160] Luo Y, Xu Y, Chen L, Luo H, Peng C, Fu J, et al. Preparative purification of anti-tumor derivatives of honokiol by high-speed counter-current chromatography. J Chromatogr A. 2008;1178(1–2):160–5. doi:10.1016/j.chroma.2007.11.072. PubMed PMID: 18082756.

[161] Luo J, Kong W, Yang M. HJC, a new arylnaphthalene lignan isolated from Justicia procumbens, causes apoptosis and caspase activation in K562 leukemia cells. J Pharmacol Sci. 2014;125(4):355–63. PubMed PMID: 25141923.

[162] Yang BH, Zhang WD, Liu RH, Li TZ, Zhang C, Zhou Y, et al. Lignans from bark of *Larix olgensis* var. koreana. J Nat Prod. 2005;68(8):1175–9. doi:10.1021/np058022s. PubMed PMID: 16124756.

[163] Youn UJ, Chen QC, Jin WY, Lee IS, Kim HJ, Lee JP, et al. Cytotoxic lignans from the stem bark of *Magnolia officinalis*. J Nat Prod. 2007;70(10):1687–9. doi:10.1021/np070388c. PubMed PMID: 17918910.

[164] Guclu-Ustundag O, Mazza G. Saponins: properties, applications and processing. Crit Rev Food Sci Nutr. 2007;47(3):231–58. doi:10.1080/10408390600698197. PubMed PMID: 17453922.

[165] Podolak I, Galanty A, Sobolewska D. Saponins as cytotoxic agents: a review. Phytochem Rev. 2010;9(3):425–74. doi:10.1007/s11101-010-9183-z. PubMed PMID: 20835386; PubMed Central PMCID: PMCPMC2928447.

[166] Nguyen VT, Darbour N, Bayet C, Doreau A, Raad I, Phung BH, et al. Selective modulation of P-glycoprotein activity by steroidal saponines from *Paris polyphylla*. Fitoterapia. 2009;80(1):39–42. doi:10.1016/j.fitote.2008.09.010. PubMed PMID: 18940238.

[167] Zhou Y, Yang J, Peng L, Li Y, Chen W. Two novel saponins of 20, 26-epoxy derivatives of pseudojujubogenin from the seeds of *Hovenia trichocarpa*. Fitoterapia. 2013;87:65–8. doi:10.1016/j.fitote.2013.03.014. PubMed PMID: 23529014.

[168] Lu YN, Cui P, Tian XQ, Lou LG, Fan CQ. Unusual cytotoxic steroidal saponins from the gorgonian *Astrogorgia dumbea*. Planta Med. 2016;82(9–10):882–7. doi:10.1055/s-0042-106168. PubMed PMID: 27352300.

[169] Shen P, Wang SL, Liu XK, Yang CR, Cai B, Yao XS. Steroidal saponins from rhizomes of *Tupistra wattii* Hook. f. Chem Pharm Bull (Tokyo). 2003;51(3):305–8. PubMed PMID: 12612416.

[170] Ye B, Yang J, Li J, Niu T, Wang S. In vitro and in vivo antitumor activities of tenacissoside C from *Marsdenia tenacissima*. Planta Med. 2014;80(1):29–38. doi:10.1055/s-0033-1360128. PubMed PMID: 24338554.

[171] Huang LJ, Wang B, Zhang JX, Yan C, Mu SZ, Hao XJ. Studies on cytotoxic pregnane sapogenins from *Cynanchum wilfordii*. Fitoterapia. 2015;101:107–16. doi:10.1016/j.fitote.2014.10.014. PubMed PMID: 25451793.

[172] Fan Y, Guo DY, Song Q, Li T. Effect of total saponin of aralia taibaiensis on proliferation of leukemia cells. Zhong Yao Cai. 2013;36(4):604–7. PubMed PMID: 24134011.

[173] Chow LM, Chui CH, Tang JC, Teo IT, Lau FY, Cheng GY, et al. *Gleditsia sinensis* fruit extract is a potential chemotherapeutic agent in chronic and acute myelogenous leukemia. Oncol Rep. 2003;10(5):1601–7. PubMed PMID: 12883747.

[174] Liu M, Zhao X, Xiao L, Liu G, Liu H, Wang X, et al. Cytotoxicity of the compounds isolated from *Pulsatilla chinensis* saponins and apoptosis induced by 23-hydroxybetulinic acid. Pharm Biol. 2015;53(1):1–9. doi:10.3109/13880209.2014.907323. PubMed PMID: 25026337.

[175] Song J, Jeon JE, Won TH, Sim CJ, Oh DC, Oh KB, et al. New cyclic cystine bridged peptides from the sponge *Suberites waedoensis*. Mar Drugs. 2014;12(5):2760–70. doi:10.3390/md12052760. PubMed PMID: 24824023; PubMed Central PMCID: PMCPMC4052314.

[176] Woo JK, Jeon JE, Kim CK, Sim CJ, Oh DC, Oh KB, et al. Gombamide A, a cyclic thiopeptide from the sponge *Clathria gombawuiensis*. J Nat Prod. 2013;76(7):1380–3. doi:10.1021/np4003367. PubMed PMID: 23799303.

[177] Li GY, Liu JZ, Zhang B, Yang M, Chen SG, Hou M, et al. Tegillarca granosa extract Haishengsu (HSS) suppresses expression of mdr1, BCR/ABL and sorcin in drug-resistant K562/ADM tumors in mice. Adv Med Sci. 2013;58(1):112–7. doi:10.2478/v10039-012-0069-8. PubMed PMID: 23729583.

[178] Li GY, Liu JZ, Chen SG, Zhang B, Wang CB, Wang LX. *Tegillarca granosa* extract Haishengsu inhibits the expression of P-glycoprotein and induces apoptosis in drug-resistant K562/ADM cells. Pharm Biol. 2010;48(5):529–33. doi:10.3109/13880200903176620. PubMed PMID: 20645795.

[179] Li GY, Liu JZ, Yu XM, Chen SF, Zhang B, Zhang WF, et al. Effect of a seashell protein Haishengsu on cell growth and expression of apoptosis genes in leukemia K562 cells. Clin Invest Med. 2008;31(4):E218–21. PubMed PMID: 18682046.

[180] Lee HS, Rho JR, Sim CJ, Shin J. New acetylenic acids from a sponge of the genus Stelletta. J Nat Prod. 2003;66(4):566–8. doi:10.1021/np020345q. PubMed PMID: 12713419.

[181] Peng K, Mei WL, Zhao YX, Tan LH, Wang QH, Dai HF. A novel degraded sesquiterpene from the fresh stem of *Aquilaria sinensis*. J Asian Nat Prod Res. 2011;13(10):951–5. doi:10.1080/10286020.2011.598860. PubMed PMID: 21972811.

[182] Sreekanth D, Arunasree MK, Roy KR, Chandramohan Reddy T, Reddy GV, Reddanna P. Betanin a betacyanin pigment purified from fruits of *Opuntia ficus*-indica induces apoptosis in human chronic myeloid leukemia Cell line-K562. Phytomedicine. 2007;14 (11):739–46. doi:10.1016/j.phymed.2007.03.017. PubMed PMID: 17482444.

[183] Xu R, Xie HQ, Deng LL, Zhang JX, Yang FM, Liu JH, et al. A new bufadienolide with cytotoxic activity from the Chinese traditional drug Ch'an Su. Chin J Nat Med. 2014;12 (8):623–7. doi:10.1016/S1875-5364(14)60095-9. PubMed PMID: 25156289.

[184] Jiang HY, Wang CF, Fan L, Yang K, Feng JB, Geng ZF, et al. Cytotoxic constituents from the stems of *Clausena lansium* (Lour.) Skeels. Molecules. 2013;18(9):10768–75. doi:10.3390/molecules180910768. PubMed PMID: 24005969.

[185] Dai HF, Gan YJ, Que DM, Wu J, Wen ZC, Mei WL. Two new cytotoxic cardenolides from the latex of *Antiaris toxicaria*. J Asian Nat Prod Res. 2009;11(9):832–7. doi:10.1080/10286020903164285. PubMed PMID: 20183332.

[186] Thanh PN, Jin W, Song G, Bae K, Kang SS. Cytotoxic coumarins from the root of *Angelica dahurica*. Arch Pharm Res. 2004;27(12):1211–5. PubMed PMID: 15646793.

[187] Reyes-Chilpa R, Estrada-Muniz E, Apan TR, Amekraz B, Aumelas A, Jankowski CK, et al. Cytotoxic effects of mammea type coumarins from *Calophyllum brasiliense*. Life Sci. 2004;75(13):1635–47. doi:10.1016/j.lfs.2004.03.017. PubMed PMID: 15261767.

[188] Gomez-Verjan JC, Estrella-Parra EA, Gonzalez-Sanchez I, Vazquez-Martinez ER, Vergara-Castaneda E, Cerbon MA, et al. Molecular mechanisms involved in the cytotoxicity induced by coumarins from *Calophyllum brasiliense* in K562 leukaemia cells. J Pharm Pharmacol. 2014;66(8):1189–95. doi:10.1111/jphp.12245. PubMed PMID: 24673519.

[189] Ge YQ, Cheng RB, Yang B, Huang Z, Chen Z. Effect of cryptotanshinone on imatinib sensitivity and P-glycoprotein expression of chronic myeloid leukemia cells. Zhongguo Zhong Yao Za Zhi. 2015;40(12):2389–95. PubMed PMID: 26591531.

[190] Ge Y, Yang B, Xu X, Dai Q, Chen Z, Cheng R. Cryptotanshinone acts synergistically with imatinib to induce apoptosis of human chronic myeloid leukemia cells. Leuk Lymphoma. 2015;56(3):730–8. doi:10.3109/10428194.2014.928934. PubMed PMID: 24884318.

[191] Wang HM, Zhang L, Liu J, Yang ZL, Zhao HY, Yang Y, et al. Synthesis and anti-cancer activity evaluation of novel prenylated and geranylated chalcone natural products and their analogs. Eur J Med Chem. 2015;92:439–48. doi:10.1016/j.ejmech.2015.01.007. PubMed PMID: 25590864.

[192] Chen G, Cui CB, Qi AD, Li CW, Tao ZW, Ren R. Polyanthumin, a novel cyclobutane chalcone trimmer from *Memecylon polyanthum*. J Asian Nat Prod Res. 2015;17(2):170–7. doi:10.1080/10286020.2014.945439. PubMed PMID: 25434469.

[193] Rajalekshmi DS, Kabeer FA, Madhusoodhanan AR, Bahulayan AK, Prathapan R, Prakasan N, et al. Anticancer activity studies of cubebin isolated from *Piper cubeba* and its synthetic derivatives. Bioorg Med Chem Lett. 2016;26(7):1767–71. doi:10.1016/j.bmcl.2016.02.041. PubMed PMID: 26916436.

[194] Huang YC, Guh JH, Teng CM. Denbinobin-mediated anticancer effect in human K562 leukemia cells: role in tubulin polymerization and Bcr-Abl activity. J Biomed Sci. 2005;12(1):113–21. doi:10.1007/s11373-004-8171-y. PubMed PMID: 15864744.

[195] Bhouri W, Skandrani I, Sghair MB, Franca MG, Ghedira K, Ghedira LC. Digallic acid from *Pistascia lentiscus* fruits induces apoptosis and enhances antioxidant activities. Phytother Res. 2012;26(3):387–91. doi:10.1002/ptr.3540. PubMed PMID: 21780210.

[196] Chen Y, Li Y, Qing C, Zhang Y, Wang L, Liu Y. 1,4,5-Trihydroxy-7-methoxy-9H-fluoren-9-one, a new cytotoxic compound from *Dendrobium chrysotoxum*. Food Chem. 2008;108(3):973–6. doi:10.1016/j.foodchem.2007.12.007. PubMed PMID: 26065760.

[197] Liao B, Ge RY, Chen X, Huangfu ZP, Qi Y, Song YP, et al. Synergistic reversal effect of Chinese medicine compound FFJZ combined with cyclosporine A on multidrug resistance of leukemia K562/VCR cell line. Zhongguo Shi Yan Xue Ye Xue Za Zhi. 2007;15(4):752–5. PubMed PMID: 17708797.

[198] Wang KW, Ju XY, Zhang L, Wang W, Shen LQ. A novel C27-steroidal glycoside sulfate from *Liriope graminifolia*. Yao Xue Xue Bao. 2012;47(5):619–23. PubMed PMID: 22812006.

[199] Trifunovic S, Vajs V, Juranic Z, Zizak Z, Tesevic V, Macura S, et al. Cytotoxic constituents of *Achillea clavennae* from Montenegro. Phytochemistry. 2006;67(9):887–93. doi:10.1016/j.phytochem.2006.02.026. PubMed PMID: 16616262.

[200] Lv C, Yan X, Tu Q, Di Y, Yuan C, Fang X, et al. Isolation and asymmetric total synthesis of perforanoid A. Angew Chem Int Ed Engl. 2016;55(26):7539–43. doi:10.1002/anie.201602783. PubMed PMID: 27167098.

[201] Aburai N, Esumi Y, Koshino H, Nishizawa N, Kimura K. Inhibitory activity of linoleic acid isolated from proso and Japanese millet toward histone deacetylase. Biosci Biotechnol Biochem. 2007;71(8):2061–4. doi:10.1271/bbb.70068. PubMed PMID: 17690455.

[202] Taher M, Susanti D, Rezali MF, Zohri FS, Ichwan SJ, Alkhamaiseh SI, et al. Apoptosis, antimicrobial and antioxidant activities of phytochemicals from *Garcinia malaccensis* Hk. f. Asian Pac J Trop Med. 2012;5(2):136–41. doi:10.1016/S1995-7645(12)60012-1. PubMed PMID: 22221758.

[203] Chen JJ, Long ZJ, Xu DF, Xiao RZ, Liu LL, Xu ZF, et al. Inhibition of autophagy augments the anticancer activity of alpha-mangostin in chronic myeloid leukemia cells. Leuk Lymphoma. 2014;55(3):628–38. doi:10.3109/10428194.2013.802312. PubMed PMID: 23734655.

[204] Mei WL, Han Z, Cui HB, Zhao YX, Deng YY, Dai HF. A new cytotoxic iridoid from *Callicarpa nudiflora*. Nat Prod Res. 2010;24(10):899–904. doi:10.1080/14786410802267544. PubMed PMID: 19753502.

[205] Yi J, Chen J, Sun J, Wei H, Shi J. Effect of parthenolide on leukemia K562 cells and its leukemia stem cells. Zhongguo Zhong Yao Za Zhi. 2010;35(2):219–22. PubMed PMID: 20394299.

[206] Sanchez-Torres LE, Torres-Martinez JA, Godinez-Victoria M, Omar JM, Velasco-Bejarano B. Perezone and its isomer isoperezone induce caspase-dependent and caspase-independent cell death. Phytomedicine. 2010;17(8–9):614–20. doi:10.1016/j.phymed.2009.12.011. PubMed PMID: 20089388.

[207] Elsebai MF, Ghabbour HA, Mehiri M. Unusual nitrogenous phenalenone derivatives from the marine-derived fungus *Coniothyrium cereale*. Molecules. 2016;21(2):178. doi:10.3390/molecules21020178. PubMed PMID: 26840293.

[208] Wu L, Li Q, Liu Y. Polyphyllin D induces apoptosis in K562/A02 cells through G2/M phase arrest. J Pharm Pharmacol. 2014;66(5):713–21. doi:10.1111/jphp.12188. PubMed PMID: 24325805.

[209] Joseph MM, Aravind SR, Varghese S, Mini S, Sreelekha TT. Evaluation of antioxidant, antitumor and immunomodulatory properties of polysaccharide isolated from fruit rind of *Punica granatum*. Mol Med Rep. 2012;5(2):489–96. doi:10.3892/mmr.2011.638. PubMed PMID: 22012001.

[210] Ji M, Shi Y, Lou H. Overcoming of P-glycoprotein-mediated multidrug resistance in K562/A02 cells using riccardin F and pakyonol, bisbibenzyl derivatives from liverworts. Biosci Trends. 2011;5(5):192–7. PubMed PMID: 22101374.

[211] Guo DX, Xiang F, Wang XN, Yuan HQ, Xi GM, Wang YY, et al. Labdane diterpenoids and highly methoxylated bibenzyls from the liverwort *Frullania inouei*. Phytochemistry. 2010;71(13):1573–8. doi:10.1016/j.phytochem.2010.05.023. PubMed PMID: 20561 654.

[212] Yan YX, Sun Y, Chen JC, Wang YY, Li Y, Qiu MH. Cytotoxic steroids from *Sarcococca saligna*. Planta Med. 2011;77(15):1725–9. doi:10.1055/s-0030-1271101. PubMed PMID: 21590651.

[213] Lu MC, Yang SH, Hwang SL, Lu YJ, Lin YH, Wang SR, et al. Induction of G2/M phase arrest by squamocin in chronic myeloid leukemia (K562) cells. Life Sci. 2006;78(20):2378–83. doi:10.1016/j.lfs.2005.09.048. PubMed PMID: 16310807.

[214] Tseng WR, Huang CY, Tsai YY, Lin YS, Hwang TL, Su JH, et al. New cytotoxic and anti–inflammatory steroids from the soft coral *Klyxum flaccidum*. Bioorg Med Chem Lett. 2016;26(14):3253–7. doi:10.1016/j.bmcl.2016.05.060. PubMed PMID: 27256910.

[215] Kim CK, Song IH, Park HY, Lee YJ, Lee HS, Sim CJ, et al. Suvanine sesterterpenes and deacyl irciniasulfonic acids from a tropical *Coscinoderma* sp. sponge. J Nat Prod. 2014;77(6):1396–403. doi:10.1021/np500156n. PubMed PMID: 24828374.

[216] Ji M, Choi J, Lee J, Lee Y. Induction of apoptosis by ar-turmerone on various cell lines. Int J Mol Med. 2004;14(2):253–6. PubMed PMID: 15254774.

[217] Woo JK, Kim CK, Ahn CH, Oh DC, Oh KB, Shin J. Additional sesterterpenes and a nortriterpene saponin from the sponge *Clathria gombawuiensis*. J Nat Prod. 2015;78 (2):218–24. doi:10.1021/np500753q. PubMed PMID: 25634623.

[218] Dai HF, Gan YJ, Que DM, Wu J, Wen ZC, Mei WL. A new cytotoxic 19-nor-cardenolide from the latex of *Antiaris toxicaria*. Molecules. 2009;14(9):3694–9. doi:10.3390/molecules14093694. PubMed PMID: 19783952.

[219] Chen F, Liu Y, Wang S, Guo X, Shi P, Wang W, et al. Triptolide, a Chinese herbal extract, enhances drug sensitivity of resistant myeloid leukemia cell lines through downregulation of HIF-1alpha and Nrf2. Pharmacogenomics. 2013;14(11):1305–17. doi:10.2217/pgs.13.122. PubMed PMID: 23930677.

[220] Ghoneim MM, Ma G, El-Hela AA, Mohammad AE, Kottob S, El-Ghaly S, et al. Biologically active secondary metabolites from *Asphodelus microcarpus*. Nat Prod Commun. 2013;8(8):1117–9. PubMed PMID: 24079182.

[221] Pan Y, Wang X, Hu X. Cytotoxic withanolides from the flowers of *Datura metel*. J Nat Prod. 2007;70(7):1127–32. doi:10.1021/np070096b. PubMed PMID: 17583953.

[222] Liu MJ, Wang Z, Li HX, Wu RC, Liu YZ, Wu QY. Mitochondrial dysfunction as an early event in the process of apoptosis induced by woodfordin I in human leukemia K562 cells. Toxicol Appl Pharmacol. 2004;194(2):141–55. PubMed PMID: 14736495.

[223] Han QB, Wang YL, Yang L, Tso TF, Qiao CF, Song JZ, et al. Cytotoxic polyprenylated xanthones from the resin of *Garcinia hanburyi*. Chem Pharm Bull (Tokyo). 2006;54 (2):265–7. PubMed PMID: 16462081.

[224] Han QB, Xiang W, Li RT, Li ML, Li SW, Sun HD. Cytotoxic ent-kaurane diterpenoids from *Isodon rubescens* var. rubescens. Planta Med. 2004;70(3):269–72. doi:10.1055/s-2004-818922. PubMed PMID: 15114509.

[225] Chen XQ, Li Y, Li KZ, Peng LY, He J, Wang K, et al. Spirocyclic acylphloroglucinol derivatives from *Hypericum beanii*. Chem Pharm Bull (Tokyo). 2011;59(10):1250–3. PubMed PMID: 21963634.

[226] Umebayashi C, Yamamoto N, Nakao H, Toi Y, Chikahisa-Muramatsu L, Kanemaru K, et al. Flow cytometric estimation of cytotoxic activity of rhodexin A isolated from *Rhodea japonica* in human leukemia K562 cells. Biol Pharm Bull. 2003;26(5):627–30. PubMed PMID: 12736502.

[227] Anuchapreeda S, Thanarattanakorn P, Sittipreechacharn S, Chanarat P, Limtrakul P. Curcumin inhibits WT1 gene expression in human leukemic K562 cells. Acta Pharmacol Sin. 2006;27(3):360–6. doi:10.1111/j.1745-7254.2006.00291.x. PubMed PMID: 16490174.

[228] Giommarelli C, Zuco V, Favini E, Pisano C, Dal Piaz F, De Tommasi N, et al. The enhancement of antiproliferative and proapoptotic activity of HDAC inhibitors by curcumin is mediated by Hsp90 inhibition. Cell Mol Life Sci. 2010;67(6):995–1004. doi:10.1007/s00018-009-0233-x. PubMed PMID: 20039095.

[229] Shi X, Chen X, Li X, Lan X, Zhao C, Liu S, et al. Gambogic acid induces apoptosis in imatinib-resistant chronic myeloid leukemia cells via inducing proteasome inhibition and caspase-dependent Bcr-Abl downregulation. Clin Cancer Res. 2014;20(1):151–63. doi:10.1158/1078-0432.CCR-13-1063. PubMed PMID: 24334603; PubMed Central PMCID: PMCPMC3938960.

[230] Zhang L, Yi Y, Chen J, Sun Y, Guo Q, Zheng Z, et al. Gambogic acid inhibits Hsp90 and deregulates TNF-alpha/NF-kappaB in HeLa cells. Biochem Biophys Res Commun. 2010;403(3–4):282–7. doi:10.1016/j.bbrc.2010.11.018. PubMed PMID: 21074517.

[231] Schillaci D, Venturella F, Venuti F, Plescia F. Antimicrobial and antiproliferative activity of *Peucedanum nebrodense* (Guss.) Strohl. J Ethnopharmacol. 2003;87(1):99–101. PubMed PMID: 12787961.

[232] Chang JS, Chiang LC, Hsu FF, Lin CC. Chemoprevention against hepatocellular carcinoma of *Cornus officinalis* in vitro. Am J Chin Med. 2004;32(5):717–25. doi:10.1142/S0192415X04002296. PubMed PMID: 15633807.

[233] Koschek PR, Alviano DS, Alviano CS, Gattass CR. The husk fiber of *Cocos nucifera* L. (Palmae) is a source of anti-neoplastic activity. Braz J Med Biol Res. 2007;40(10):1339–43. PubMed PMID: 17713650.

[234] Mishra KP, Padwad YS, Dutta A, Ganju L, Sairam M, Banerjee PK, et al. Aqueous extract of Rhodiola imbricata rhizome inhibits proliferation of an erythroleukemic cell line K-562 by inducing apoptosis and cell cycle arrest at G2/M phase. Immunobiology. 2008;213(2):125–31. doi:10.1016/j.imbio.2007.07.003. PubMed PMID: 18241696.

[235] Park YK, Do YR, Jang BC. Apoptosis of K562 leukemia cells by Abnobaviscum F(R), a European mistletoe extract. Oncol Rep. 2012;28(6):2227–32. doi:10.3892/or.2012.2026. PubMed PMID: 22972372.

[236] Wang T, Yuan Y, Wang J, Han C, Chen G. Anticancer activities of constituents from the stem of *Polyalthia rumphii*. Pak J Pharm Sci. 2012;25(2):353–6. PubMed PMID: 22459461.

[237] Ravi A, Mallika A, Sama V, Begum AS, Khan RS, Reddy BM. Antiproliferative activity and standardization of *Tecomella undulata* bark extract on K562 cells. J Ethnopharmacol. 2011;137(3):1353–9. doi:10.1016/j.jep.2011.07.067. PubMed PMID: 21843623.

[238] Rizzo LY, Longato GB, Ruiz AL, Tinti SV, Possenti A, Vendramini-Costa DB, et al. In vitro, in vivo and in silico analysis of the anticancer and estrogen-like activity of guava leaf extracts. Curr Med Chem. 2014;21(20):2322–30. PubMed PMID: 24438525.

[239] Tayarani-Najaran Z, Sareban M, Gholami A, Emami SA, Mojarrab M. Cytotoxic and apoptotic effects of different extracts of *Artemisia turanica* Krasch. on K562 and HL-60 cell lines. Sci World J. 2013;2013:628073. doi:10.1155/2013/628073. PubMed PMID: 24288497; PubMed Central PMCID: PMCPMC3830890.

[240] Teh SS, Ee GC, Mah SH, Yong YK, Lim YM, Rahmani M, et al. In vitro cytotoxic, antioxidant, and antimicrobial activities of *Mesua beccariana* (Baill.) Kosterm., *Mesua*

ferrea Linn., and *Mesua congestiflora* extracts. Biomed Res Int. 2013;2013:517072. doi:10.1155/2013/517072. PubMed PMID: 24089682; PubMed Central PMCID: PMCPMC3780478.

[241] Ebrahimnezhad Darzi S, Amirghofran Z. Dichloromethane fraction of *Melissa officinalis* induces apoptosis by activation of intrinsic and extrinsic pathways in human leukemia cell lines. Immunopharmacol Immunotoxicol. 2013;35(3):313–20. doi:10.3109/08923973.2013.768268. PubMed PMID: 23432355.

[242] Jin W, Shi Q, Hong C, Cheng Y, Ma Z, Qu H. Cytotoxic properties of thiophenes from *Echinops grijissi* Hance. Phytomedicine. 2008;15(9):768–74. doi:10.1016/j.phymed.2007.10.007. PubMed PMID: 18068965.

[243] Samet I, Han J, Jlaiel L, Sayadi S, Isoda H. Olive (*Olea europaea*) leaf extract induces apoptosis and monocyte/macrophage differentiation in human chronic myelogenous leukemia K562 cells: insight into the underlying mechanism. Oxid Med Cell Longev. 2014;2014:927619. doi:10.1155/2014/927619. PubMed PMID: 24803988; PubMed Central PMCID: PMCPMC3997986.

[244] Asmaa MJ, Al-Jamal HA, Ang CY, Asan JM, Seeni A, Johan MF. Apoptosis induction in MV4–11 and K562 human leukemic cells by *Pereskia sacharosa* (Cactaceae) leaf crude extract. Asian Pac J Cancer Prev. 2014;15(1):475–81. PubMed PMID: 24528077.

[245] Campos JF, dos Santos UP, Macorini LF, de Melo AM, Balestieri JB, Paredes-Gamero EJ, et al. Antimicrobial, antioxidant and cytotoxic activities of propolis from *Melipona orbignyi* (Hymenoptera, Apidae). Food Chem Toxicol. 2014;65:374–80. doi:10.1016/j.fct.2014.01.008. PubMed PMID: 24412556.

[246] Hwang YJ, Kim J, Park DS, Hwang KA. Study on the immunomodulation effect of *Isodon japonicus* extract via splenocyte function and NK anti-tumor activity. Int J Mol Sci. 2012;13(4):4880–8. doi:10.3390/ijms13044880. PubMed PMID: 22606016; PubMed Central PMCID: PMCPMC3344252.

[247] de FNSD, Yunes RA, Schaab EH, Malheiros A, Cechinel Filho V, Franchi GC, Jr., et al. Evaluation of the anti-proliferative effect the extracts of *Allamanda blanchetti* and *A. schottii* on the growth of leukemic and endothelial cells. J Pharm Pharm Sci. 2006;9(2):200–8. PubMed PMID: 16959189.

[248] Quispe-Mauricio A, Callacondo D, Rojas J, Zavala D, Posso M, Vaisberg A. Cytotoxic effect of physalis peruviana in cell culture of colorectal and prostate cancer and chronic myeloid leukemia. Rev Gastroenterol Peru. 2009;29(3):239–46. PubMed PMID: 19898596.

[249] Sadeghi H, Yazdanparast R. Effect of Dendrostellera lessertii on the intracellular alkaline phosphatase activity of four human cancer cell lines. J Ethnopharmacol. 2003;86(1):11–4. PubMed PMID: 12686435.

[250] Tsolmon S, Han J, Isoda H. Inhibition of cell growth by *Stellera chamaejasme* extract is associated with induction of autophagy and differentiation in chronic leukemia K562

cells. J Biosci Bioeng. 2010;110(2):262–8. doi:10.1016/j.jbiosc.2010.02.006. PubMed PMID: 20547324.

[251] Cheung S, Tai J. Anti-proliferative and antioxidant properties of rosemary *Rosmarinus officinalis*. Oncol Rep. 2007;17(6):1525–31. PubMed PMID: 17487414.

[252] Gao X, Zhang G, Zhou M, Luo D, Li B. Antiproliferative activity of *Goldfussia psilostachys* ethanolic extract on K562 leukemia cells. Fitoterapia. 2004;75(7–8):639–44. doi:10.1016/j.fitote.2004.06.008. PubMed PMID: 15567238.

[253] Castaneda DM, Pombo LM, Uruena CP, Hernandez JF, Fiorentino S. A gallotannin-rich fraction from *Caesalpinia spinosa* (Molina) Kuntze displays cytotoxic activity and raises sensitivity to doxorubicin in a leukemia cell line. BMC Complement Altern Med. 2012;12:38. doi:10.1186/1472-6882-12-38. PubMed PMID: 22490328; PubMed Central PMCID: PMCPMC3353181.

[254] Bigovic D, Savikin K, Jankovic T, Menkovic N, Zdunic G, Stanojkovic T, et al. Antiradical and cytotoxic activity of different *Helichrysum plicatum* flower extracts. Nat Prod Commun. 2011;6(6):819–22. PubMed PMID: 21815418.

[255] Amirghofran Z, Bahmani M, Azadmehr A, Javidnia K. Induction of apoptosis in leukemia cell lines by *Linum persicum* and *Euphorbia cheiradenia*. J Cancer Res Clin Oncol. 2006;132(7):427–32. doi:10.1007/s00432-006-0084-x. PubMed PMID: 16477442.

[256] Amirghofran Z, Bahmani M, Azadmehr A, Javidnia K. Anticancer effects of various Iranian native medicinal plants on human tumor cell lines. Neoplasma. 2006;53(5):428–33. PubMed PMID: 17013538.

[257] Soumaya KJ, Zied G, Nouha N, Mounira K, Kamel G, Genvieve FD, et al. Evaluation of in vitro antioxidant and apoptotic activities of *Cyperus rotundus*. Asian Pac J Trop Med. 2014;7(2):105–12. doi:10.1016/S1995-7645(14)60004-3. PubMed PMID: 24461 522.

[258] Al-Salahi OS, Ji D, Majid AM, Kit-Lam C, Abdullah WZ, Zaki A, et al. Anti-tumor activity of *Eurycoma longifolia* root extracts against K-562 cell line: in vitro and in vivo study. PLoS One. 2014;9(1):e83818. doi:10.1371/journal.pone.0083818. PubMed PMID: 24409284; PubMed Central PMCID: PMCPMC3883656.

[259] Yeap SK, Omar AR, Ho WY, Beh BK, Ali AM, Alitheen NB. *Rhaphidophora korthalsii* modulates peripheral blood natural killer cell proliferation, cytokine secretion and cytotoxicity. BMC Complement Altern Med. 2013;13:145. doi:10.1186/1472-6882-13-145. PubMed PMID: 23800124; PubMed Central PMCID: PMCPMC3701493.

[260] Brito SV, Sales DL, Costa JG, Rodrigues FF, Ferreira FS, Angelico EC, et al. Investigation of the cytocidal potential of *Rhinella jimi* skin methanol extracts. Pharm Biol. 2012;50 (8):1026–30. doi:10.3109/13880209.2012.655858. PubMed PMID: 22775420.

[261] Roscetti G, Franzese O, Comandini A, Bonmassar E. Cytotoxic activity of *Hypericum perforatum* L. on K562 erythroleukemic cells: differential effects between methanolic

extract and hypericin. Phytother Res. 2004;18(1):66–72. doi:10.1002/ptr.1369. PubMed PMID: 14750204.

[262] Matic IZ, Aljancic I, Zizak Z, Vajs V, Jadranin M, Milosavljevic S, et al. In vitro antitumor actions of extracts from endemic plant *Helichrysum zivojinii*. BMC Complement Altern Med. 2013;13:36. doi:10.1186/1472-6882-13-36. PubMed PMID: 23414290; PubMed Central PMCID: PMCPMC3585823.

[263] Aguiar JS, Araujo RO, Rodrigues Mdo D, Sena KX, Batista AM, Guerra MM, et al. Antimicrobial, antiproliferative and proapoptotic activities of extract, fractions and isolated compounds from the stem of Erythroxylum caatingae plowman. Int J Mol Sci. 2012;13(4):4124–40. doi:10.3390/ijms13044124. PubMed PMID: 22605969; PubMed Central PMCID: PMCPMC3344205.

[264] Predes FS, Ruiz AL, Carvalho JE, Foglio MA, Dolder H. Antioxidative and in vitro antiproliferative activity of *Arctium lappa* root extracts. BMC Complement Altern Med. 2011;11:25. doi:10.1186/1472-6882-11-25. PubMed PMID: 21429215; PubMed Central PMCID: PMCPMC3073957.

[265] Fong WF, Wang C, Zhu GY, Leung CH, Yang MS, Cheung HY. Reversal of multidrug resistance in cancer cells by *Rhizoma Alismatis* extract. Phytomedicine. 2007;14(2–3):160–5. doi:10.1016/j.phymed.2006.03.004. PubMed PMID: 16713217.

[266] Kumarappan CT, Mandal SC. Antitumor activity of polyphenolic extract of *Ichnocarpus frutescens*. Exp Oncol. 2007;29(2):94–101. PubMed PMID: 17704739.

[267] Renno MN, Barbosa GM, Zancan P, Veiga VF, Alviano CS, Sola-Penna M, et al. Crude ethanol extract from babassu (*Orbignya speciosa*): cytotoxicity on tumoral and non-tumoral cell lines. An Acad Bras Cienc. 2008;80(3):467–76. PubMed PMID: 18797799.

[268] Lin CC, Ng LT, Hsu FF, Shieh DE, Chiang LC. Cytotoxic effects of *Coptis chinensis* and *Epimedium sagittatum* extracts and their major constituents (berberine, coptisine and icariin) on hepatoma and leukaemia cell growth. Clin Exp Pharmacol Physiol. 2004;31 (1–2):65–9. PubMed PMID: 14756686.

[269] Rossi D, Bruni R, Bianchi N, Chiarabelli C, Gambari R, Medici A, et al. Evaluation of the mutagenic, antimutagenic and antiproliferative potential of *Croton lechleri* (Muell. Arg.) latex. Phytomedicine. 2003;10(2–3):139–44. doi:10.1078/094471103321659843. PubMed PMID: 12725567.

[270] Amirghofran Z, Bahmani M, Azadmehr A, Ashouri E, Javidnia K. Antitumor activity and apoptosis induction in human cancer cell lines by *Dionysia termeana*. Cancer Invest. 2007;25(7):550–4. doi:10.1080/07357900701518487. PubMed PMID: 18027150.

[271] Muller CI, Kumagai T, O'Kelly J, Seeram NP, Heber D, Koeffler HP. Ganoderma lucidum causes apoptosis in leukemia, lymphoma and multiple myeloma cells. Leuk Res. 2006;30 (7):841–8. doi:10.1016/j.leukres.2005.12.004. PubMed PMID: 16423392.

[272] Cheng XD, Hou CH, Zhang XJ, Xie HY, Zhou WY, Yang L, et al. Effects of Huangqi (Hex) on inducing cell differentiation and cell death in K562 and HEL cells. Acta Biochim Biophys Sin (Shanghai). 2004;36(3):211–7. PubMed PMID: 15202506.

[273] da Silva DA, Alves VG, Franco DM, Ribeiro LC, de Souza MC, Kato L, et al. Antiproliferative activity of *Luehea candicans* Mart. et Zucc. (Tiliaceae). Nat Prod Res. 2012;26 (4):364–9. doi:10.1080/14786411003752102. PubMed PMID: 21432719.

[274] Turan N, Akgun-Dar K, Kuruca SE, Kilicaslan-Ayna T, Seyhan VG, Atasever B, et al. Cytotoxic effects of leaf, stem and root extracts of *Nerium oleander* on leukemia cell lines and role of the p-glycoprotein in this effect. J Exp Ther Oncol. 2006;6(1):31–8. PubMed PMID: 17228522.

[275] Wagh V, Mishra P, Thakkar A, Shinde V, Sharma S, Padigaru M, et al. Antitumor activity of NPB001–05, an orally active inhibitor of Bcr-Abl tyrosine kinase. Front Biosci (Elite Ed). 2011;3:1349–64. PubMed PMID: 21622141.

[276] Liu JJ, Huang RW, Lin DJ, Wu XY, Lin Q, Peng J, et al. Antiproliferation effects of ponicidin on human myeloid leukemia cells in vitro. Oncol Rep. 2005;13(4):653–7. PubMed PMID: 15756438.

[277] Zhang XJ, Xu XF, Gao RL, Xu JF. Rubus parvifolius L. inhibited the growth of leukemia K562 cells in vitro and in vivo. Chin J Integr Med. 2014;20(1):36–42. doi:10.1007/s11655-013-1537-0. PubMed PMID: 24242132.

[278] Tayarani-Najaran Z, Mousavi SH, Vahdati-Mashhadian N, Emami SA, Parsaee H. *Scutellaria litwinowii* induces apoptosis through both extrinsic and intrinsic apoptotic pathways in human promyelocytic leukemia cells. Nutr Cancer. 2012;64(1):80–8. doi:10.1080/01635581.2012.630162. PubMed PMID: 22098153.

[279] Roy S, Banerjee B, Vedasiromoni JR. Cytotoxic and apoptogenic effect of *Swietenia mahagoni* (L.) Jacq. leaf extract in human leukemic cell lines U937, K562 and HL-60. Environ Toxicol Pharmacol. 2014;37(1):234–47. doi:10.1016/j.etap.2013.11.008. PubMed PMID: 24366058.

[280] Urech K, Scher JM, Hostanska K, Becker H. Apoptosis inducing activity of viscin, a lipophilic extract from *Viscum album* L. J Pharm Pharmacol. 2005;57(1):101–9. doi:10.1211/0022357055083. PubMed PMID: 15638998.

[281] https://clinicaltrials.gov/ct2/show/NCT00114959?term=chronic+myeloid +leukemia&rank=5.

[282] https://clinicaltrials.gov/ct2/results?term=NCT00100997&cond=%22Chronic+Myeloid +Leukemia%22.

[283] https://clinicaltrials.gov/ct2/show/NCT00003230?term=NCT00003230&rank=1.

6

The Challenging Triad: Microbiota, Immune System and Anticancer Drugs

Andreea Letitia Arsene, Cristina Manuela Dragoi, Alina Crenguta Nicolae, Daniela Elena Popa, George T.A. Burcea-Dragomiroiu, Ion Bogdan Dumitrescu, Olivia Carmen Timnea and Denisa Ioana Udeanu

Abstract

Gut microbiota is essential for the development of the intestinal immune system, protecting the host against pathogens and harmful inflammatory processes. Germ-free animals have smaller Peyer's patches, fewer immune cells and impaired immunoglobulin A (IgA) secretion, fewer intraepithelial lymphocytes, as well as compromised production of antimicrobial peptides. Mucositis (mucosal barrier injury) is a major oncological problem caused by chemotherapeutic agents. Intestinal mucositis translates into a broad spectra of clinical symptoms (diarrhea, vomiting) and can be worsened by neutropenia and antibiotics. Since IECs do not regulate intestinal homeostasis by themselves, but require symbiotic coordination with commensal bacteria and local gut leukocytic cells, the role of intestinal microbiota in the development and severity of mucositis induced by chemotherapeutic products became an issue. The present chapter reviews the interplay between microbiota, immune system, and anticancer therapy. The published researches in this field showed that microbiota has immunomodulatory effect on the anticancer immune response, both in the presence and in the absence of chemotherapy. Animal and human studies evoked that the anticancer response depends on microbiota variability.

Keywords: microbiota, immune system, anticancer therapy, efficacy, toxicity

1. Introduction

The relationship between cancer and microbiota was recognized and challenged since the nineteenth century when William Coley, a surgical oncologist, developed a mixture consisting of killed bacteria of species *Streptococcus pyogenes* and *Serratia marcescens*, also known as "Coley's toxin," as a treatment for cancer.

Ever since, experimental and clinical researchers tried to isolate microbial agents or products to treat malignant disease, such as treatment of superficial bladder cancer based on an attenuated form of *Mycobacterium bovis*, an oncolytic herpes virus for the treatment of melanoma, or the treatment of pancreatic cancer with *Listeria monocytogenes* [1].

The present chapter reviews the interplay between microbiota, immune system, and anticancer therapy. The published researches in this field showed that microbiota has immunomodulatory effect on the anticancer immune response, both in the presence and in the absence of the chemotherapy. Animal and human studies evoked that the anticancer response depends on microbiota variability. In initiating an efficient chemotherapy, the following aspects should be considered:

- The interactions between microbiota and cancer progression.
- The influence of the microbiota on the chemotherapy response.
- The microbiota imbalance influences drugs bioavailability, efficacy and toxicity.

2. Microbiota, health and diseases

Microbiota affects many physiological processes, while its alteration is thought to render a number of pathologies.

The growing evidence regarding the importance of the microbiome for health and disease and the host-microbe symbiosis at the immunological and metabolic levels become highly challenging for a better understanding of immunopathologies such as autoimmune and inflammatory disorders. Microbiome changes were correlated with a variety of diseases such as inflammatory bowel disease, obesity, type 2 diabetes, autism, and allergies.

Crohn's disease (CD) and ulcerative colitis (UC) are the most prevalent forms of inflammatory bowel disease (IBD), characterized by chronic relapsing inflammation affecting the intestinal mucosa. The etiology of these diseases is unknown, but there are increasing scientific evidences that microbiota influences the pathogenesis of IBD [2].

Patients exhibit a decrease in microbial population and functional diversity, with a decrease of *Firmicutes*, an increase in *Bacteroidetes*, and facultative anaerobes such as *Enterobacteriaceae* [3–5].

The intestinal microbiota was also implicated in several other gastrointestinal-related diseases, such as obesity, type 2 diabetes, celiac disease, and colorectal cancer. The last two of these were associated with changes in microbiota composition, but interestingly, no pattern of alteration was demonstrated [6–10]. Recent studies showed that the expression of the leukocyte antigen DQ2 is a strong risk factor for the development of celiac disease. It seemed that children possessing this haplotype also had an altered microbiota composition (compared to non-HLA DQ2 individuals) prior to clinically apparent disease [11].

On the other hand, there is a bidirectional functional relationship between the intestine and the kidneys, the urinary pH influencing the intestinal microbiota metabolism, while microbial-related metabolites are involved in the development of the kidney pathologies [12].

Several studies focused on the possibility that the intestinal microbiota may influence the hypothalamus-pituitary-adrenal (HPA) axis, and, therefore, the cognitive function and behavior. HPA is a pathway activated in response to infection and perturbed by psychological stressors (the "gut-brain axis"). There are publications that evoke a direct relationship between enteric infections on one hand and anxiety, depression, and cognitive dysfunctions, on the other hand [13–16].

3. Microbiota and cancer

Microbial communities inhabiting human body represent so far unknown environmental factors that seem to have a role in carcinogenesis.

Cancer susceptibility, development, and progression result from a complex interplay between gene regulation and the environment.

For decades, the researches on the interaction of the microbes with human organism were focused almost exclusively on the effects of **the single pathogenic microbial infection**.

Several mechanisms regarding the cancer development were described for some microbial species.

The direct carcinogen class usually comprises viruses which may produce cancer by genetic mechanisms [17, 18].

Researches on molecular mechanisms revealed that most of the oncoproteins encoded by human viruses target generally the tumor suppressor proteins: retinoblastoma RB1 and p53, which play major roles in cellular anticancer protection.

Other targets reported for carcinogenesis induce by viruses involved interaction with complex pathways of interferon signaling, transcription factors like nuclear factor-κB (NF-κB), telomerase complex, or cell adhesion molecules.

The Epstein-Barr virus (EBV), hepatitis C virus, and human papilloma virus are only a few examples of the most studied oncogenic viruses.

The Epstein-Barr virus (EBV) or human herpes virus 4 (HHV-4) is one of the most common viruses in humans and also the first discovered to be involved in tumorigenesis. The EBV infects immune system cells (lymphocyte B) and epithelial cells, and the infections were correlated with some lymphoma, gastric cancer, anogenital and oropharyngeal carcinomas and with certain autoimmune diseases [19].

Hepatitis C virus is one of the major etiologic agents of hepatocellular carcinoma [20]. Researches on HCV-specific proteins revealed that they exert multiple functions during the life cycle of the virus. Due to their ability to adopt different structural conformations, the viral proteins are capable of various interactions with cellular proteins interfering in signaling pathways essential to cell functions. HCV causes genome instability suggesting that cooperation of both viral and host factors plays a role in developing the disease [21, 22].

Human papillomavirus (HPV) belongs to the DNA class viruses and is capable to infect keratinocytes of the skin and the mucosa. There are over 170 types of HPV described, and about dozen types are considered high-risk human carcinogen producing at least six types of cancer: cervix, penis, vulva, vagina, anus, and oropharynx [23].

The E6 and E7 genes of HPV have been identified as oncogenes involved in promoting tumor growth and transformation to malignancy. The E6 protein is involved in ubiquitination of p53, marking this protein for proteasomal degradation, while the protein E7 is involved in competing the retinoblastoma protein for binding and favors the cell cycle to continue.

The E6 and E7 deregulate the host innate immune defense required for the recruitment of the effector immune cells. Both proteins cooperate for the downregulation of the proinflammatory interleukins: IL-18 and IL-8 and of some chemoattractants like MCP-1 and MIP3α. Also, proteins E6 and E7 interfere in the intracellular signaling pathways NF-κB and interferon regulatory factors inhibiting the activation of these major antiviral transcription factors [24].

Although molecular mechanism of cancerogenesis has been explained for some pathogenic viruses, it is too simplistic to consider these microbes the only cause of tumorigenesis. Cancer is a complex multistep process which evolves over time and involves many signaling pathways and molecular interactions to generate a particular cellular phenotype.

Indirect carcinogen mechanisms comprise the injury of the epithelial barrier or inflammation associated to some infections produced by bacterial species like *Helicobacter pylori* or *Chlamydia trachomatis*.

Helicobacter pylori is a gram-negative pathogen which infects about half of humans all over the world and represents the main cause for gastric cancer. The *H. pylori* virulence factors, vacuolating cytotoxin (VacA) and CagA protein encoded by cytotoxin-associated gene-pathogenicity island, are identified as major antigens. These microbial proteins interact with several host receptors like toll-like receptor 2 (TLR2), NOD-like receptor family member NLRP3, and caspase-1 promoting the activation of the inflammasome.

The host cellular dysfunctions on secretory system, apoptosis, and immune inhibition were other mechanisms described as consequences of the *H. pylori* infection [25].

Chlamydia trachomatis infects both men and women, but it is commonly found in the reproductive system of women. The chronic infection causes pelvic inflammation with severe consequences like infertility. The incidence of infections is significant among patients with cervical cancer, but no proof exists to demonstrate that *Chlamydia* itself promotes cancer. Research proved that a common association with HPV favors cancer growth. Further studies in this direction are necessary for confirmation.

Other experiments indicate a correlation between some commensals, the production of oxygen-reactive species, and colon cancer. Thus, superoxide-producing *Enterococcus faecalis* was demonstrated to cause colonic epithelial cell DNA damage [26].

Recent years' researches focused on obesity as a risk factor for different types of cancer. Gut microbiota plays an important role in developing obesity. Some *Clostridium* spp. are microorganisms overrepresented in obese intestine and were directly correlated with liver and colorectal cancers. These commensals convert primary bile acids into deoxycholic acid (DCA), a carcinogen that can cause DNA damage via the production of free radicals [27].

For a long time, scientific research describes many other potential microorganisms involved in cancer promoting, but several questions about the main cause of tumorigenesis were raised because of a low incidence of cancer among infected patients with susceptible agents.

Recent researches have changed the perspective on many human diseases. Many scientific publications in the last years sustain the fact that global changes in our microbiome are the main causes of disease and not only a single opportunistic pathogen development.

Increased communities of *Capnocytophaga gingivalis, Capnocytophaga ochracea, Eubacterium sabureum, Leptotrichia buccalis,* and *Streptococcus mitis* present in saliva were observed in patients with oral squamous cell carcinoma.

Human esophageal cancer was associated in some cases with an increased presence of *Streptococcus anginosus, Streptococcus mitis, Treponema denticola,* or some *Campylobacter spp.*

Salmonella typhi and *S. paratyphi* were increased in some bile samples collected from patients with gall bladder cancer.

Colorectal cancer is one of the most studied regarding the microbial imbalance and molecular mechanisms of the disease.

Cohort studies demonstrated that samples collected from patients with colon cancer presented feces bacterial diversity with increased communities of pro-inflammatory species of *Fusobacterium* and *Porphyromonas* and a decreased presence of *Lactobacillus, Microbacterium, Anoxybacillus,* and *Akkermansia muciniphila.*

In colon cancer cases induced by a preexisting inflammatory colitis, microbiota played an important role in influencing inflammation or innate immunity, genomic stability of intestinal epithelial cells (IECs), or the release of some metabolites functioning as histone deacetylase inhibitors. Studies performed in gnotobiotic or in antibiotic-treated mice revealed the implication of microbes in tumorigenesis driven or not by inflammation.

4. Microbiota and immune functions

In the last years, many scientific studies demonstrated that the commensal is an important participant to the host metabolism, inflammatory process, and immune response.

Nowadays, gut microbiota is particularly the most studied, and it has been proven to be essential for the development of the intestinal immune system, protecting the host against pathogens and harmful inflammatory processes. Germ-free animals have smaller Peyer's patches, fewer immune cells and impaired immunoglobulin A (IgA) secretion, fewer intraepithelial lymphocytes, as well as compromised production of antimicrobial peptides [28–30].

Gut microbiota is involved in the immune responses and inflammatory processes both local and systemic. The link between inflammation and cancer is well known raising the questions about the potential interference of microbiota. This area of research is new, and astonishing recent results revealed that microbiota is a key player in the immunomodulatory mechanisms of cancer and impact of the therapeutic responsiveness [31–35].

The present knowledge sustains that the presence and the quality of gut microbiota may induce inflammation and promote cancer or may induce tumor-destructive immune responses and favor anticancer treatment. Most studies involved experimental animal model of transplantable tumors, and only few data are sustained by clinical evidence.

The inflammation induced by microbiota may contribute to cancer by stimulating the release of cytokines involved in the cell proliferation and apoptosis inhibition pathways.

In a study regarding a hepatocellular carcinoma mouse model, the intestinal microbiota was essential for the promotion and initiation of cancer by signaling pathways involving toll-like receptor 4 (TLR4), a surface immune cell receptor, which senses the microbial molecular patterns. The activation of this receptor induced an increased level of a hepatomitogen, which mediates the proliferative and antiapoptotic effects in tumors [36].

The beneficial immunomodulatory effect in cancer regression is supported by the use of some microbial in anticancer therapy. The intravesical *bacillus Calmette-Guerin* (BCG) therapy is one of the standard methods of management of intermediate- and high-risk non-muscle invasive bladder cancer. Also, intratumoral inoculation of heat-killed *Propionibacterium acnes* in subcutaneous melanoma promotes local and systemic Th1 and Tc1 responses associated with tumor regression.

More other evidences are presented and discussed by the scientific literature about the key role of microbiota and the possibility to modulate it. However, the specific mechanisms are far to be elucidated due to the complex composition and the multifactorial interaction between gene and environment.

5. Microbiota and chemotherapy

The intestinal epithelium is a single-cell layer, which functions as the largest barrier of the human body. It is characterized by a selective permeability for the nutrients, electrolytes, and water and has an effective role in defense against toxins and enteric microbiota. Intestinal epithelial cells maintain the local environmental balance by facilitating the interaction between commensal and the host immune cells [37].

In order to obtain the best anticancer drug bioavailability, the formulation must consider besides the physicochemical properties or drug adjuvants, the permeability of the intestinal barrier.

Mucositis (mucosal barrier injury) is a major oncological problem caused by chemotherapeutic agents. Intestinal mucositis translates into a broad spectra of clinical symptoms (diarrhea, vomiting) and can be worsened by neutropenia and antibiotics. Since IECs do not regulate intestinal homeostasis by themselves, but require symbiotic coordination with commensal bacteria and local gut leukocytic cells, the role of intestinal microbiota in the development and severity of mucositis induced by chemotherapeutic products became an issue [38].

5.1. Cyclophosphamide (CTX)

Cyclophosphamide (CTX) is an alkylating agent commonly used in combination with other therapies to target cancer cells.

The importance of gut microbiota in efficacy of the treatment is sustained by studies involving germ-free (GF) mice and specific-pathogen-free (SPF) mice with transplantable MCA205 sarcomas. A significant decrease effect of the CTX treatment was obtained in case of GF animals in comparison with SPF mice [22].

Similar effects comparing to untreated control groups were obtained in case of the animal treatment with vancomycin A, an antibiotic that destroys the gram-positive bacteria. The results indicate that the presence of some bacteria creates an immunologic local environment essential for the therapeutic effect of CTX [39].

5.2. CpG oligodeoxynucleotides

The cytosine phosphodiester-linked guanine (CpG) oligodeoxynucleotides (CpG-ODN) are synthetic compounds with immunostimulatory effect used for enhancing the anticancer treatments. Preclinical and clinical study demonstrated a synergy between these drugs and monoclonal antibody and can be safely administrated together for a better therapeutic response [40–42].

The microbial DNA contains unmethylated cytosine phosphodiester-linked guanine (CpG) motifs which are recognized by specific immune receptors of the host-like human toll-like receptor 9 (TLR9) present on the surface of different immune cell types. Activation of these receptors enhances the expression of proinflammatory cytokines.

Researches on mouse models with transplantable tumors revealed that the intratumoral administration of the CpG-ODN and a monoclonal antibody (anti-interleukin-10 antibodies) induce hemorrhagic necrosis. This stimulatory immune response was mediated by tumor necrosis factor (TNF) and other inflammatory cytokines [40].

A study published in 2013 in Science using experimental model of tumor-infiltrating myeloid-derived cells on antibiotic-treated and GF mice remarkably revealed that the animals were refractory to therapy with CpG-ODN and anti-IL-10 antibody and presented low levels of TNF and cytokines required for promoting the hemorrhagic necrosis. A therapeutic response was obtained after the administration of lipopolysaccharides, a ligand for the TLR9 receptors-like. No response was obtained on TLR9-deficient mice [39].

Furthermore, study on the composition of mouse microbiota demonstrated that *Alistipes shahii* is positively correlated with TNF production in the tumor, whereas the abundance of *Lactobacillus fermentum* negatively correlated with it.

Thus, the research sustains the importance of the intact commensal microbiota for an optimal responses to cancer therapy required for the modulation myeloid-derived cell functions in the tumor microenvironment [22, 41].

5.3. Platinum salts

Platinum salts are coordination complexes of platinum used as chemotherapeutic drugs. Cisplatin and oxaliplatin interfere with DNA repair mechanism inducing intrastrand cross-link adducts activating the proapoptotic pathways. The platinum compound effect depends also by the presence of reactive oxygen species (ROS) for an apoptotic response and DNA damage.

Lida et al. presented evidence in the same study involving CpG-ODN that the therapeutic effect of the platinum salts on transplanted subcutaneous tumor depends on the presence of mice microbiota. The authors sustained that the ROS required for the genotoxic effect of these chemotherapies are produced in vivo by inflammatory cells associated to the tumor [41].

GF mice and antibiotic treatment attenuated the pharmacological effect and reduced the expression of ROS-responsive genes.

Moreover, using transgenic mice deficient for the myeloid NADPH oxidase NOX2 (Cybb_/_) with a low ROS response, the effect of oxaliplatin was attenuated.

The study highlights the importance of commensal on an efficient therapy by its contribution to tumor reduction.

5.4. Immune checkpoint blockade therapy

The problem of the therapeutic response variability was the starting point of recent researches which deal with the importance of microbiota in case of the patients treated with monoclonal antibodies involved in the immune checkpoint blockade.

Ipilimumab is an immunoglobulin G1 targeting the cytotoxic T-lymphocyte-associated protein 4 (CTLA4), which is a receptor protein involved in the immune checkpoint system and downregulation of the immune response.

The efficacy of the CTLA4 blockade was associated with T-lymphocyte responses induced by *Bacteroides thetaiotaomicron* and *Bacteroides fragilis* in both experimental models and human. No tumoral response was noticed after the treatment with ipilimumab in case of antibiotic treatment and germ-free mice. Exposure to *B. fragilis*, its polysaccharides, or its specific T cells reversed the response and favored the anticancer effect. The author of the study concluded that some *Bacteroides* spp. may play an important role and that the colitis may even antagonize the therapeutic efficacy [42].

Anti-PD-L1 is a monoclonal antibody successfully used for the treatment of several solid tumors, which target the protein programmed death-ligand 1 (PD-L1).

PD-L1 is a transmembrane protein, which acts as suppressor of the immune system and plays a role in escaping the cancer cells to immune system.

Sivan et al. demonstrated in their study that the commensal *Bifidobacterium* may have an unexpected role in enhancing antitumor immunity in vivo [43].

The authors used for research an experimental model of subcutaneous B16.SIY melanoma growth in genetically similar C57BL/6 mice. The animals were provided by two different animal facilities. After the anti-PD-L1 treatment, the results differ according to the animal provider. The *Bifidobacterium* spp. were identified by sequencing of the 16S ribosomal RNA and were correlated with the antitumor response therapy. The oral administration of bacteria improved tumor control to the same degree as anti-PD-L1, and the association of the microorganisms with this drug nearly abolished tumor outgrowth [22–43].

6. Conclusions

Even though there are increasing evidences regarding the close relationship between tumor development, chemotherapy, microbiota, and the immune system, it is still difficult and speculative to consider the microbes when deciding the therapeutic strategy for patients. However, modulating microbiota may enhance drug efficacy or diminish chemotherapy's toxicity.

Acknowledgements

This study was partially funded by the University of Medicine and Pharmacy "Carol Davila", through the research project "Young Researchers" number 33886/11.11.2014.

Author details

Andreea Letitia Arsene[1*], Cristina Manuela Dragoi[2], Alina Crenguta Nicolae[2], Daniela Elena Popa[3], George T.A. Burcea-Dragomiroiu[3], Ion Bogdan Dumitrescu[4], Olivia Carmen Timnea[5] and Denisa Ioana Udeanu[6]

*Address all correspondence to: andreeanitulescu@hotmail.com

1 Department of General and Pharmaceutical Microbiology, Faculty of Pharmacy, University of Medicine and Pharmacy "Carol Davila", Bucharest, Romania

2 Department of Biochemistry, Faculty of Pharmacy, University of Medicine and Pharmacy "Carol Davila", Bucharest, Romania

3 Department of Drug Control, Faculty of Pharmacy, University of Medicine and Pharmacy "Carol Davila", Bucharest, Romania

4 Department of Pharmaceutical Physics and Informatics, Faculty of Pharmacy, University of Medicine and Pharmacy "Carol Davila", Bucharest, Romania

5 Department of Medical Sciences, Faculty of Physical Education and Sports, Ecologic University of Bucharest, Romania

6 Department of Clinical Laboratory and Food Safety, Faculty of Pharmacy, University of Medicine and Pharmacy "Carol Davila", Bucharest, Romania

References

[1] Mittrucker, H. W., Seidel, D., Bland, P. W., Zarzycka, A., Kaufmann, S. H., Visekruna, A. and Steinhoff, U. Lack of microbiota reduces innate responses and enhances adaptive immunity against *Listeria monocytogenes* infection. Eur J Immunol. 2014. **44**: 1710–1715

[2] Ng, S. C., Plamondon, S., Kamm, M. A., et al. Immunosuppressive effects via human intestinal dendritic cells of probiotic bacteria and steroids in the treatment of acute ulcerative colitis. Inflamm Bowel Dis. 2010. **16**: 1286–1298.

[3] Yang, H., Liu, A., Zhang, M., et al. Oral administration of live Bifidobacterium substrains isolated from centenarians enhances intestinal function in mice. Curr Microbiol. 2009. **59**: 439–445.

[4] Smith, P. M., Howitt, M. R., Panikov, N., Michaud, M., Gallini, C. A., Bohlooly, Y. M., Glickman, J. N., et al. The microbial metabolites, short chain fatty acids, regulate colonic Treg cell homeostasis. Science. 2013. **341**: 569–573.

[5] Allegretti, J. R. Hamilton, M. J. Restoring the gut microbiome for the treatment of inflammatory bowel diseases. World J Gastroenterol. 2014. **20**: 3468–3474.

[6] Carroll, I. M., Chang, Y. H., Park, J., Sartor, R. B., Ringel, Y. Luminal and mucosal-associated intestinal microbiota in patients with diarrhea-predominant irritable bowel syndrome. Gut Pathog. 2010. **2**: 19.

[7] Krogius-Kurikka, L., Lyra, A., Malinen, E., Aarnikunnas, J., Tuimala, J., Paulin, L., et al. Microbial community analysis reveals high level phylogenetic alterations in the overall gastrointestinal microbiota of diarrhoea-predominant irritable bowel syndrome sufferers. BMC Gastroenterol. 2009. **9**: 95.

[8] Salonen, A., de Vos, W. M., Palva, A., Gastrointestinal microbiota in irritable bowel syndrome: present state and perspectives. Microbiology. 2010. **156**: 3205–3215.

[9] De Palma, G., Nadal, I., Medina, M., Donat, E., Ribes-Koninckx, C., Calabuig, M., et al. Intestinal dysbiosis and reduced immunoglobulin-coated bacteria associated with coeliac disease in children. BMC Microbiol. 2010. **10**: 63.

[10] Shen, X. J., Rawls, J. F., Randall, T., Burcal, L., Mpande, C. N., Jenkins, N., et al. Molecular characterization of mucosal adherent bacteria and associations with colorectal adenomas. Gut Microbes. 2010. **1**: 138–147.

[11] Olivares M, Neef A, Castillejo G, Palma GD, Varea V, Capilla A, et al. The HLA-DQ2 genotype selects for early intestinal microbiota composition in infants at high risk of developing coeliac disease. Gut. 2015. 64(3), 406–407.

[12] Evenepoel P, Meijers BKI, Bammens BRM, Verbeke K. Uremic toxins originating from colonic microbial metabolism. Kidney Int Suppl. 2009. **76**: S12–S19.

[13] Gaykema R, Goehler LE, Lyte M. Brain response to cecal infection with Campylobacter jejuni: analysis with Fos immunohistochemistry. Brain Behav Immun. 2004. **18**: 238–245.

[14] Goehler, L. E., Gaykema, R., Opitz, N., Reddaway, R., Badr, N., Lyte, M. Activation in vagal afferents and central autonomic pathways: early responses to intestinal infection with Campylobacter jejuni. Brain Behav Immun. 2005. **19**: 334–344.

[15] Goehler, L. E., Park, S. M., Opitz, N., Lyte, M., Gaykema, R. Campylobacter jejuni infection increases anxiety-like behavior in the holeboard: possible anatomical substrates for viscerosensory modulation of exploratory behavior. Brain Behav Immun. 2008. **22**: 354–366.

[16] Lyte, M., Li, W., Opitz, N., Gaykema, R., Goehler, L. E. Induction of anxiety-like behavior in mice during the initial stages of infection with the agent of murine colonic hyperplasia Citrobacter rodentium. Physiol Behav. 2006. **89**: 350–357.

[17] McLaughlin-Drubin, M. Munger, K., Viruses associated with human cancer, BBA – Mol Basis Dis. 2008. **1782**(3): 127–150.

[18] zur Hausen H. Oncogenic DNA viruses. Oncogene. 2001. **20**(54): 7820–7823.

[19] Taylor, G. S., Long, H. M., Brooks, J. M., Rickinson, A. B., Hislop, A. D. The immunology of Epstein-Barr virus-induced disease. Annu Rev Immunol. 2015. **33**: 787–821.

[20] Lin, M. V., King, L. Y., Chung, R. T. Hepatitis C virus-associated cancer. Annu Rev Pathol Mech Dis. 2015. **10**: 345–370.

[21] Moradpour, D., Penin, F., Hepatitis C virus proteins: from structure to function. In: Ralf Bartenschlager, editors. Hepatitis C Virus: From Molecular Virology to Antiviral Therapy, Springer Berlin Heidelberg, 2013. 113–142.

[22] Perez-Chanona, E., Trinchieri, G. The role of microbiota in cancer therapy. Curr Opin Immunol. 2016. **39**: 75–81.

[23] Forman, D., de Martel, C., Lacey, C. J., Soerjomataram, I., Lortet-Tieulent, J., Bruni, L., Franceschi, S. Global burden of human papillomavirus and related diseases. Vaccine. 2012. **30**: F12–F23.

[24] Richards, K. H., Wasson, C. W., Watherston, O., Doble, R., Blair, G. E., Wittmann, M., Macdonald, A. The human papillomavirus (HPV) E7 protein antagonises an Imiquimod-induced inflammatory pathway in primary human keratinocytes. Sci Rep. 2015. **5**.

[25] Pachathundikandi, S. K., Müller, A., Backert, S. Inflammasome activation by *Helicobacter pylori* and its implications for persistence and immunity. In: Steffen Beckert, editors. Inflammasome Signaling and Bacterial Infections. Springer International Publishing; 2016. p. 117–131.

[26] Huycke, M. M., Gaskins, H. R. Commensal bacteria, redox stress, and colorectal cancer: mechanisms and models. Exp Biol Med. 2004. **229**(7): 586–597.

[27] Yoshimoto, S., et al. Obesity-induced gut microbial metabolite promotes liver cancer through senescence secretome. Nature. 2013. **499**: 97–101.

[28] Hooper, L. V., Littman, D. R., Macpherson, A. J. Interactions between the microbiota and the immune system. Science. 2012. **336**(6086): 1268–1273.

[29] Cebra J. J. Influences of microbiota on intestinal immune system development. Am J Clin Nutr. 1999. **69**(5), 1046s–1051s.

[30] Maynard, C. L., Elson, C. O., Hatton, R. D., Weaver, C. T. Reciprocal interactions of the intestinal microbiota and immune system. Nature. 2012. **489**(7415): 231–241.

[31] Zitvogel, L., Galluzzi, L., Viaud, S., Vétizou, M., Daillère, R., Merad, M., Kroemer, G. Cancer and the gut microbiota: an unexpected link. Sci Trans Med. 2015. **7**(271): 271ps1–271ps1.

[32] Sekirov, I., Russell, S. L., Antunes, L. C. M., Finlay, B. B. Gut microbiota in health and disease, Physiol Rev. 2010. **90**(3): 859–904.

[33] Nakata, K., Yamamoto, M., Inagawa, H., Soma, G. I. Effects of interactions between intestinal microbiota and intestinal macrophages on health. Anticancer Res. 2013. **33**(7): 2849–2853.

[34] Fenga, C., Costa, C., Caruso, E., Raffa, L., Alibrando, C., Gangemi, S., Docea, A.O., Tsatsakis, A. M. Current evidence on the protective effect of dietary polyphenols on breast cancer. Farmacia. 2016. **64**(1): 1–12.

[35] Hashemzaei, M., Karami, S. P., Delaramifar, A., Sheidary, A. R., Tabrizian, K., Rezaee, R., Shahsavand, S., Arsene, A. L., Tsatsakis, A. M., Taghdisi, S. M. Anticancer effects of co-administration of daunorubicin and resveratrol in MOLT-4, U266 B1 and RAJI cell lines. Farmacia. 2016. **64**(1): 36–42.

[36] Dapito, D. H., et al. Promotion of hepatocellular carcinoma by the intestinal microbiota and TLR4. Cancer Cell. 2012. **21**: 504–516.

[37] Molloy, M. J., Bouladoux, N., Belkaid, Y. Intestinal microbiota: shaping local and systemic immune responses. Semin Immunol. 2012. **24**(1): 58–66.

[38] Stringer, A. M., Logan, R. M. The role of oral flora in the development of chemotherapy-induced oral mucositis. J Oral Pathol Med. 2015. **44**(2): 81–87.

[39] Viaud, S., Saccheri, F., Mignot, G., Yamazaki, T., Daillere, R., Hannani, D., Enot, D. P., Pfirschke, C., Engblom, C., Pittet, M. J. et al. The intestinal microbiota modulates the anticancer immune effects of cyclophosphamide. Science. 2013. **342**: 971–976.

[40] Vicari, A. P., Chiodoni, C., Vaure, C., Aït-Yahia, S., Dercamp, C., Matsos, F., O'Garra, A. Reversal of tumor-induced dendritic cell paralysis by CpG immunostimulatory oligonucleotide and anti–interleukin 10 receptor antibody. J Exp Med. 2002. **196**(4): 541–549.

[41] Lida, N., Dzutsev, A., Stewart, C. A., Smith, L., Bouladoux, N., Weingarten, R. A., et al. Commensal bacteria control cancer response to therapy by modulating the tumor microenvironment. Science. 2013. **342**(6161): 967–970.

[42] Vétizou, M., Pitt, J. M., Daillère, R., Lepage, P., Waldschmitt, N., Flament, C., Poirier-Colame, V. Anticancer immunotherapy by CTLA-4 blockade relies on the gut microbiota. Science. 2015. **350**(6264): 1079–1084.

[43] Sivan, A., Corrales, L., Hubert, N., Williams, J. B., Aquino-Michaels, K., Earley, Z. M., Benyamin, F. W., Lei, Y. M., Jabri, B., Alegre, M. L., et al. Commensal Bifidobacterium promotes antitumor immunity and facilitates anti-PD-L1 efficacy. Science. 2015. **350**: 1084–1089.

7

Approaches to Endow Ribonucleases with Antitumor Activity: Lessons Learned from the Native Cytotoxic Ribonucleases

Jessica Castro, Marc Ribó, Antoni Benito and Maria Vilanova

Abstract

Typical antitumor drugs disrupt the flow of biochemical information from DNA to proteins with the aim of precluding uncontrolled cell proliferation and inducing cancer cell apoptosis. However, most of the currently used small antitumor drugs are genotoxic because they act over DNA. Pharmaceutical industry is now searching for a new line of cancer chemotherapeutics without genotoxic effects. Ribonucleases (RNases) are small basic proteins, present in all life forms, which belong to this kind of chemotherapeutics. Some of them present with remarkable selective antitumor activity linked to their ability to destroy RNA, a powerful way to control gene expression, leaving DNA unharmed. In the last two decades, the knowledge gained on the cytotoxic mechanism of these RNases has been used to engineer more powerful and selective variants to kill cancer cells. In this chapter, we describe the advances reached in endowing an RNase with antitumor abilities.

Keywords: ribonucleases, antitumor activity, protein engineering, mechanism of antitumor action, delivery

1. Introduction

In their review, Hanahan and Weinberg [1] described ten hallmarks of cancer cells: genome instability and mutation, sustaining proliferative signaling, evading growth suppressors, resisting cell death, enabling replicative immortality, tumor-promoting inflammation, inducing angiogenesis, activating invasion and metastasis, reprogramming of energy metabolism, and evading immune destruction. Involved in these metaprocesses, there is a deregulation of gene expression. A significant part of the current chemotherapeutic compounds used to treat cancer patients target different over- or under-expressed genes that take part in the abovementioned processes that drive to malignant cell transformation and/or metastasis.

1.1. Why target RNA to treat cancer diseases?

Control of gene expression can be carried out at different levels in the flow of genetic information from DNA to proteins (**Figure 1**).

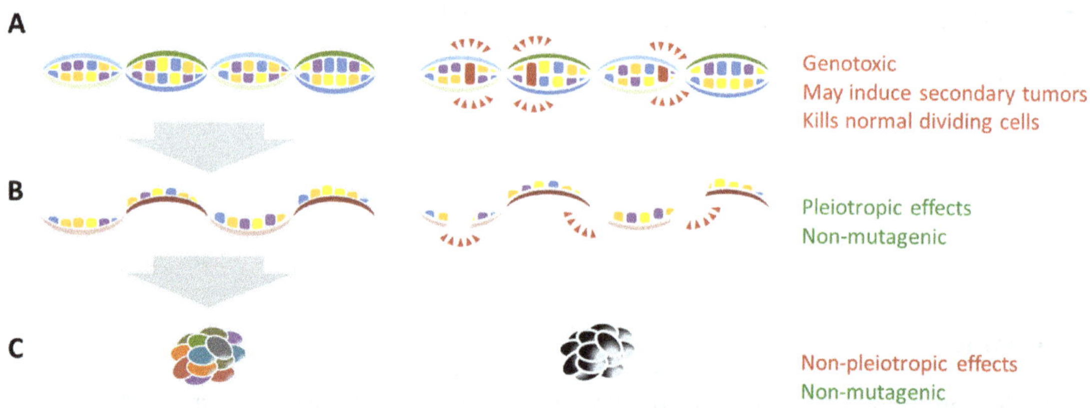

Figure 1. Targets of genotoxic and non-mutagenic antitumoral drugs along the information pathway. Transmission of biological information in tumor cells occurs from DNA to RNA and proteins that exert their biological function. (A) Classical antitumor therapies like radiotherapy and chemotherapy affect DNA inhibiting cell replication but may also kill normal dividing cells, and since they are genotoxic, they may induce secondary tumors. (B) Alternative damaging RNA therapies inhibit gene expression and its regulation. These therapies exert pleiotropic effects because they affect multiple RNA substrates and are not mutagenic. (C) Therapies affecting a single protein or pathway of the cell are highly specific but sometimes cannot cope with the multifactorial nature of cancer although are also non-mutagenic.

Drugs that act over DNA have the drawback of being mutagenic and are responsible for the appearance of new cancers, time after the patients have been cured of or controlled their first cancer disease [2]. Instead, drugs that destroy or inactivate RNA are similarly powerful without the associated risk of genotoxicity. In addition, drugs that specifically target a single protein or pathway have the advantage of being highly specific, but they are often insufficient to cope with the multifactorial complexity of the cancer phenotype. Several approaches are used to target RNAs, the use of antisense oligonucleotides, small interfering RNA (siRNAs), and the use of ribozymes or proteins with ribonucleolytic activity [3]. In the present chapter, we will focus on ribonucleases (RNases) as antitumor agents and how the knowledge gained so far about their mechanism of action has inspired researchers in the design of more powerful and selective RNases that can overcome tumor resistance as well as minimize the toxic effects to normal cells, properties strongly desired for any antitumor drug.

RNases are enzymes present in all life kingdoms that degrade RNA and in cells are responsible for RNA turnover [4]. Their interest as antitumor agents started early in the fifties of the last century when the bovine pancreatic ribonuclease (RNase A) demonstrated to have antitumor activity both *in vitro* and *in vivo* [5–10] although with contradictory results [11]. This interest vanished until the discovery of non-engineered RNases with natural anticancer activity when used at much lower concentrations than RNase A. Among them we can find prokaryotic and eukaryotic RNases [12], from microbe [13, 14], plants [15], or vertebrates. The latter belong to the known vertebrate-secreted ribonuclease family [16] from which RNase A is the paradigm [17]. Recently, in animal models, even RNases that natively are not cytotoxic, like RNase A, are shown to have antimetastatic properties when ultralow doses are administered everyday. It is suggested that this effect is related to its ability to degrade circulating noncoding RNAs assuming that in blood plasma the enzyme is not inhibited (see below) [18].

1.2. What makes a ribonuclease selectively cytotoxic for cancer cells?

Although some RNases have reached clinical trials for treatment of different types of cancer [19–25], their mechanism of action is not well understood. Nevertheless, RNases share some steps of cell intoxication with most cytotoxins.

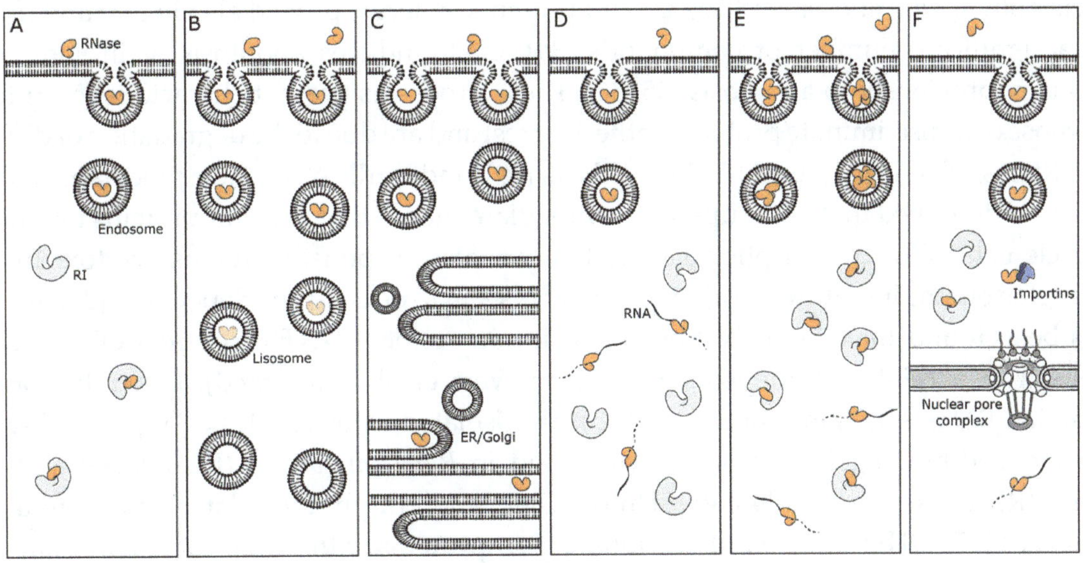

Figure 2. Multifactorial causes of RNase cytotoxicity. Some RNases are able to reach the cytosol but are not cytotoxic because they are unable to evade the action of the RI (A). Other RNases are not cytotoxic because they cannot reach the cytosol, either because they are degraded during its internalization (B) or because they follow an intracellular pathway that does not allow them to reach this compartment (C). Some RNases are cytotoxic because they reach the cytosol and are not inhibited by the RI (D). Other RNases are cytotoxic although they do not evade the RI either because they reach the cytosol with high efficiency allowing to saturate the RI present in the cytosol (E) or because they can reach the nucleus where the RI cannot inhibit them (F).

To be cytotoxic an RNase has to reach the tumor cells. This implies two basic steps: to attain target cells from the administration point (RNases are mainly administered i.v.) and to be able to enter these cells. The first step means that the RNase has to be stable enough in blood to reach their target cells and not to be cleared rapidly from circulation through glomerular filtration. The second step [26–28] implies an interaction with a specific or a nonspecific component of the target cell surface in order to be endocytosed. Then, during its journey, at some point of the endocytic pathway (**Figure 2B**), the RNase has to translocate to the cytosol to avoid lysosomal degradation and, obviously, follow a productive endocytic pathway. Once in the cytosol, it has to be stable and resistant to proteases, and at the same time, it has to evade the ribonuclease inhibitor (RI) to preserve its ribonucleolytic activity and therefore be able to degrade RNAs and induce cell death by apoptosis. The RI is a protein present in the cytosol of mammalian cells that binds to some RNases with high affinity [29]. It is hypothesized that the RI acts as a safeguard for the potential entry of any external RNase [30]. Alternatively to the evasion strategy, an RNase can also have the ability to enter the cell very efficiently to saturate the RI and to leave free RNase molecules able to degrade RNAs. Finally, an RNase can also be driven to any organelle devoid of RI where it can degrade RNAs, for instance, the cell nucleus [31] (**Figure 2F**).

The paradigmatic native cytotoxic RNase that evades the RI is onconase (ONC), a member of the vertebrate-secreted RNase family of amphibian origin (isolated from oocytes and early embryos of *Rana pipiens*). ONC reached phases II/IIIb for treatment of malignant pleural mesothelioma [21] although it presents renal toxicity that is reversed when the treatment is discontinued [32]. It exhibits selective cytostatic and cytotoxic activities against many tumor models both *in vitro* and *in vivo* [22, 33] and presents synergy, proved also *in vivo* and *in vitro*, with a significant number of compounds [34]. ONC induces apoptosis or in some cases autophagy previously to apoptosis [35, 36]. These processes present characteristics different from those of indiscriminate protein synthesis arrest and are due to the degradation of different target RNAs, rRNAs [37], mRNAs [38], tRNAs [39], and miRNAs or their precursors [40–42]. It has been described that ONC up- or downregulates genes that code for proteins involved in cell cycle control or transcription factors that are also responsible for its cytotoxicity [43]. Although from the literature the apoptotic effects seem to be cell-type dependent [34], recently it has been found that the activating transcription factor 3 (ATF3) controls ONC-induced apoptosis in a cell-type independent manner (Vert et al., submitted). Other tumoricidal amphibian RNases are Amphinase (Amph), also isolated from oocytes of *R. pipiens* [44] and the sialic acid-binding lectins (leczymes) found in *Rana catesbeiana* (RC-RNase) and *Rana japonica* (RJ-RNase) oocytes [45, 46]. Unlike ONC and Amph, these latter ones agglutinate cancer cells [47–49] binding to cell membrane glycoproteins with a high content of sialic acids [47, 49]. It is also proposed, like for ONC and Amph, that these leczymes require an internalization process to trigger apoptosis [50]; however compared to them, clinical trials and studies on animal models are needed to unveil their mechanism of antitumor activity and clinical potential.

The critical process of ONC internalization is still an open question. This is not a minor issue because it is strongly related to the RNase cytotoxic selectivity for cancer cells. For ONC it has been described both the existence of a specific receptor [37] and an entry through a non-saturable process [51] as well as an entry through the clathrin/AP-2-mediated endocytic pathway [52] and a non-dynamin-dependent pathway [51]. These discrepancies may be explained by the model cell lines used in the different works. In addition, electrostatics are described as necessary for the cellular uptake of ONC, while for other RNases, an specific interaction with cell surface structures seems to contribute more decisively to their internalization [53]. Essentially, RNases are cationic proteins, and since the surface of most cancer cells is more electronegative [54] than that of normal cells, the electrostatic interactions that they establish may dictate their selectivity. Very recently, both RNase A and its human counterpart, the human pancreatic ribonuclease (HP-RNase), have been described to interact with a neutral hexasaccharide glycosphingolipid, Globo H [55], a component of a glycolipid or a glycoprotein located on the outer membrane of epithelial cells and detected in high levels in the outer membrane of several tumor cells [56]. The authors suggest that this interaction is not only substantial for the internalization of these RNases but for their release from the lumen of endosomes allowing for the access to the cytosol [55], although if they are not engineered to avoid the RI, they are not cytotoxic (see below). In addition, for RNase A, it has been described a multipathway of internalization that involves both clathrin-coated vesicles and macropinosomes [57]. Finally, through an *in silico* study by sliding-window hydrophobicity analysis, it has been hypothesized that some cytotoxic RNases have a hydrophobic segment sterically available for a hydrophobic interaction with both tumor cell and endosomal membranes that would facilitate their internalization [58]. The more it is known about the membrane structures that are recognized by RNases or the productive pathway, by which they enter the cell, the better they can be engineered to increase their selectivity and potency.

Another RNase that naturally shows antitumor activity by RI evasion is bovine seminal ribonuclease (BS-RNase), present in the bull seminal plasma. In this case the quaternary structure attained by this enzyme is responsible for its low RI affinity due to steric hindrance, while the monomeric form is strongly inhibited by the RI [59]. BS-RNase exists as a mixture of two dimeric forms, M=M and MxM, each monomer being a structural homolog of RNase A [60]. The MxM dimer exchanges the N-terminal α-helices forming a 3D-swapped structure and is the form that even in the reducing conditions of the cell cytosol is cytotoxic [61] (for a comparative review on the RNase structures, see [62, 63]). BS-RNase binds to the extracellular matrix, and this interaction seems to be important for its cytotoxic effect [64, 65] even though it does not bind to cell membranes, suggesting an adsorption cell entry mechanism [66]. BS-RNase has been localized in endosomes and its cytotoxicity is blocked by inhibition of this energy-dependent entry mechanism [65]. It has also been localized in the trans-Golgi network of treated malignant cells, which may be indicative that this organelle is an effective site for translocation providing an explanation for its selectivity [65, 67]. Although, it has been described that BS-RNase can destabilize artificial membranes [68, 69], it is not exactly known how BS-RNase permeates the trans-Golgi membranes. Like for ONC, rRNA is a target of BS-RNase and its cleavage induces apoptosis [64], but the enzyme has also been found in the nucleolus of cancer cells [65], and although it is not known how it reaches the cell nucleus, a correlation between cytotoxicity and a decrease of telomerase activity and its associated RNA has been found [70]. Recently, it has been described that BS-RNase triggers Beclin1-mediated autophagy in treated cancer cells being ineffective in normal cells, suggesting that autophagy more than apoptosis can be the mechanism of cancer cell death induced by BS-RNase [71]. Comparable to ONC, this selective autophagy for cancer cells seems to be related to the basic charge distribution in the surface of these RNases [36, 71].

Apart from RNases of animal origin, it is worth mentioning that there are a vast array of RNases from fungal, bacterial, and plant origin that natively present remarkable cytotoxic properties. Among them we can mention mushroom RNases [72, 73]; microbial RNases such as α-sarcin from *Aspergillus*; the two well-known T1 ribonuclease members from *Bacillus*, binase (*B. intermedius*), and barnase (*B. amyloliquefaciens*); and RNase Sa (*S. aureofaciens*) [28, 74] as well as plant RNases from ginseng, wheat leaf, mung bean, black pine pollen, seeds of bitter gourd, tomato, and hop [12, 15, 75–79]. Although adverse effects due to immunogenicity and nonspecific binding [12] have been described for some of them, others are described to have a lower immunogenicity than ONC [28]. In addition, they have a remarkable resistance to RI, and in some cases, the cytotoxic effect is comparable to that of ONC. However, in terms of knowledge of their cytotoxic mechanism and clinical applications, they are still lagging behind when compared to the animal counterparts. In the last years, especially for binase, a significant advance has been attained in the understanding of its mechanism of cell intoxication. The cytotoxic effect of binase is effected via induction of both intrinsic and extrinsic apoptotic pathways [80], and evidence is provided that targets KIT and AML1-ETO oncogenes in human leukemia Kasumi-1 cells [81]. It has also shown a positive effect on the liver of tumor-bearing mice, articulated as a tumor reduction in the volume of destructive changes in the live parenchyma as well as of being effective in tumor growth suppression [82].

2. How to endow a ribonuclease with selective antitumor activity

In the last two decades, the knowledge gained on the cytotoxic mechanism of natively tumoricidal RNases, described in the previous section, as well as in the references therein, has been used to engineer more powerful and selective RNase variants able to kill cancer cells. From this knowledge, it is clear that RNases will be cytotoxic if they are able to reach the cytosol avoiding lysosomal degradation or nonproductive intracellular pathways and if, once in the cytosol, they can evade the action of RI (**Figure 2A–C**). Consequently, an RNase will be cytotoxic either if it can avoid the RI inhibition or it can efficiently reach the cytosol saturating all the RI present in this compartment (**Figure 2D–F**). Several approaches have been used to fulfill these requirements that will be reviewed in this section and are summarized in **Figure 3**.

2.1. Engineered RNases that evade the RI

In the literature two main approaches used to engineer noncytotoxic RNases to render them resistant to the RI and endow them with cytotoxicity are described: The most evident one consists of precluding RNase-RI complex formation through steric hindrance or coulombic repulsion. The variant's design is based on the known 3D structure of the RI-RNase A complex described by Kobe and Deisenhofer [83]. However, another approach is to hide RNases from the inhibitor. This is accomplished by targeting monomeric RNases to an organelle free of RI making needless neither the RI evasion nor the RI saturation.

2.1.1. *RNases in a monomeric form*

The first reported approaches to endow an RNase with the ability to evade the RI were carried out by Raines and coworkers, who introduced single or few amino acid changes in wild-type noncytotoxic RNase A that created steric hindrance to decrease RI binding [84]. Replacement of Gly 88 of RNase A by bulky charged residues, like Arg or Asp, resulted in a variant with 10^4-fold less affinity for the RI and which was only about 20-fold less cytotoxic than ONC. Similar approaches were used on HP-RNase [85, 86] or monomeric BS-RNase [87, 88]. This first approach was concomitant or followed by the introduction of other changes that disturbed the electrostatic interaction between the RNase and the RI [89–92] creating new variants each time more cytotoxic. For instance, the RNase A variant Asp38Arg/Arg39Asp/Asn67Arg/Gly88Arg had 5.9×10^9-fold lower affinity for the RI keeping the activity and stability of the parental enzyme with a cytotoxicity equivalent to that of ONC [91]. Although this approach has attained success, in some cases the use of the same rationale has not worked to get variants with the expected properties [89, 93]. This is due to the fact that the replacement of some residues to disrupt the RNase-RI interaction at the same time alters other factors important for the enzyme cytotoxicity, such as the catalytic activity or the stability of the enzyme that counterbalances the obtained gain on RI evasion. Nevertheless, one of the engineered RNases to evade the RI has reached clinical trials. The QBI-139 RNase variant (Evade™ ribonucleases from Quintessence Biosciences Inc. (http://www.quintbio.com/) is now in Phase I of clinical

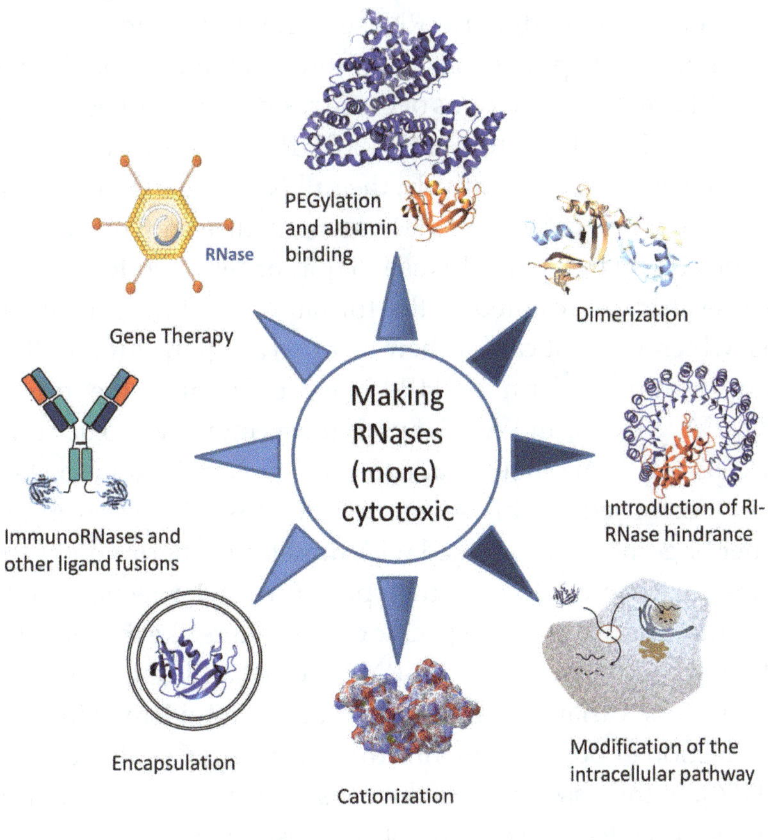

Figure 3. Strategies to create cytotoxic RNases or to improve its antitumor activity. Two groups of strategies are considered: those allowing the RNase to avoid the inhibition by the RI (dark blue arrows) and those that improve the delivery of the RNase into the cell (light blue arrows). Some of the indicated strategies can be included in both groups.

trials for the treatment of solid tumors [25]. On the other hand, different strategies have been carried out to avoid some of the non-desired side effects. The Gly88Arg RI-evading RNase A, described above, was engineered to introduce nonnative disulfide bonds to increase its conformational stability [94], resulting in a more cytotoxic variant. Also, an increase in stability has also been attained by the glycosylation of the protein. For instance, the production of ONC in *Pichia pastoris* yields a glycosylated protein more stable and 50-fold more cytotoxic [95].

2.1.2. RNase dimerization or oligomerization

The formation of oligomeric structures, such as the BS-RNase dimers, has inspired the design and production of new RNase variants with the aim of precluding their binding to the RI by steric hindrance mimicking the way of action of BS-RNase [96, 97]. The pursuit of dimeric or oligomeric variants is very attractive because they are more cationic proteins and can potentially strongly interact with the negative surfaces of cancer cells gaining selectivity and, at the same time, reducing kidney clearance due to the increase of molecular mass. As stated in Section 1.2, the current model for BS-RNase cytotoxicity is that in the reducing conditions of the cell citosol, the unswapped isomer from (M=M) dissociates into monomers, which are strongly inhibited by the RI, whereas the swapped isomer (M×M) remains as a non-covalent dimer able to evade the RI [64, 98]. In addition, analysis of the structure of the non-covalent dimer of BS-RNase [61] and different mutated forms [99] suggested that it adopts a compact quaternary structure that is critical for the RI interaction, explaining its trapping. One of the first approaches to get cytotoxic dimeric RNase variants was to reproduce the structural determinants of BS-RNase swapping [62] in different members of the vertebrate-secreted RNase family. Thus, different combinations of those residues identified as responsible of dimer formation (Cys31, Cys32, Leu28, Gly16, Ser80) of BS-RNase were introduced in the sequence of either HP-RNase or RNase A. Alternatively, the full N-terminal hinge sequence (the peptide that links the N-terminal α-helix of V-shaped RNase structure with the rest of the protein body) of RNase A was replaced by that of BS-RNase [63] in order to endow RNase A with dimerization abilities. These changes resulted in the formation of different ratios of swapped and unswapped forms, which was critical for their cytotoxicity [63]. Among these constructs it is remarkable that of a dimeric form of HP-RNase containing the mutations Glu111Gly, Gln28Leu, Arg31Cys, Arg32Cys, and Asn34Lys that was more cytotoxic and selective than BS-RNase for cancer cells [100]. As another approach, covalent linkers to stabilize the dimeric structures have also been used. In this sense, first cytotoxic RNase A dimers [101, 102] and more recently higher oligomers cross-linked with dimethyl suberimidate [103] were obtained. Although these constructs were cytotoxic, they presented heterogeneity, a drawback for their use as antitumor agents. The use of more specific cross-linkers like the introduction of thioether bonds between different Cys residues of BS-RNase [104] and RNase A [105], in some cases, allowed the production of variants with an increased cytotoxicity. Finally, an evaluation of cross-linkers and selection of positions to introduce different Cys was carried out in the work of Rutkoski et al. [106]. In this case, some of the constructs were as cytotoxic as the RI-evading RNases. However, as far as we know, none of the described constructs has reached clinical trials yet. An interesting and different way to get dimeric RNases consists in the fusion of two RNase genes using a linker to get a tandem RNase [107]. This construct although inhibited by the RI showed a cytotoxicity of the same order of that shown by BS-RNase. Modeling studies of this tandem RNase bound to the RI revealed that the engineered enzyme binds the RI with a 1:1 stoichiometry, and the authors suggested that the cytotoxic effect was due to an improved endocytosis efficiency [108] likely due to a higher cationization (see below).

Finally, related with the formation of oligomeric structures, it is worth mentioning that RNase A can form 3D domain-swapped multimers, ranging from trimers to hexamers [109, 110] and up to decatetramers [111]. These oligomers are enzymatically and biologically active [110, 112] and what is more interesting they exhibit cytotoxicity [99, 113]. The study of these oligomeric structures could reveal new scaffolds for the design of potential antitumor RNase variants [63].

2.1.3. *Targeting organelle RI-free*

The tumor cell nucleus is the final destination of multiple conventional antitumor drugs [114, 115] as well as a critical compartment for suicide gene therapy [116]. In addition, drugs that do not have a native tendency to accumulate in the cell nucleus have been conjugated/engineered/encapsulated by different means to reach this compartment. Literature is full of examples, for instance, drugs that have been modified by the introduction of a nuclear localization signal (NLS) as a modular component of a construct [117–119] and that have been encapsulated in nanoparticles directed to the cell nucleus [120] or the viral-based vectors, which are an elegant choice as vehicles to deliver DNA that encodes therapeutic proteins or RNAs to this organelle [121–123]. Based on this, an alternative strategy to bypass the RI action was to guide the RNases to the cell nucleus, which is described as free of RI [124] or at least the nucleolus [125]. Initially, an HP-RNase variant was produced, namely PE5, that carries a noncontiguous extended bipartite NLS [31, 126]. Although this variant is inhibited by the RI, at the same time it is recognized by α-importin [126] and cleaves nuclear but not cytoplasmic RNA *in vivo* [127]. At present, the mechanism by which the engineered HP-RNase reaches the cell nucleus is different from the one described above for BS-RNase (Section 1.2). It is postulated that the concentrations of RI and α-importin are similar in the cytosol. Thus, the affinity of PE5 for each protein will determine to which it will mainly bind. However, those RNase molecules captured by the α-importin will be released into the nucleus and, therefore, removed from the two competing equilibriums, and PE5 will progressively accumulate into the nucleus [128]. PE5 kills the cells by apoptosis mediated by the induction of $p21^{WAF/CIP1}$ and inactivation of JNK and increases the number of cells in the S-G_2/M-phases of cell cycle [129]. Moreover, the cytotoxic mechanism of PE5 is not prevented by a mutated p53 or a multidrug-resistant (MDR) phenotype [129], and it is synergic with doxorubicin [130] on doxorubicin-resistant NCI/ADR-RES cell line [130]. Very recently, using microarray-derived transcriptional profiling, it has been shown that PE5 remarkably downregulates multiple genes that code for enzymes involved in the deregulated metabolic pathways in cancer cells [131], one of the hallmarks of cancer. In addition, new cytotoxic RNase variants directed to the cell nucleus, collectively named ND-RNases, have been engineered either by reverting some of PE5 changes to render the variant more similar to wild-type enzyme or by the addition of an extra NLS to its N-terminus. In the latter case, a tenfold more cytotoxic enzyme than PE5 [132] has been obtained. Due to their cytotoxic mechanism, which differs from that of RNases that exert its action on the cell's cytosol, ND-RNases are very interesting antitumor agents that can cope with the complexity of cancer cell phenotype, and their multiple effects allow anticipating synergism with many currently clinically used antitumor agents. In *in vivo* studies with animal models, the ND-RNases have shown very low toxicity (it has not been possible to calculate the maximum tolerated doses (MTD) but the maximum feasible dose (MFD) which is of 80 mg/kg) (Castro et al., results not published).

2.2. Engineered RNases that might saturate the intracellular RI and/or gain selectivity

The efficiency of cell internalization is another important determinant of the cytotoxicity of the RNases because an RI-sensitive RNase is still a potential danger provided that enough enzyme molecules reach the cell cytosol. The most basic strategy to increase the internalization of RNases is their cationization by chemical or genetic modification, that is, to make the RNases even more basic to increase their interaction with the anionic membranes of tumor cells. As stated above, this fact may also increase their selectivity for cancer cells [133]. Several examples of this approach can be found in the literature. The chemical modification of the carbonyl groups of RC-RNase with a water-soluble carbodiimide in the presence of nucleophiles or the amidation with ethylenediamine, 2-aminoethanol, taurine, or ethylenediamine of HP-RNase and RNase A increases their cytotoxicity [134–136]. The preparation of RNase A and noncytotoxic cross-linked dimers of RNase A, both covalently linked to polyspermine to increase their basicity, slightly increased their cytotoxicity [137]. In general, the higher cationic variants were more efficiently internalized into the cells. However, in some cases, the chemical modifications seriously compromised the ribonucleolytic activity of the modified enzymes [134, 135] and generated heterogeneous products difficult to use as antitumor drugs. RC-RNase and RNase Sa variants were engineered substituting acidic residues by Asn, Gln, or Arg [138] or by positively charged residues [139, 140], respectively, showing antitumor activity and enhanced internalization. Gly38Lys-BS-RNase that bears an enforced cluster of positive charges at the N-terminal surface also presented an increased cytotoxicity relative to its parental RNase and a higher membrane interaction capability [141]. Fuchs et al. [142] replaced two residues of a cytotoxic variant of RNase A to create a patch of Arg residues on its surface that rendered a threefold increase in cytotoxicity and added a protein translocation domain (nona-arginine) to a previously cytotoxic RNase variant that increased their cytotoxicity [142, 143]. However, the same group has proposed that the internalization of pancreatic RNases by cationization can be counterbalanced by an increased affinity for the anionic RI in the cytosol [92]. Like for RI evasion, one has to be very cautious in the design of these variants in order to not counterbalance the increased internalization by the loss of other important characteristics responsible for the RNase cytotoxicity. In the same line but with a different approach, co-treating cells with a cationic 2 poly(amidoamine) dendrimer [144] increase the cytotoxicity of the RNase probably by increasing its translocation from the endosomes without affecting its ribonucleolytic activity or conformational stability observed upon cationization of some RNases.

In addition to merely increasing the positive charge of an RNase, other approaches that can enhance its delivery to the cytosol or to a specific organelle are related to the construction of targeted RNases either by chemical conjugation or fusion with a specific component that directs them to cancer cells. These procedures have been used with other drugs combining a targeting molecule, mainly antibodies, with an effector moiety getting what has been called immunotoxins (see below) [145, 146]. Small molecule drugs are still the modality of choice for addressing intracellular targets due to the barriers to cell entry that proteins have to face. Nevertheless, despite the considerable research efforts and advances attained, there remain many protein-protein interactions that small molecules cannot modulate effectively [147], and proteins have a lower propensity for off-targets. Thus, the strategies described below include both small molecules and proteins as drivers of payload RNases, including that nonsensitive to the RI.

2.2.1. Intracellular pathway

The engineering of RNases to amend the intracellular pathway, apart from the ND-RNases described in Section 2.1.3 that have a different goal, is the less explored approach. This is likely because the productive intracellular route followed by cytotoxic RNases is the part of the intoxication process that looks like more as a black box. Nevertheless, there are some examples to deliver RNases to cellular compartments other than the cytosol. The KDEL consensus sequence, which drives proteins to the endoplasmic reticulum (ER), was added to the C-terminal end of BS-RNase resulting in a loss of cytotoxicity compared to the parental enzyme [65] indicating that this compartment is not an essential intracellular station for the arrival of BS-RNase to the cell cytosol. In addition, it has been tried to decrease the lysosomal degradation of one of the cytotoxic Evade™ RNases, the Gly88Arg variant, by introducing the change Lys7Arg in the Lys-Phe-Glu-Arg-Gln sequence that targets proteins to the lysosomes. In this case, Lys7Arg/Gly88Arg RNase A is nearly tenfold more cytotoxic than Gly88Arg RNase A variant but has more than tenfold less affinity for RI [90]. Once again, the changes introduced to enhance one of the aspects of RNase cytotoxicity affect other important features of this process precluding a clear conclusion.

2.2.2. Chemical conjugation

Targeting RNase molecules to tumor cells was early carried out by chemical conjugation of both RNase A to transferrin (Tf) or mAb against Tf receptor (TfR) [148] as well as to the T-cell antigen CD5 [149] and ONC to anti-Tf receptor mAb 5E9 [150]. These studies showed that the antibody conjugates were more efficient than Tf conjugates and that ONC and RNase A conjugated to antibodies by a reducible disulfide bond were equally potent (IC_{50} values in the nM range). However, ONC conjugates showed increased efficiency likely due to the fact that ONC is not inhibited by the RI, while RNase A might not be able to saturate it even when conjugated to a particular cell driver [151]. In these primary studies also, ONC was conjugated to CD22-specific mAb LL2 and RFB4, which resulted in a several thousand-fold increase in cytotoxicity comparable to that of anti-CD22 immunotoxin conjugated to plant or bacterial toxin cargoes [152]. These results confirmed that RNases are as potent as these toxins when properly targeted. Nevertheless, although these chemical conjugates reduced the tumor size in animal models while not showing appreciable toxicity, their lot-to-lot heterogeneity was a serious drawback for further development [153]. ONC was also conjugated to P-glycoprotein (P-gp) neutralizing mAb MRK16. This construct increased ONC cytotoxicity and at the same time sensitized the multidrug-resistant cancer cells that overexpress MDR1 gene to vincristine [154]. These results may be explained by both the mAb binding to P-gp that diminishes its drug-expelling ability and its ability to internalize ONC.

More recently, the amino groups of Lys side chains of RNase A and variant Lys41Arg (Lys41 is an amino acid critical for the ribonucleolytic activity of the enzyme [155]) were randomly conjugated to folate since folate receptors are overexpressed on the surface of many types of cancer [156, 157]. However, the results showed an abolition of the catalytic activity of RNase A, while the variant Lys41Arg only retained 54 % of its catalytic activity. In the same work, a folate analogue was designed, produced, and used to specifically S-alkylate Cys residues introduced by site-directed mutagenesis at positions 19 or 88. Only those proteins modified at positions that endow them with the ability to evade the RI were able to diminish cell proliferation. Thus, even in this case, enhanced internalization had to be accompanied by an RI evasion [158].

2.2.3. *Fusion RNases and ImmunoRNases*

The progress attained in the technology of construction and production of recombinant fusion proteins particularly using antibodies [145, 146] has been applied to RNases. Several RNases have been used either as scaffold onto which a targeting domain is engineered or fused, including antibodies. In the latter case, several antibody constructs such as scFv, diabodies, scFv-Fc, and $F(ab)_2$ antibody fragments were used as a fusion partner [159]. Generally speaking, small antibody constructs are best suited to penetrate and distribute into solid tumors. However, the smaller the construct, the faster it disappears from blood circulation. Thus, a compromise in the molecular mass has been agreed, between 60 and 120 kDa for a therapeutic protein in order to ensure a good pharmacokinetics [160]. On the other hand, when choosing a particular RNase to be fused to an antibody or any targeting domain, it has to be taken into account the connecting linker and the orientation of the RNase relative to the carrier molecule in order not to alter some of the previously described RNase properties important for their cytotoxicity.

Primarily, HP-RNase as well as other members of the same family [161] such as angiogenin (ANG) and other RNases such as eosinophil-derived neurotoxin (EDN) and some engineered variants of them were tested in experimental sets of RNase-antibody fusion targeting Tf. They showed about 10^3 times more potency than the respective chemically conjugated RNase-antibody (Section 2.2.2) [149, 162]. The main concern with these constructs was the host selected for production indicating that the final yield was dependent on the expression system used [154]. To overcome production concerns and to get more specific clinical targets, different immunoRNases have been produced directed to antigens expressed on certain types of leukemia but not in hematopoietic stem cells, such as CD22 and CD30 or the ErbB2 that showed significant advantages over the equivalent chemical conjugates [153]. As alternatives, ANG,

HP-RNase, or RapLR1 (*R. pipiens* liver RNase 1), a close relative of ONC, were fused to two CD22-specific scFV antibody fragments generated either by reengineering the variable domain core structure of mAb LL2 or grafting the complementary-determining regions (CDR) of the clinically established mAb RF4B into consistent human scFv scaffolds [163–165]. Some of them were successfully produced and exhibited potent cytotoxicity (IC_{50} in the nM range) [164] which drove to a second generation of anti-CD22 immunoRNases in diabody format fusing LL2 or humRFB4 to ANG or RapLRI. Bivalent anti-CD22 immunoRNases showed a superior cytotoxicity toward $CD22^+$ tumor cells when compared to their monovalent counterparts due to antigen binding by avidity and enhanced internalization [163, 164]. Different CD30-targeting constructs have also been produced fusing HP-RNase or ANG to CD30-specific murine or human scFvs that inhibited tumor growth [166], but the entirely human bivalent scFv-Fc-HP-RNase showed better properties and inhibited the growth of $CD30^+$ Hodgkin lymphoma cells [167]. Even better results were obtained for immunoRNases resulting from the fusion of CD30-specific scFv Ki4 to ANG [168]. Recently, a humanized anti-epidermal growth factor receptor (EGFR) scFV was used to target ONC to EGFR-expressing tumor cell lines [169]. Fusion was accomplished by a flexible linker $(G_4S)_3$, but the construct resulted in very poor cytotoxicity, likely due to endosomal accumulation and lysosomal degradation. To avoid this drawback, the authors substituted the linker by a peptide from dengue virus that has been reported to be involved in the endosomal escape of the virus. The modified immunoRNase exhibited exceptionally high cytotoxicity toward EGFR-expressing head and neck cancer cell lines without affecting specificity. More recently, the same research group constructed a derived diabody fragment with the specificity of the clinically established mAb Cetuximab to deliver ONC to EGFR-expressing tumor cells. The dimeric immunoRNase was several orders of magnitude more cytotoxic toward EGFR-expressing tumor cell lines than its monomeric counterpart and exhibited significant antitumor activity in a murine A431 xenograft model, but in this case, the linker was $(G_4S)_3$ [170]. Thus, not only the linker between the ONC and the antibody fragment is important but the structure of the antibody moiety.

An ONC variant with a modified putative N-glycosylation site (Asn69Gln) has also fused to humanized antibody hRS7 raised against Trop-2, a cell surface glycoprotein expressed in a variety of epithelial cancers [171]. The construct contained two ONC molecules fused to each of the N-terminus of light chains of the antibody and was produced in stably transfected myeloma cells. The purified immunoRNase inhibited the proliferation of Trop-2-expressing cell lines with an IC_{50} in the nM range and was able to suppress tumor growth in a prophylactic model of nude mice bearing Calu-3 human non-small cell lung cancer xenografts with an increase of the median survival time from 55 to 96 days [172]. More recently, a second generation of these immunoRNases has been produced by the dock-and-lock (DNL) method. This methodology consists in the use of a pair of distinct protein domains that are involved in the natural association between protein kinase A (PKA; cyclic AMP-dependent protein kinase) and A-kinase-anchoring proteins. The dimerization and docking domain (DDD) found in the regulatory subunit of PKA and the anchoring domain (AD) of an interactive-A-kinase anchoring protein are each attached to a biological entity through specific linkers and the resulting derivatives, when combined, readily form a stably tethered complex of defined composition that fully retains the functions of individual constituents. That is, the docked complex can be made irreversible using a pair of linker modules that introduce Cys residues into both the DDD and the AD domains at strategic positions that facilitate the formation of disulfide bridges [173]. The integration of genetic engineering and conjugation chemistry of the DNL method has been used to get two constructs containing four ONC molecules linked to either the C_H3 or C_K C-termini of hRS7 that have been evaluated as potential therapeutics for triple-negative breast cancer (TNBC). Both constructs showed specific cell-binding and rapid internalization in MDA-MB-486, a Trop-2-expressing TNBC, and displayed potent *in vitro* cytotoxicity against diverse breast cancer cell lines. In addition, both seemed well tolerated at clinically relevant concentrations. However, C_K-based construct exhibited superior Fc-effector functions *in vitro*, as well as improved pharmacokinetics, stability, and activity *in vivo*. Further studies are needed regarding their immunogenicity although they are potentially a new class of immunoRNases that warrant future research [174].

Not only animal RNases have been used to construct immunoRNases. For instance, the construct formed by two barnase molecules fused serially to scFv of humanized 4D5 antibody directed to the extracellular domain of epidermal growth factor receptor 2 (HER2 or ErbB2) was produced [175]. This scFv 4D5-dibarnase showed cytotoxicity *in vitro* and significant *in vivo* inhibition of human breast cancer xenografts in nude mice without severe side effects [176].

The first entirely human immunoRNase was produced fusing HP-RNase to an ErbB2-specific scFv named Erbicin [177, 178]. The construct recognizes an epitope distinct to that of trastuzumab and pertuzumab [179], the two humanized antibodies currently used to treat $HER2^+$ metastatic mammary carcinomas [180, 181] and do not induce cardiac dysfunction as the other two do [182–184]. Although this immunoRNase was inhibited by the RI to an extent comparable to that of HP-RNase, the quantity that entered the cell cytosol saturated the RI, and it exhibited a clear RNA degradation ability [185]. Due to this limitation, a second generation of immunoRNases was obtained by fusing an RI-insensitive HP-RNase variant (Arg39Asp/Asn67Asp/Asn88Ala/Gly89Asp/Arg91Asp) [186] to ErbB2-specific scFv showing resistance to RI inhibition and the ability to kill mammary $ErbB2^+$ tumor cells more efficiently [187]. This variant does not show cardiotoxic effects *in vitro* and does not impair cardiac function in mouse models [188]. In addition, since bivalent immunoRNases are more powerful than monovalent ones, a dimeric variant of HP-RNase was fused to two Erbicin molecules, one per subunit [189]. The new construct was able to bind to ErbB2-positive cancer cell lines with an increased avidity with respect to the monovalent variant and was a more cytotoxic, likely due to an increased RI evasion.

2.2.4. Delivery strategies

Although RNases have reached clinical trials, one important aspect that researchers have still to cope with is to improve their tissue delivery. This means, to enhance the RNases circulating half-live in the blood and to avoid a high glomerular filtration rate. These factors contribute to an optimal pharmacokinetics and biodistribution. Related to these issues, some formulations have been carried out. One of the ways to increase persistence in circulation of small proteins such as RNases is PEGylation. Early, RNase A-PEG conjugates were randomly made [190–194]. However, although they presented increased persistence in circulation, they showed a significant reduced catalytic efficiency due to modification of the critical catalytic residue Lys 41 that abolished their cytotoxic properties. More recently, previously acylated RNase A [195] or HP-RNase [196] has been PEGylated at specific positions (Gly88Cys in RNase A and Gly89Cys in HP-RNase). Although the conjugates show a significantly reduced cytotoxicity *in vitro*, they are effective in inhibiting tumors in xenograft mouse models, likely because the diminished renal clearance *in vivo* compensates the potential loss of cytotoxicity due to the PEG moiety. Due to the efficacy of this approach, mono-PEGylation of RNase A has been studied using two chemicals, N-hydroxysuccinimide ester of S-acetylthioacetic acid (SATA) and 2-iminothiolane (IT). Both react with primary amino groups to introduce thiol groups, a process followed by PEGylation using maleimide chemistry. Interestingly, by thiolation, the original positive charges of RNase A can be conserved, an important feature in order not to lose the cationic residues. In addition, in both cases the enzymatic activity of the RNase A was essentially maintained [197].

Another method to increase the half-life of a protein in the blood is its conjugation with bovine serum albumin (BSA) [198]. However, depending on the way used to get the conjugate, albumin can decrease the enzymatic activity of RNase A. Thus, different strategies have been described to prepare RNase A-BSA conjugates to keep the bioactivity of the enzyme, although the pharmacokinetic and pharmacodynamic properties still need to be determined [199].

In an attempt to get an ONC that can circumvent renal clearance, improve tumor cell targeting, and gain endosomal escape, a modular construct has recently been described. ONC was fused to human serum albumin (HSA) through its C-terminus, and this former construct was also C-terminus appended to scFv 4D5MOCB, which targets epithelial cell adhesion molecule (EpCAM), a validated target for anticancer therapy [200] (construct Onc-HSA-4D5MOCB). In addition, in the same work, the link between ONC and the rest of the construct was also carried out through a cleavable disulfide linker (construct Onc-SS-HSA-4D5MOCB) that potentially enables the release of ONC from its carrier after endocytosis and avoids HSA inactivation of ONC catalytic activity. Although both constructs overcame most of the *in vitro* barriers, *in vivo* toxicity studies with animal models showed that they increased liver toxicity while ONC is described to produce renal toxicity [32]. Unfortunately, only the construct Onc-SS-HSA-4D5MOCB showed a reduction of tumor growth, but it was similar to that of ONC alone, and the tumor started to regrowth when treatment was discontinued [201]. Nevertheless, this all-in-one drug delivery system may inspire other constructs that can accomplish the pursued goal.

The genetic delivery of ONC using oncolytic adenovirus has just been tested. A combination of viral oncolysis with intratumoral genetic delivery of an EGFR-binding scFv antibody fragment fused to ONC (ONC_{EGFR}) has demonstrated feasible. ONC_{EGFR} expression by oncolytic viruses is possible with an optimized, replication-dependent gene expression strategy. Very interestingly, virus-encoded ONC_{EGFR} induced a potent and EGFR-dependent bystander killing of tumor cells. That is, some of the non-transformed cells die by the entry of ONC_{EGFR} released from transfected cells. Thus, ONC_{EGFR}-encoding oncolytic adenovirus showed dramatically increased cytotoxicity specifically to EGFR-positive tumor cells *in vitro* and significantly enhanced therapeutic activity in a mouse xenograft tumor model. The authors claim that this virus-antibody therapy platform can be further developed for personalized therapy by exploiting antibody diversity to target further established or emerging tumor markers or combination of thereof [202].

Finally, to avoid cerebellar neuronal toxicity while affecting glioma cells, ONC has been encapsulated in biodegradable poly(ricinoleic-co-sebacic acid) for local controlled delivery in the parietal lobe of the brain [203]. In this way ONC was released in a controlled manner and was cytotoxic against 9L glioma cells xenograft into the brain while evading neurotoxicity in the cerebellum.

3. Conclusion

The efforts to construct, produce, and characterize RNase variants to get more potent and selective non-genotoxic antitumor drugs have been successful because both natural and engineered RNases have reached clinical trials for the treatment of different types of cancer. RNases do not cleave a specific RNA molecule. Instead, their effects on gene expression are pleiotropic. This ensures a broad spectrum of synergistic interactions with other chemotherapeutics and, as stand-alone compounds, makes difficult the appearance of resistance to the drug by treated cancer cells. Thus, RNases are considered a new class of modern antitumor drugs very interesting for the pharmaceutical industry with fewer side effects than conventional chemotherapeutic treatments.

Acknowledgements

This work is supported by grants BIO2013-435217 from Ministerio de Economia y Competitividad (MINECO), Spain; SGR2014-70 from Generalitat de Catalunya, Spain; and MPCUdG2016-18 from Universitat de Girona. We are indebted to Dr. Pere Tubert for the design of **Figure 2**.

Author details

Jessica Castro[1,2], Marc Ribó[1,2], Antoni Benito[1,2] and Maria Vilanova[1,2*]

*Address all correspondence to: maria.vilanova@udg.edu

1 Protein Engineering Laboratory, Department of Biology, Faculty of Sciences, University of Girona, Girona, Spain

2 Institute of Biomedical Research of Girona "Dr. Josep Trueta" (IdIBGi), Girona, Spain

References

[1] Hanahan D, Weinberg RA. Hallmarks of cancer: the next generation. Cell. 2011;144:646–674. DOI: 10.1016/j.cell.2011.02.013

[2] Gurova K. New hopes from old drugs: revisiting DNA-binding small molecules as anticancer agents. Future Oncology. 2009;5:1685–1704. DOI: 10.2217/fon.09.127

[3] Tafech A, Bassett T, Sparanese D, Lee CH. Destroying RNA as a therapeutic approach. Current Medicinal Chemistry. 2006;13:863–881. DOI: 10.2174/092986706776361021

[4] Li WM, Barnes T, Lee CH. Endoribonucleases-enzymes gaining spotlight in mRNA metabolism. FEBS Journal. 2010;277:627–641. DOI: 10.1111/j.1742-4658.2009.07488.x

[5] Ledoux L, Baltus E. The effects of ribonuclease on cells of Ehrlich carcinoma. Experientia 1954;10:500–501. DOI: 10.1007/BF02166182

[6] Ledoux L. Action of ribonuclease on two solid tumours *in vivo*. Nature. 1955;176:36–37. DOI: 10.1038/175258b0

[7] Ledoux L, Revell SH. Action of ribonuclease on neoplastic growth. I. Chemical aspects of normal tumour growth: the Landschütz ascites tumour. Biochimica et Biophysica Acta. 1955;18:416–426

[8] Ledoux L. Action of ribonuclease on neoplastic growth. II. Action on Landschütz ascites cells *in vitro*. Biochimica et Biophysica Acta. 1956;20:369–377

[9] Aleksandrowicz J. Intracutaneous Ribonuclease in chronic myelocytic leukaemia. Lancet. 1958;272:420. DOI: 10.1016/S0140-6736(58)90139-9

[10] Telford IR, Kemp JF, Taylor EF, Yeaman MW. Effect of ribonuclease on survival of ascites tumor bearing mice. Proceedings of the Society for Experimental Biology and Medicine. 1959;100:829–831.

[11] Roth JS. Ribonuclease activity and cancer: a review. Cancer Research. 1963;23:657–666.

[12] Fang EF, Ng TB. Ribonucleases of different origins with a wide spectrum of medicinal applications. Biochimica et Biophysica Acta—Reviews on Cancer. 2011;1815:65–74. DOI: 10.1016/j.bbcan.2010.09.001

[13] Irie M. RNase T1/RNase T2 Family RNases. In: D'Alessio G, Riordan JF, editors. Ribonucleases: Structures and Functions. New York: Academic Press; 1997. p. 101–130. DOI: 10.1016/B978-012588945-2/50004-2

[14] Yoshida H. The ribonuclease T1 family. Methods in Enzymology. 2001;341:28–41. DOI: 10.1016/S0076-6879(01)41143-8

[15] Matousek J, Podzimek T, Pouckova P, Stehlik J, Skvor J, Lipovova P, et al. Antitumor activity of apoptotic nuclease TBN1 from *L. esculentum*. Neoplasma. 2010;57:339–348. DOI: 10.4149/neo_2010_04_339

[16] D'Alessio G. The Superfamily of Vertebrate-Secreted Ribonucleases. In: Nicholson AW, editor. Nucleic Acids Mol. Biol. 26. Springer Berlin Heidelberg; 2011. p. 1–34. DOI: 10.1007/978-3-642-21078-5_1

[17] Cuchillo CM, Vilanova M, Nogués MV. Pancreatic Ribonucleases. In: D'Alessio G, Riordan JF, editors. Ribonucleases: Structures and Functions. New York: Academic Press; 1997. p. 271–304.

[18] Patutina O, Mironova N, Ryabchikova E, Popova N, Nikolin V, Kaledin V, et al. Inhibition of metastasis development by daily administration of ultralow doses of RNase A and DNase I. Biochimie. 2011;93:689–696.DOI: 10.1016/j.biochi.2010.12.011

[19] Costanzi J, Sidransky D, Navon A, Goldsweig H. Ribonucleases as a novel pro-apoptotic anticancer strategy: review of the preclinical and clinical data for ranpirnase. Cancer Investigation. 2005;23:643–650. DOI: 10.1080/07357900500283143

[20] Favaretto A. Overview on ongoing or planned clinical trials in Europe. Lung Cancer. 2005;49 Suppl 1:S117–S121. DOI: 10.1016/j.lungcan.2005.03.022

[21] Pavlakis N, Vogelzang NJ. Ranpirnase-an antitumour ribonuclease: its potential role in malignant mesothelioma. Expert Opinion on Biological Therapy. 2006;6:391–399. DOI: 10.1517/14712598.6.4.391

[22] Beck AK, Pass HI, Carbone M, Yang H. Ranpirnase as a potential antitumor ribonuclease treatment for mesothelioma and other malignancies. Future Oncology. 2008;4:341–349. DOI: 10.2217/14796694.4.3.341

[23] Lee JE, Raines RT. Ribonucleases as novel chemotherapeutics: the ranpirnase example. BioDrugs. 2008;22:53–58. DOI: 10.2165/00063030-200822010-00006

[24] Porta C, Paglino C, Mutti L. Ranpirnase and its potential for the treatment of unresectable malignant mesothelioma. Biologics: Targets & Therapy. 2008;2:601–609. DOI: https://dx.doi.org/10.2147/BTT.S2383

[25] Strong LE, Kink JA, Baigen M, Shahan MN, Raines RT. First-in-human phase I clinical trial of QBI-139, a human ribonuclease variant, in solid tumors. In: ASCO Annual Meeting, editor. J. Clin. Oncol. Chicago, Illinois: ASCO University; 2012. p. suppl; abstr TPS3113.

[26] Benito A, Ribó M, Vilanova M. On the track of antitumour ribonucleases. Molecular BioSystems. 2005;1:294–302. DOI: 10.1039/b502847g

[27] Benito A, Vilanova M, Ribó M. Intracellular routing of cytotoxic pancreatic-type ribonucleases. Current Pharmaceutical Biotechnology. 2008;9:169–179.DOI: 10.2174/138920108784567281

[28] Makarov AA, Kolchinsky A, Ilinskaya ON. Binase and other microbial RNases as potential anticancer agents. Bioessays. 2008;30:781–790. DOI: 10.1002/bies.20789

[29] Rutkoski TJ, Raines RT. Evasion of ribonuclease inhibitor as a determinant of ribonuclease cytotoxicity. Current Pharmaceutical Biotechnology. 2008;9:185–189. DOI: 10.2174/138920108784567344

[30] Haigis MC, Kurten EL, Raines RT. Ribonuclease inhibitor as an intracellular sentry. Nucleic Acids Research. 2003;31:1024–1032. DOI: 10.1093/nar/gkg163

[31] Bosch M, Benito A, Ribó M, Puig T, Beaumelle B, Vilanova M. A nuclear localization sequence endows human pancreatic ribonuclease with cytotoxic activity. Biochemistry. 2004;43:2167–2177. DOI: 10.1021/bi035729+

[32] Vasandani VM, Burris JA, Sung C. Reversible nephrotoxicity of onconase and effect of lysine pH on renal onconase uptake. Cancer Chemotherapy and Pharmacology 1999;44:164–169. DOI: 10.1007/s002800050962

[33] Ardelt W, Shogen K, Darzynkiewicz Z. Onconase and amphinase, the antitumor ribonucleases from *Rana pipiens* oocytes. Current Pharmaceutical Biotechnology. 2008;9:215–225. DOI: 10.2174/138920108784567245

[34] Ribó M, Benito A, Vilanova M. Antitumor Ribonucleases. In: Nicholson AW, editor. Nucleic Acids and Molecular Biology 26. Heidelberg: Springer Berlin Heidelberg; 2011. p. 55–88. DOI: 10.1007/978-3-642-21078-5_3

[35] Michaelis M, Cinatl J, Anand P, Rothweiler F, Kotchetkov R, Deimling A Von, et al. Onconase induces caspase-independent cell death in chemoresistant neuroblastoma cells. Cancer Letters. 2007;250:107–116. DOI: 10.1016/j.canlet.2006.09.018

[36] Fiorini C, Cordani M, Gotte G, Picone D, Donadelli M. Onconase induces autophagy sensitizing pancreatic cancer cells to gemcitabine and activates Akt/mTOR pathway in a ROS-dependent manner. Biochimimica et biophysica acta. 2015;1853:549–560. DOI: 10.1016/j.bbamcr.2014.12.016

[37] Wu Y, Mikulski SM, Ardelt W, Rybak SM, Youle RJ. A cytotoxic ribonuclease. Study of the mechanism of onconase cytotoxicity. The Journal of Biological Chemistry. 1993;268:10686–10693.

[38] Goparaju CM, Blasberg JD, Volinia S, Palatini J, Ivanov S, Donington JS, et al. Onconase mediated NFKβ downregulation in malignant pleural mesothelioma. Oncogene. 2011;30:2767–2777. DOI: 10.1038/onc.2010.643

[39] Saxena SK, Sirdeshmukh R, Ardelt W, Mikulski SM, Shogen K, Youle RJ. Entry into cells and selective degradation of tRNAs by a cytotoxic member of the RNase A family. The Journal of Biological Chemistry 2002;277:15142–15146. DOI: 10.1074/jbc.M108115200

[40] Ardelt B, Ardelt W, Darzynkiewicz Z. Cytotoxic ribonucleases and RNA interference (RNAi). Cell Cycle. 2003;2:22–24. DOI: 10.4161/cc.2.1.232

[41] Zhao H, Ardelt B, Ardelt W, Shogen K, Darzynkiewicz Z. The cytotoxic ribonuclease onconase targets RNA interference (siRNA). Cell Cycle. 2008;7:3258–3261.DOI: 10.4161/cc.7.20.6855

[42] Qiao M, Zu L-D, He X-H, Shen R-L, Wang Q-C, Liu M-F. Onconase downregulates microRNA expression through targeting microRNA precursors. Cell Research 2012;22:1199–1202. DOI: 10.1038/cr.2012.67

[43] Altomare DA, Rybak SM, Pei J, Maizel J V, Cheung M, Testa JR, et al. Onconase responsive genes in human mesothelioma cells: implications for an RNA damaging therapeutic agent. BMC Cancer. 2010;10:34. DOI: 10.1186/1471-2407-10-34

[44] Singh UP, Ardelt W, Saxena SK, Holloway DE, Vidunas E, Lee HS, et al. Enzymatic and structural characterisation of amphinase, a novel cytotoxic ribonuclease from *Rana pipiens* oocytes. Journal of Molecular Biology 2007;371:93–111. DOI: 10.1016/j.jmb.2007.04.071

[45] Youle RJ, D'Alessio G. Antitumor RNases. In: D'Alessio G, Riordan JF, editors. Ribonucleases: Structures and Functions. New York: Elsevier; 1997. p. 491–514. DOI: 10.1016/B978-012588945-2/50016-9

[46] Irie M, Nitta K, Nonaka T. Biochemistry of frog ribonucleases. Cellullar and Molecular Life Sciences 1998;54:775–784. DOI: 10.1007/s000180050206

[47] Sakakibara F, Kawauchi H, Takayanagi G, Ise H. Egg lectin of *Rana japonica* and its receptor glycoprotein of Ehrlich tumor cells. Cancer Research. 1979;39:1347–1352.

[48] Okabe Y, Katayama N, Iwama M, Watanabe H, Ohgi K, Irie M, et al. Comparative base specificity, stability, and lectin activity of two lectins from eggs of *Rana catesbeiana* and *R. japonica* and liver ribonuclease from *R. catesbeiana*. Journal of Biochemistry. 1991;109:786–790.

[49] Nitta K, Ozaki K, Ishikawa M, Furusawa S, Hosono M, Kawauchi H, et al. Inhibition of cell proliferation by *Rana catesbeiana* and *Rana japonica* lectins belonging to the ribonuclease superfamily. Cancer Research. 1994;54:920–927.

[50] Tatsuta T, Sugawara S, Takahashi K, Ogawa Y, Hosono M, Nitta K. Leczyme: a new candidate drug for cancer therapy. BioMed Research International. 2014;2014:421415. DOI: 10.1155/2014/421415

[51] Haigis MC, Raines RT. Secretory ribonucleases are internalized by a dynamin-independent endocytic pathway. Journal of Cell Science. 2003;116:313–324. DOI: 10.1242/jcs.00214

[52] Rodríguez M, Torrent G, Bosch M, Rayne F, Dubremetz J-F, Ribó M, et al. Intracellular pathway of Onconase that enables its delivery to the cytosol. Journal of Cell Science. 2007;120:1405–1411. DOI: 10.1242/jcs.03427

[53] Sundlass NK, Eller CH, Cui Q, Raines RT. Contribution of electrostatics to the binding of pancreatic-type ribonucleases to membranes. Biochemistry. 2013;52:6304–6312. DOI 10.1021/bi400619m

[54] Ran S, Downes A, Thorpe PE. Increased exposure of anionic phospholipids on the surface of tumor blood vessels. Cancer Research. American Association for Cancer Research; 2002;62:6132–6140. DOI: 10.3109/09687689409160430

[55] Eller CH, Chao T-Y, Singarapu KK, Ouerfelli O, Yang G, Markley JL, et al. Human cancer antigen Globo H is a cell-surface ligand for human ribonuclease 1. ACS Central Science 2015;1:181–190. DOI: 10.1021/acscentsci.5b00164

[56] Zhang S, Cordon-Cardo C, Zhang HS, Reuter VE, Adluri S, Hamilton WB, et al. Selection of tumor antigens as targets for immune attack using immunohistochemistry: I. Focus on gangliosides. International Journal of Cancer. 1997;73:42–49. DOI: 10.1002/(SICI)1097-0215(19970926)73:1<42::AID-IJC8>3.0.CO;2-1

[57] Chao T-Y, Raines RT. Mechanism of ribonuclease A endocytosis: analogies to cell-penetrating peptides. Biochemistry. 2011;50:8374–8382. DOI: 10.1021/bi2009079

[58] Shirshikov F V., Cherepnev G V., Ilinskaya ON, Kalacheva N V. A hydrophobic segment of some cytotoxic ribonucleases. Medical Hypotheses. 2013;81:328–334. DOI: 10.1016/j.mehy.2013.04.006

[59] Murthy BS, Sirdeshmukh R. Sensitivity of monomeric and dimeric forms of bovine seminal ribonuclease to human placental ribonuclease inhibitor. Biochemical Journal. 1992;281:343–348. DOI: 10.1042/bj2810343

[60] D'Alessio G, Di Donato A, Mazzarella L, Piccoli R. Seminal ribonuclease: the importance of diversity. ribonucleases: structures and functions. New York: Academic Press; 1997. p. 383–423.

[61] Sica F, Di Fiore A, Merlino A, Mazzarella L. Structure and stability of the non-covalent swapped dimer of bovine seminal ribonuclease: an enzyme tailored to evade ribonuclease protein inhibitor. The Journal of Biological Chemistry. 2004;279:36753–36760. DOI: 10.1074/jbc.M405655200

[62] Benito A, Laurents D V, Ribó M, Vilanova M. The structural determinants that lead to the formation of particular oligomeric structures in the pancreatic-type ribonuclease family. Current Protein and Peptide Science 2008;9:370–393. DOI: 10.2174/138920308785132695

[63] Gotte G, Laurents D V., Merlino A, Picone D, Spadaccini R. Structural and functional relationships of natural and artificial dimeric bovine ribonucleases: new scaffolds for potential antitumor drugs. FEBS Letters. 2013;587:3601–3608. DOI: 10.1016/j.febslet.2013.09.038

[64] Mastronicola MR, Piccoli R, D'Alessio G. Key extracellular and intracellular steps in the antitumor action of seminal ribonuclease. European Journal of Biochemistry. 1995;230:242–249. DOI: 10.1111/j.1432-1033.1995.0242i.x

[65] Bracale A, Spalletti-Cernia D, Mastronicola M, Castaldi F, Mannucci R, Nitsch L, et al. Essential stations in the intracellular pathway of cytotoxic bovine seminal ribonuclease. Biochemical Journal. 2002;362:553–560. DOI: 10.1042/bj3620553

[66] Kim JS, Soucek J, Matousek J, Raines RT. Mechanism of ribonuclease cytotoxicity. The Journal of Biological Chemistry. 1995;270:31097–31102. DOI: 10.1074/jbc.270.52.31097

[67] Wu Y, Saxena SK, Ardelt W, Gadina M, Mikulski SM, De Lorenzo C, et al. A study of the intracellular routing of cytotoxic ribonucleases. The Journal of Biological Chemistry. 1995;270:17476–17481. DOI: 10.1074/jbc.270.29.17476

[68] Mancheno JM, Gasset M, Onaderra M, Gavilanes JG, Dalessio G. Bovine Seminal Ribonuclease Destabilizes Negatively Charged Membranes. Biochemical Biophysical Research Communications. 1994;199:119–124. DOI: 10.1006/bbrc.1994.1202

[69] Notomista E, Mancheño JM, Crescenzi O, Di Donato A, Gavilanes J, D'Alessio G. The role of electrostatic interactions in the antitumor activity of dimeric RNases. FEBS Journal. 2006;273:3687–3697. DOI: 10.1111/j.1742-4658.2006.05373.x

[70] Viola M, Libra M, Callari D, Sinatra F, Spada D, Noto D, et al. Bovine seminal ribonuclease is cytotoxic for both malignant and normal telomerase-positive cells. International Journal of Oncology. 2005;27:1071–1077. DOI: 10.3892/ijo.27.4.1071

[71] Fiorini C, Gotte G, Donnarumma F, Picone D, Donadelli M. Bovine seminal ribonuclease triggers Beclin1-mediated autophagic cell death in pancreatic cancer cells. Biochimica et Biophysica Acta—Molecular Cell Research 2014;1843:976–984. DOI: 10.1016/j.bbamcr.2014.01.025

[72] Ng T. Peptides and proteins from fungi. Peptides. 2004;25:1055–1073. DOI: 10.1016/j.peptides.2004.03.013

[73] Wong JH, Ng TB, Cheung RCF, Ye XJ, Wang HX, Lam SK, et al. Proteins with antifungal properties and other medicinal applications from plants and mushrooms. Applied Microbiology and Biotechnology. 2010;87:1221–1235. DOI: 10.1007/s00253-010-2690-4

[74] Hameş EE, Demir T. Microbial ribonucleases (RNases): production and application potential. World Journal of Microbiology and Biotechnology. 2015;31:1853–1862. DOI: 10.1007/s11274-015-1945-8

[75] Skvor J, Lipovová P, Poucková P, Soucek J, Slavík T, Matousek J. Effect of wheat leaf ribonuclease on tumor cells and tissues. Anticancer Drugs. 2006;17:815–823. DOI: 10.1097/01.cad.0000217430.75078.cc

[76] Soucek J, Skvor J, Poucková P, Matousek J, Slavík T, Matousek J. Mung bean sprout (*Phaseolus aureus*) nuclease and its biological and antitumor effects. Neoplasma. 2006;53:402–409.

[77] Lipovova P, Podzimek T, Orctova L, Matousek J, Pouckova P, Soucek J, et al. Antitumor and biological effects of black pine (*Pinus nigra*) pollen nuclease. Neoplasma. 2008;55:158–164.

[78] Matousek J, Matousek J. Plant ribonucleases and nucleases as antiproliferative agens targeting human tumors growing in mice. Recent Patents on DNA and Gene Sequences. 2010;4:29–39. DOI:10.2174/187221510790410813

[79] Fang EF, Zhang CZY, Fong WP, Ng TB. RNase MC2: a new Momordica charantia ribonuclease that induces apoptosis in breast cancer cells associated with activation of MAPKs and induction of caspase pathways. Apoptosis. 2012;17:377–387. DOI:10.1007/s10495-011-0684-z

[80] Mironova NL, Petrushanko IY, Patutina OA, Sen'kova A V, Simonenko O V, Mitkevich VA, et al. Ribonuclease binase inhibits primary tumor growth and metastases via apoptosis induction in tumor cells. Cell Cycle. 2013;12:2120–2131.DOI: 10.4161/cc.25164

[81] Mitkevich VA, Petrushanko IY, Spirin P V, Fedorova T V, Kretova O V, Tchurikov NA, et al. Sensitivity of acute myeloid leukemia Kasumi-1 cells to binase toxic action depends on the expression of KIT and AML1-ETO oncogenes. Cell Cycle. 2011;10:4090–4097. DOI: 10.4161/cc.10.23.18210

[82] Sen'kova AV, Mironova NL, Patutina OA, Mitkevich VA, Markov OV, Petrushanko IY, et al. Ribonuclease binase decreases destructive changes of the liver and restores its regeneration potential in mouse lung carcinoma model. Biochimie. 2014;101:256-259. DOI: 10.1016/j.biochi.2014.02.006

[83] Kobe B, Deisenhofer J. Mechanism of ribonuclease inhibition by ribonuclease inhibitor protein based on the crystal structure of its complex with ribonuclease A. Journal of Molecular Biology. 1996;264:1028–1043. DOI: 10.1006/jmbi.1996.0694

[84] Leland PA, Schultz LW, Kim B-M, Raines RT. Ribonuclease A variants with potent cytotoxic activity. Proceedings of the National Academy of Sciences. 1998;95:10407–10412. DOI: 10.1073/pnas.95.18.10407

[85] Leland PA, Staniszewski KE, Kim BM, Raines RT. Endowing human pancreatic ribonuclease with toxicity for cancer cells. The Journal of Biological Chemistry. 2001;276:43095–43102. DOI:10.1074/jbc.M106636200

[86] Gaur D, Swaminathan S, Batra JK. Interaction of human pancreatic ribonuclease with human ribonuclease inhibitor. Generation of inhibitor-resistant cytotoxic variants. The Journal of Biological Chemistry. 2001;276:24978–24984. DOI: 10.1074/jbc.M102440200

[87] Antignani A, Naddeo M, Cubellis M V, Russo A, D'Alessio G. Antitumor action of seminal ribonuclease, its dimeric structure, and its resistance to the cytosolic ribonuclease inhibitor. Biochemistry. 2001;40:3492–3496. DOI: 10.1021/bi002781m

[88] Lee JE, Raines RT. Cytotoxicity of bovine seminal ribonuclease: monomer versus dimer. Biochemistry. 2005;44:15760–15767. DOI: 10.1021/bi051668z

[89] Bretscher LE, Abel RL, Raines RT. A ribonuclease A variant with low catalytic activity but high cytotoxicity. The Journal of Biological Chemistry. 2000;275:9893–9896. DOI: 10.1074/jbc.275.14.9893

[90] Haigis MC, Kurten EL, Abel RL, Raines RT. KFERQ sequence in ribonuclease A-mediated cytotoxicity. The Journal of Biological Chemistry. 2002;277:11576–11581. DOI: 10.1074/jbc.M112227200

[91] Rutkoski TJ, Kurten EL, Mitchell JC, Raines RT. Disruption of shape-complementarity markers to create cytotoxic variants of ribonuclease A. Journal of Molecular Biology. 2005;354:41–54. DOI: 10.1016/j.jmb.2005.08.007

[92] Johnson RJ, Chao TY, Lavis LD, Raines RT. Cytotoxic ribonucleases: the dichotomy of Coulombic forces. Biochemistry. 2007;46:10308–10316. DOI: 10.1021/bi700857u

[93] Dickson KA, Dahlberg CL, Raines RT. Compensating effects on the cytotoxicity of ribonuclease A variants. Archives of Biochemistry and Biophysics. 2003;415:172–177. DOI: 10.1016/S0003-9861(03)00214-5

[94] Klink TA, Raines RT. Conformational stability is a determinant of ribonuclease A cytotoxicity. The Journal of Biological Chemistry. 2000;275:17463–17467. DOI: 10.1074/jbc.M001132200

[95] Kim B-M, Kim H, Raines RT, Lee Y. Glycosylation of onconase increases its conformational stability and toxicity for cancer cells. Biochemical and Biophysical Research Communications. 2004;315:976–983. DOI: 10.1016/j.bbrc.2004.01.153

[96] Libonati M. Biological actions of the oligomers of ribonuclease A. Cellular and Molecular Life Sciences. 2004;61:2431–2436. DOI: 10.1007/s00018-004-4302-x

[97] Libonati M, Gotte G, Vottariello F. A novel biological actions acquired by ribonuclease through oligomerization. Current Pharmaceutical Biotechnology. 2008;9:200–209. DOI: 10.2174/138920108784567308

[98] Cafaro V, De Lorenzo C, Piccoli R, Bracale A, Mastronicola MR, Di Donato A, et al. The antitumor action of seminal ribonuclease and its quaternary conformations. FEBS Letters. 1995;359:31–34. DOI: 10.1016/0014-5793(94)01450-F

[99] Merlino A, Ercole C, Picone D, Pizzo E, Mazzarella L, Sica F. The buried diversity of bovine seminal ribonuclease: shape and cytotoxicity of the swapped non-covalent form of the enzyme. Journal of Molecular Biology 2008;376:427–437. DOI: 10.1016/j.jmb.2007.11.008

[100] Di Gaetano S, D'alessio G, Piccoli R. Second generation antitumour human RNase: significance of its structural and functional features for the mechanism of antitumour action. Biochemical Journal. 2001;358:241–247. DOI: 10.1042/bj3580241

[101] Bartholeyns J, Baudhuin P. Inhibition of tumor cell proliferation by dimerized ribonuclease. Proceedings of the National Academy of Sciences of the United States of America. 1976;73:573–576.

[102] Tarnowski GS, Kassel RL, Mountain IM, Blackburn P, Wilson G, Wang D. Comparison of antitumor activities of pancreatic ribonuclease and its cross-linked dimer. Cancer Research. 1976;36:4074–4078.

[103] Gotte G, Testolin L, Costanzo C, Sorrentino S, Armato U, Libonati M. Cross-linked trimers of bovine ribonuclease A: activity on double-stranded RNA and antitumor action. FEBS Letters. 1997;415:308–312. DOI: 10.1016/S0014-5793(97)01147-2

[104] Kim JS, Soucek J, Matousek J, Raines RT. Catalytic activity of bovine seminal ribonuclease is essential for its immunosuppressive and other biological activities. Biochemical Journal. 1995;308:547–550. DOI: 10.1042/bj3080547

[105] Suzuki M, Saxena SK, Boix E, Prill RJ, Vasandani VM, Ladner JE, et al. Engineering receptor-mediated cytotoxicity into human ribonucleases by steric blockade of inhibitor interaction. Nature Biotechnology. 1999;17:265–270. DOI: 10.1038/7010

[106] Rutkoski TJ, Kink J.A., Strong LE, Schilling CI, Raines RT. Antitumor activity of ribonuclease multimers created by site-specific covalent tethering. Bioconjugate Chemistry. 2010;21:1691–1702. DOI: 10.1021/bc100292x

[107] Leich F, Köditz J, Ulbrich-Hofman R, Arnold U. Tandemization endows bovine pancreatic ribonuclease with cytotoxic activity. Journal of Molecular Biology. 2006;358:1305–1313. DOI: 10.1016/j.jmb.2006.03.007

[108] Arnold U, Leich F, Neumann P, Lilie H, Ulbrich-Hofmann R. Crystal structure of RNase A tandem enzymes and their interaction with the cytosolic ribonuclease inhibitor. FEBS Journal. 2011;278:331–340. DOI: 10.1111/j.1742-4658.2010.07957.x

[109] Gotte G, Bertoldi M, Libonati M. Structural versatility of bovine ribonuclease A. Distinct conformers of trimeric and tetrameric aggregates of the enzyme. European Journal of Biochemistry 1999;265:680–687. DOI: 10.1046/j.1432-1327.1999.00761.x

[110] Gotte G, Laurents D V., Libonati M. Three-dimensional domain-swapped oligomers of ribonuclease A: identification of a fifth tetramer, pentamers and hexamers, and detection of trace heptameric, octameric and nonameric species. Biochimica et Biophysica Acta—Proteins Proteomics. 2006;1764:44–54. DOI: 10.1016/j.bbapap.2005.10.011

[111] López-Alonso JP, Gotte G, Laurents DV. Kinetic analysis provides insight into the mechanism of Ribonuclease A oligomer formation. Archives of Biochemistry and Biophysics. 2009;489:41–47. DOI: 10.1016/j.abb.2009.07.013

[112] Matousek J, Gotte G, Pouckova P, Soucek J, Slavik T, Vottariello F, et al. Antitumor activity and other biological actions of oligomers of ribonuclease A. The Journal of Biological Chemistry. 2003;278:23817–23822. DOI: 10.1074/jbc.M302711200

[113] Cafaro V, Bracale A, Di Maro A, Sorrentino S, D'Alessio G, Di Donato A. New muteins of RNase A with enhanced antitumor action. FEBS Letters. 1998;437:149–152. DOI: 10.1016/S0014-5793(98)01221-6

[114] Balderas-Renteria I, Gonzalez-Barranco P, Garcia A, Banik BK, Rivera G. Anticancer drug design using scaffolds of β-lactams, sulfonamides, quinoline, quinoxaline and natural products. Drugs advances in clinical trials. Current Medicinal Chemistry. 2012;19:4377–4398. DOI: 10.2174/092986712803251593

[115] Schapira M. Pharmacogenomics opportunities in nuclear receptor targeted cancer therapy. Current Cancer Drug Targets. 2002;2:243–256.

[116] Vassaux G, Martin-Duque P. Use of suicide genes for cancer gene therapy: study of the different approaches.Expert Opinion on Biological Therapy. 2004; 4:519–530. DOI: 10.1517/14712598.4.4.519

[117] Kuusisto H V, Wagstaff KM, Alvisi G, Roth DM, Jans DA. Global enhancement of nuclear localization-dependent nuclear transport in transformed cells. FASEB Journal. 2012;26:1181–1193. DOI: 10.1096/fj.11-191585

[118] Costantini DL, Chan C, Cai Z, Vallis KA, Reilly RM. 111In-Labeled Trastuzumab (Herceptin) Modified with Nuclear Localization Sequences (NLS): an Auger Electron-Emitting Radiotherapeutic Agent for HER2/neu-Amplified Breast Cancer. Journal Nuclear Medicine, Society of Nuclear Medicine. 2007;48:1357–1368.DOI: 10.2967/jnumed.106.037937

[119] Costantini DL, McLarty K, Lee H, Done SJ, Vallis KA, Reilly RM. Antitumor effects and normal-tissue toxicity of 111In-nuclear localization sequence-trastuzumab in athymic mice bearing HER-positive human breast cancer xenografts. Journal of Nuclear Medicine. 2010;51:1084–1091. DOI: 10.2967/jnumed.109.072389

[120] Misra R, Sahoo SK. Intracellular trafficking of nuclear localization signal conjugated nanoparticles for cancer therapy. European Journal of Pharmaceutical Sciences. 2010;39:152–163. DOI: 10.1016/j.ejps.2009.11.010

[121] Arís A, Villaverde A. Engineering nuclear localization signals in modular protein vehicles for gene therapy. Biochemistry and Biophysical Research Communications. 2003;304:625–631. DOI: 10.1016/S0006-291X(03)00644-2

[122] Akhlynina T V, Jans DA, Statsyuk N V, Balashova IY, Toth G, Pavo I, et al. Adenoviruses synergize with nuclear localization signals to enhance nuclear delivery and photodynamic action of internalizable conjugates containing chlorin e6. International Journal of Cancer. 1999;81:734–740. DOI: 10.1002/(SICI)1097-0215(19990531)81:5<734::AID-IJC12>3.0.CO;2-J

[123] Akhlynina T V, Jans DA, Rosenkranz AA, Statsyuk N V, Balashova IY, Toth G, et al. Nuclear targeting of chlorin e6 enhances its photosensitizing activity. The Journal of Biological Chemistry. 1997;272:20328–20331. DOI: 10.1074/jbc.272.33.20328

[124] Roth JS, Juster H. On the absence of ribonuclease inhibitor in rat liver nuclei. Biochimica et Biophysica Acta—Nucleic Acids Protein Synthesis. 1972;287:474–476. DOI: 10.1016/0005-2787(72)90291-2

[125] Furia A, Moscato M, Calì G, Pizzo E, Confalone E, Amoroso MR, et al. The ribonuclease/angiogenin inhibitor is also present in mitochondria and nuclei. FEBS Letters. 2011;585:613–617. DOI: 10.1016/j.febslet.2011.01.034

[126] Rodríguez M, Benito A., Tubert P, Castro J, Ribó M, Beaumelle B, et al. A cytotoxic ribonuclease variant with a discontinuous nuclear localization signal constituted by basic residues scattered over three areas of the molecule. Journal of Molecular Biology 2006;360:548–557. DOI: 10.1016/j.jmb.2006.05.048

[127] Tubert P, Rodríguez M, Ribó M, Benito A, Vilanova M. The nuclear transport capacity of a human-pancreatic ribonuclease variant is critical for its cytotoxicity. Investigational New Drugs. 2011;29:811–817. DOI: 10.1007/s10637-010-9426-2

[128] Castro J, Ribó M, Benito A, Vilanova M. Mini-review: nucleus-targeted ribonucleases as antitumor drugs. Current Medicinal Chemistry. 2013;20:1225–1231. DOI: 10.2174/0929867311320100003

[129] Castro J, Ribó M, Navarro S, Nogués MV, Vilanova M, Benito A. A human ribonuclease induces apoptosis associated with p21WAF1/CIP1 induction and JNK inactivation. BMC Cancer. 2011;11:9. DOI: 10.1186/1471-2407-11-9

[130] Castro J, Ribó M, Puig T, Colomer R, Vilanova M, Benito A. A cytotoxic ribonuclease reduces the expression level of P-glycoprotein in multidrug-resistant cell lines. Investigational New Drugs. 2012;30:880–888. DOI: 10.1007/s10637-011-9636-2

[131] Vert A, Castro J, Ribó M, Benito A, Vilanova M. A nuclear-directed human pancreatic ribonuclease (PE5) targets the metabolic phenotype of cancer cells. Oncotarget. 2016;7:18309–18324. DOI: 10.18632/oncotarget.7579

[132] Vert A, Castro J, Ruiz-Martínez S, Tubert P, Escribano D, Ribó M, et al. Generation of new cytotoxic human ribonuclease variants directed to the nucleus. Molecular Pharmaceutics 2012;9:2894–2902. DOI: 10.1021/mp300217b

[133] Chao T-Y, Lavis LD, Raines RT. Cellular uptake of ribonuclease A relies on anionic glycans. Biochemistry. 2010;49:10666–10673. DOI: 10.1021/bi1013485

[134] Futami J, Maeda T, Kitazoe M, Nukui E, Tada H, Seno M, et al. Preparation of potent cytotoxic ribonucleases by cationization: enhanced cellular uptake and decreased interaction with ribonuclease inhibitor by chemical modification of carboxyl groups. Biochemistry. 2001;40:7518–7524. DOI: 10.1021/bi010248g

[135] Futami J, Nukui E, Maeda T, Kosaka M, Tada H, Seno M, et al. Optimum modification for the highest cytotoxicity of cationized ribonuclease. Journal of Biochemistry. 2002;132:223–228.

[136] Iwama M, Ogawa Y, Sasaki N, Nitta K, Takayanagi Y, Ohgi K, et al. Effect of modification of the carboxyl groups of the sialic acid binding lectin from bullfrog (Rana catesbeiana) oocyte on anti-tumor activity. Biological and Pharmaceutical Bulletin. 2001;24:978–981. DOI: http://doi.org/10.1248/bpb.24.978

[137] Poučková P, Morbio M, Vottariello F, Laurents D V., Matoušek J, Souček J, et al. Cytotoxicity of polyspermine-ribonuclease A and polyspermine-dimeric ribonuclease A. Bioconjugate Chemistry. 2007;18:1946–1955. DOI: 10.1021/bc700253c

[138] Ogawa Y, Iwama M, Ohgi K, Tsuji T, Irie M, Itagaki T, et al. Effect of replacing the aspartic acid/glutamic acid residues of bullfrog sialic acid binding lectin with asparagine/glutamine and arginine on the inhibition of cell proliferation in murine leukemia P388 cells. Biological and Pharmaceutical Bulletin. 2002;25:722–727. DOI: http://doi.org/10.1248/bpb.25.722

[139] Ilinskaya ON, Dreyer F, Mitkevich VA, Shaw KL, Pace CN, Makarov AA. Changing the net charge from negative to positive makes ribonuclease Sa cytotoxic. Protein Science 2002;11:2522–2525. DOI: 10.1110/ps.0216702.toward

[140] Ilinskaya ON, Koschinski A, Mitkevich VA, Repp H, Dreyer F, Pace CN, et al. Cytotoxicity of RNases is increased by cationization and counteracted by KCa channels. Biochemical and Biophysical Research Communications. 2004;314:550–554. DOI: 10.1016/j.bbrc.2003.12.110

[141] D'Errico G, Ercole C, Lista M, Pizzo E, Falanga A, Galdiero S, et al. Enforcing the positive charge of N-termini enhances membrane interaction and antitumor activity of bovine seminal ribonuclease. Biochimimica et Biophysica Acta—Biomembranes 2011;1808:3007–3015. DOI: 10.1016/j.bbamem.2011.08.009

[142] Fuchs SM, Rutkoski TJ, Kung VM, Groeschl RT, Raines RT. Increasing the potency of a cytotoxin with an arginine graft. Protein Engineering, Design and Selection. 2007;20:505–509. DOI: 10.1093/protein/gzm051

[143] Fuchs SM, Raines RT. Polyarginine as a multifunctional fusion tag. Protein Science. 2005;14:1538–1544. DOI: 10.1110/ps.051393805

[144] Ellis GA, Hornung ML, Raines RT. Potentiation of ribonuclease cytotoxicity by a poly(amidoamine) dendrimer. Bioorganic & Medicinal Chemistry Letters. 2011;21:2756-2758 DOI: 10.1016/j.bmcl.2010.11.028

[145] Dübel S. Handbook of Therapeutic Antibodies. Dübel S, Reichert JM, editors. Weinheim, Germany: Wiley-VCH Verlag GmbH & Co. KGaA; 2014. 2188 p. DOI: 10.1002/9783527682423

[146] Guillard S, Minter RR, Jackson RH. Engineering therapeutic proteins for cell entry: the natural approach. Trends in Biotechnology. 2015;33:163–171. DOI: 10.1016/j.tibtech. 2014.12.004

[147] Arkin MR, Tang Y, Wells JA. Small-molecule inhibitors of protein-protein interactions: progressing toward the reality. Chemistry and Biology. 2014;21:1102–1114.DOI: 10.1016/j.chembiol.2014.09.001

[148] Rybak SM, Saxena SK, Ackerman EJ, Youle RJ. Cytotoxic potential of ribonuclease and ribonuclease hybrid proteins. The Journal of Biological Chemistry. 1991;266:21202–21207.

[149] Newton DL, Ilercil O, Laske DW, Oldfield E, Rybak SM, Youle RJ. Cytotoxic ribonuclease chimeras. Targeted tumoricidal activity *in vitro* and *in vivo*. The Journal of Biological Chemistry. 1992;267:19572–19578.

[150] Rybak SM, Newton DL, Mikulski SM, Viera A, Youle RJ. Cytotoxic onconase and ribonuclease a chimeras: comparison and *in vitro* characterization. Drug Delivery. 1993;1:3–10. DOI: 10.3109/10717549309031335

[151] Rybak SM. Antibody-onconase conjugates: cytotoxicity and intracellular routing. Current Pharmaceutical Biotechnolology. 2008;9:226–230. DOI: 10.2174/138920108784567272

[152] Newton DL, Hansen HJ, Mikulski SM, Goldenberg DM, Rybak SM. Potent and specific antitumor effects of an anti-CD22-targeted cytotoxic ribonuclease: Potential for the treatment of non-Hodgkin lymphoma. Blood. 2001;97:528–535. DOI: 10.1182/blood.V97.2.528

[153] Schirrmann T, Krauss J, Arndt MAE, Rybak SM, Dübel S. Targeted therapeutic RNases (ImmunoRNases). Expert Opinion on Biological Therapy. 2009;9:79–95. DOI: 10.1517/14712590802631862

[154] Newton DL, Pollock D, DiTullio P, Echelard Y, Harvey M, Wilburn B, et al. Antitransferrin receptor antibody-RNase fusion protein expressed in the mammary gland of transgenic mice. Journal of Immunological Methods. 1999;231:159–167. DOI: 10.1016/S0022-1759(99)00154-4

[155] Cuchillo CM, Nogués MV, Raines RT. Bovine pancreatic ribonuclease: fifty years of the first enzymatic reaction mechanism. Biochemistry. 2011;50:7835–7841. DOI: 10.1021/bi201075b

[156] Garin-Chesa P, Campbell I, Saigo PE, Lewis JL, Old LJ, Rettig WJ. Trophoblast and ovarian cancer antigen LK26. Sensitivity and specificity in immunopathology and molecular identification as a folate-binding protein. The American journal of pathology. 1993;142:557–567.

[157] Ross JF, Chaudhuri PK, Ratnam M. Differential regulation of folate receptor isoforms in normal and malignant tissues *in vivo* and in established cell lines. Physiologic and

clinical implications. Cancer. 1994;73:2432–2443. DOI: 10.1002/1097-0142(19940501)73:9<2432::AID-CNCR2820730929>3.0.CO;2-S

[158] Smith BD, Higgin JJ, Raines RT. Site-specific folate conjugation to a cytotoxic protein. Bioorganic & Medicinal Chemistry Letters. 2011;21:5029-5032. DOI: 10.1016/j.bmcl. 2011.04.081

[159] Rybak SM, Newton DL. Immunotoxins and beyond: targeted RNases. In: Dübel S, editor. Handbook of Therapeutic Antibodies. Weinheim, Germany: Wiley-VCH Verlag GmbH; 2007. p. 379–410. DOI: 10.1002/9783527619740.ch16

[160] Hudson PJ, Souriau C. Engineered antibodies. Nature Medicine. 2003;9:129–134.DOI: 10.1038/nm0103-129

[161] Sorrentino S. The eight human "canonical" ribonucleases: Molecular diversity, catalytic properties, and special biological actions of the enzyme proteins. FEBS Letters. 2010;584:2194–2200. DOI: 10.1016/j.febslet.2010.04.018

[162] Newton DL, Nicholls PJ, Rybak SM, Youle RJ. Expression and characterization of recombinant human eosinophil-derived neurotoxin and eosinophil-derived neurotox-in-anti-transferrin receptor sFv. The Journal of Biological Chemistry. 1994;269:26739–26745.

[163] Arndt MAE, Krauss J, Vu BK, Newton DL, Rybak SM. A dimeric angiogenin immuno-fusion protein mediates selective toxicity toward CD22+ tumor cells. Journal of Immunotherapy. 2005;28:245–251.

[164] Krauss J, Arndt MAE, Vu BK, Newton DL, Seeber S, Rybak SM. Efficient killing of CD22+ tumor cells by a humanized diabody–RNase fusion protein. Biochemical and Biophysical Research Communications. 2005;331:595–602. DOI: 10.1016/j.bbrc. 2005.03.215

[165] Krauss J, Arndt MAE, Vu BK, Newton DL, Rybak SM. Targeting malignant B-cell lymphoma with a humanized anti-CD22 scFv-angiogenin immunoenzyme. British Journal of Haematology. 2005;128:602–609. DOI: 10.1111/j. 1365-2141.2005.05356.x

[166] Braschoss S, Hirsch B, Dübel S, Stein H, MD HD. New anti-CD30 human pancreatic ribonuclease-based immunotoxin reveals strong and specific cytotoxicity *in vivo*. Leukemia & Lymphoma. 2009;48:1179-1186. DOI: 10.1080/10428190701272264

[167] Menzel C, Schirrmann T, Konthur Z, Jostock T, Dübel S. Human antibody RNase fusion protein targeting CD30+ lymphomas. Blood. 2008;111:3830–3837.DOI: 10.1182/ blood-2007-04-082768

[168] Stöcker M, Tur MK, Sasse S, Krüßmann A, Barth S, Engert A. Secretion of functional anti-CD30-angiogenin immunotoxins into the supernatant of transfected 293T-cells. Protein Expression and Purification. 2003;28:211–219. DOI: 10.1016/ S1046-5928(02)00709-X

[169] Kiesgen S, Liebers N, Cremer M, Arnold U, Weber T, Keller A, et al. A fusogenic dengue virus-derived peptide enhances antitumor efficacy of an antibody-ribonuclease fusion protein targeting the EGF receptor. Protein Engineering, Design and Selection. 2014;27:331–337. DOI: 10.1093/protein/gzu040

[170] Kiesgen S, Arndt MAE, Körber C, Arnold U, Weber T, Halama N, et al. An EGF receptor targeting Ranpirnase-diabody fusion protein mediates potent antitumour activity *in vitro* and *in vivo*. Cancer Letters. 2015;357:364–373. DOI: 10.1016/j.canlet.2014.11.054

[171] Rapani E, Sacchetti A, Corda D, Alberti S. Human TROP-2 is a tumor-associated calcium signal transducer. International Journal of Cancer. 1998;76:671–676. DOI: 10.1002/(SICI)1097-0215(19980529)76:5<671::AI

[172] Chang C-H, Gupta P, Michel R, Loo M, Wang Y, Cardillo TM, et al. Ranpirnase (frog RNase) targeted with a humanized, internalizing, anti-Trop-2 antibody has potent cytotoxicity against diverse epithelial cancer cells. Molecular Cancer Therapeutics; 2010;9:2276–2286. DOI: 10.1158/1535-7163.MCT-10-0338

[173] Chang C-H, Rossi EA, Goldenberg DM. The dock and lock method: a novel platform technology for building multivalent, multifunctional structures of defined composition with retained bioactivity. Clinical Cancer Research; 2007;13:5586s –5591s. DOI: 10.1158/1078-0432.CCR-07-1217

[174] Liu D, Cardillo TM, Wang Y, Rossi EA, Goldenberg DM, Chang C-H, et al. Trop-2-targeting tetrakis-ranpirnase has potent antitumor activity against triple-negative breast cancer. Molecular Cancer. 2014;13:53. DOI: 10.1186/1476-4598-13-53

[175] Glinka EM, Edelweiss EF, Sapozhnikov AM, Deyev SM. A new vector for controllable expression of an anti-HER2/neu mini-antibody-barnase fusion protein in HEK 293T cells. Gene. 2006;366:97–103. DOI: 10.1016/j.gene.2005.06.042

[176] Balandin TG, Edelweiss E, Andronova N V., Treshalina EM, Sapozhnikov AM, Deyev SM. Antitumor activity and toxicity of anti-HER2 immunoRNase scFv 4D5-dibarnase in mice bearing human breast cancer xenografts. Investigational New Drugs. 2011;29:22–32. DOI: 10.1007/s10637-009-9329-2

[177] De Lorenzo C, Palmer DB, Piccoli R, Ritter MA, D'Alessio G. A new human antitumor immunoreagent specific for ErbB2. Clinical Cancer Research; 2002;8:1710–1719. DOI: 10.1038/319230a0

[178] De Lorenzo C, Arciello A, Cozzolino R, Palmer DB, Laccetti P, Piccoli R, et al. A fully human antitumor immunoRNase selective for ErbB-2-positive carcinomas. Cancer Research. 2004;64:4870–4874. DOI: 10.1158/0008-5472.CAN-03-3717

[179] Troise F, Monti M, Merlino A, Cozzolino F, Fedele C, Russo Krauss I, et al. A novel ErbB2 epitope targeted by human antitumor immunoagents. FEBS Journal. 2011;278:1156–1166.DOI: 10.1111/j.1742-4658.2011.08041.x

[180] Romond EH, Perez EA, Bryant J, Suman VJ, Geyer CEJ, Davidson NE, et al. Trastuzumab plus Adjuvant Chemotherapy for Operable HER2-Positive Breast Cancer. The New England journal of medicine. 2005;353: 1673-1684 DOI: 10.1056/NEJMoa052122

[181] Chung C, Lam MSH. Pertuzumab for the treatment of human epidermal growth factor receptor type 2-positive metastatic breast cancer. American Journal of Health-System Pharmacy. 2013;70:1579–1587. DOI: 10.2146/ajhp120735

[182] Gelardi T, Damiano V, Rosa R, Bianco R, Cozzolino R, Tortora G, et al. Two novel human anti-ErbB2 immunoagents are active on trastuzumab-resistant tumours. British Journal of Cancer. 2010;102:513–519. DOI: 10.1038/sj.bjc.6605499

[183] Perez EA, Suman VJ, Davidson NE, Martino S, Kaufman PA, Lingle WL, et al. HER2 testing by local, central, and reference laboratories in specimens from the north central cancer treatment group n9831 intergroup adjuvant trial. Journal of Clinical Oncology. 2006;24:3032–3038. DOI: 10.1200/JCO.2005.03.4744

[184] Lenihan D, Suter T, Brammer M, Neate C, Ross G, Baselga J. Pooled analysis of cardiac safety in patients with cancer treated with pertuzumab. Annals of Oncology. 2012;23:791–800. DOI: 10.1093/annonc/mdr294

[185] De Lorenzo C, Di Malta C Di, CalÌ G, Troise F, Nitsch L, D'Alessio G. Intracellular route and mechanism of action of ERB-hRNase, a human anti-ErbB2 anticancer immunoagent. FEBS Letters. 2007;581:296–300. DOI: 10.1016/j.febslet.2006.12.034

[186] Johnson RJ, McCoy JG, Bingman CA, Phillips GN, Raines RT. Inhibition of human pancreatic ribonuclease by the human ribonuclease inhibitor protein. Journal of Molecular Biology 2007;368:434–449. DOI: 10.1016/j.jmb.2007.02.005

[187] Riccio G, D'avino C, Raines RT, De Lorenzo C. A novel fully human antitumor ImmunoRNase resistant to the RNase inhibitor. Protein Engineering, Design and Selection. 2013;26:243–248.DOI: 10.1093/protein/gzs101

[188] D'Avino C, Paciello R, Riccio G, Coppola C, Coppola M, Laccetti P, et al. Effects of a second-generation human anti-ErbB2 ImmunoRNase on trastuzumab-resistant tumors and cardiac cells. Protein Engineering, Design and Selection. 2014;27:83–88. DOI: 10.1093/protein/gzt065

[189] Riccio G, Borriello M, D'Alessio G, De Lorenzo C. A novel human antitumor dimeric immunoRNase. Journal of Immunotherapy. 2008;31:440–445. DOI: 10.1097/CJI.0b013e31816bc769

[190] Veronese FM, Largajolli R, Boccù E, Benassi CA, Schiavon O. Surface modification of proteins. Activation of monomethoxy-polyethylene glycols by phenylchloroformates and modification of ribonuclease and superoxide dismutase. Applied Biochemistry and Biotechnology. 1985;11:141–152. DOI: 10.1007/BF02798546

[191] Caliceti P, Schiavon O, Veronese FM, Chaiken IM. Effects of monomethoxypoly(ethylene glycol) modification of ribonuclease on antibody recognition, substrate accessibility and conformational stability. Journal of Molecular Recognition. 1990;3:89–93. DOI: 10.1002/jmr.300030206

[192] Schiavon O, Caliceti P, Sartore L, Veronese FM. Surface modification of enzymes for therapeutic use: monomethoxypoly (ethylene glycol) derivatization of ribonuclease. Il Farmaco. 1991;46:967–978.

[193] Matoušek J, Poučková P, Souček J, Škvor J. PEG chains increase aspermatogenic and antitumor activity of RNase A and BS-RNase enzymes. Journal of Controled Release. 2002;82:29–37. DOI: 10.1016/S0168-3659(02)00082-2

[194] Matoušek J, Poučková P, Hloušková D, Zadinová M, Souček J, Škvor J. Effect of hyaluronidase and PEG chain conjugation on the biologic and antitumor activity of RNase A. Journal of Controled Release. 2004;94:401–410. DOI: 10.1016/j.jconrel.2003.10.025

[195] Rutkoski TJ, Kink JA, Strong LE, Raines RT. Site-specific PEGylation endows a mammalian ribonuclease with antitumor activity. Cancer Biology and Therapy. 2011;12:208–214. DOI: 10.4161/cbt.12.3.15959

[196] Rutkoski TJ, Kink JA, Strong LE, Raines RT. Human ribonuclease with a pendant poly(ethylene glycol) inhibits tumor growth in mice. Translational Oncology. 2013;6:392–397. DOI: 10.1593/tlo.13253

[197] Liu S, Sun L, Wang J, Ma G, Su Z, Hu T. Mono-PEGylation of ribonuclease A: high PEGylation efficiency by thiolation with small molecular weight reagent. Process Biochemistry. 2012;47:1364–1370. DOI: 10.1016/j.procbio.2012.05.003

[198] Kratz F. Albumin as a drug carrier: design of prodrugs, drug conjugates and nanoparticles. Journal of Controled Release. 2008;132:171–183. DOI: 10.1016/j.jconrel.2008.05.010

[199] Li C, Lin Q, Wang J, Shen L, Ma G, Su Z, et al. Preparation, structural analysis and bioactivity of ribonuclease A-albumin conjugate: Tetra-conjugation or PEG as the linker. Journal of Biotechnology. 2012;162:283–288. DOI: 10.1016/j.jbiotec.2012.09.008

[200] van der Gun BTF, Melchers LJ, Ruiters MHJ, de Leij LFMH, McLaughlin PMJ, Rots MG. EpCAM in carcinogenesis: the good, the bad or the ugly. Carcinogenesis. 2010;31:1913–1921. DOI: 10.1093/carcin/bgq187

[201] Zhao HL, Xue C, Du JL, Ren M, Xia S, Cheng YG, et al. Sustained and cancer cell targeted cytosolic delivery of Onconase results in potent antitumor effects. Journal of Controled Release. 2012;159:346–352. DOI: 10.1016/j.jconrel.2012.02.019

[202] Fernández-Ulibarri I, Hammer K, Arndt MAE, Kaufmann JK, Dorer D, Engelhardt S, et al. Genetic delivery of an immunoRNase by an oncolytic adenovirus enhances

anticancer activity. International Journal of Cancer. 2015;136:2228–2240. DOI: 10.1002/ijc.29258

[203] Slager J, Tyler B, Shikanov A, Domb AJ, Shogen K, Sidransky D, et al. Local controlled delivery of anti-neoplastic RNAse to the brain. Pharmaceutical Research. 2009;26:1838–1846. DOI: 10.1007/s11095-009-9893-3

8

Liver Cancer Treatment by Chinese Medicines and their Active Compounds

Ming Hong, Ning Wang and Yibin Feng

Abstract

Recent studies have indicated that traditional Chinese medicines (CMs) and their active compounds play an important role in liver cancer treatment by preventing tumor formation, inhibiting tumor growth, metastasis and recurrence as well as improving the quality of life and reducing side effects of radiotherapy and chemotherapy. Mechanism studies have proved the advantage of multicomponent, multitarget and multipathway combinational regulation by CMs in liver cancer treatment. This chapter emphatically introduces the molecular mechanisms underlying liver cancer treatment by CMs. In addition, we also put forward discussion on existing obstacles and prospect of the future development on liver cancer treatment using CMs, in terms of providing a comprehensive understanding of action of CMs in liver cancer treatment.

Keywords: TCM, Chinese medicines, Chinese herbal medicines, Anticancer, Antimetastasis, Antiangiogenesis, adjuvant therapy, complementary, alternative treatment

1. Introduction

Primary liver cancer is a serious disease threatening human health. It was the sixth most frequent cancer, and the second leading cause of cancer death worldwide according to the reports from the International Liver Cancer Association in 2014 [1]. The most common type of liver cancer is hepatocellular carcinoma (HCC), which is originated from hepatocyte. Other types of liver cancer, such as hepatoblastoma and intrahepatic cholangiocarcinoma, are relatively uncommon. Recognized risk factors for liver cancer include viral hepatitis B or C infection, obesity and alcohol abuse. In developing countries such as African countries and China, Hepatitis B or C is the major cause of liver cancer, whereas in developed countries such as the European Union and United States, the predominant cause of liver cancer is cirrhosis caused by alcohol abuse or obesity [2]. In addition, inherited factor may also increase the risk of liver cancer. Recent studies have found that some patients developed liver cancer with inherited susceptible genes from their parents [3]. Usually, liver cancer has no symptoms at the early stages; with the tumor progression, symptoms such as yellow skin, abdominal pain, abdominal mass, nausea or liver dysfunction appear and rapidly deteriorate. Generally, the prognosis of liver cancer is poor, because only 10–20% patients with early detection can receive curative resection surgery. In addition, surgical resection is unavailable for cirrhotic patients as increased risk of fatal complications may occur during resection on cirrhotic livers [4]. Other conventional cancer treatment options such as radiation and chemotherapy are not routinely used for liver cancer as the liver is chemotherapy-refractory and not tolerant to radiation [5, 6]. In recent decades, several novel targeted therapies have been developed for liver cancer treatment. The National Comprehensive Cancer Network (NCCN) guidelines recommend sorafenib as the standard frontline therapy for patients with unresectable HCC but with well-preserved liver function [7, 8]. Other locoregional or adjuvant therapies such as the percutaneous ablation (ethanol injection and radiofrequency ablation), intra-arterial radiolabeled lipiodol, intra-arterial chemotherapy, transarterial chemoembolization (TACE), interferon, adoptive immunotherapy and complementary and alternative medicine are recommended for providing opportunity for liver transplantation or extending disease-free survival and improving survival quality. For patients who are diagnosed with early stage liver cancer, the 5-year survival rate is about 31%. If the tumor has invaded to the surrounding organs or lymph nodes, the 5-year survival rate will decrease to 11%. If the cancer has metastasized to distant organs, the 5-year survival rate is only 3% [9].

Traditional Chinese medicine (TCM) is one of the most popular complementary and alternative medicine in cancer patients worldwide. In China, TCM is based on the foundation of about 2500 years of folk medical practice, which have been covered by the National Health Insurance Program and supported by the government in both Mainland of China and Taiwan. Different from the western medicines that are based on modern human anatomy and pathology, TCM is mainly focused on the identification of functional entities. In the view of TCM, health is based on the harmonious interaction of the internal functional entities and the external environment. The primary functional entities used by TCM include gas (Qi), blood (Xie), internal organs (Zang-fu) and the meridians (Jing-luo) that are main channels of communication of Qi and Xie in the body and link Zang-Fu with the superficial areas of the body [10, 11]. There are various forms of TCM, which have been used for cancer patients, such as the herbal remedies, acupuncture, moxibustion, breathing exercise and dietary therapy. These therapies may have potential in improving the overall survival in cancer patients and the survival quality.

2. The understanding of liver cancer in traditional Chinese medicine

In TCM, liver cancer is associated with the presence of an "abdominal mass" called "zheng jia" (癥瘕). "Zheng" (癥) means fixed mass in the abdomen with fixed pain, while "Jia" (瘕)

refers to abdominal mass occurs intermittently with no fixed pain. According to TCM literature, the symptoms of liver cancer include abdominal distention, jaundice, abdominal fullness and oppression. Those symptoms can be concluded as "Jiju" (积聚), which means syndromes caused by abdominal lump with pain or swelling. In TCM, the causes of liver cancer can be divided into internal factors and external factors. The internal factors include individual congenital constitution and emotional conditions. The emotions are considered as the major internal causes of liver cancer in TCM. Emotions are regarded as internal, normal, physiological response to stimulus from the external factors. The negative emotions with high intensity and prolonged duration may cause serious damage to the internal organs and influence the healthy condition of the whole body. External factors include unhealthy dietary habits and lifestyle such as alcohol beverage and contaminated food or over exhaustion. These factors can lead to spleen and body disharmony. Other external factors such as the environment also play an important role in the process of tumorigenesis. For example, the wet climate is considered as an induction factor for liver cancer in TCM. Both internal and external factors may cause stagnation of qi, spleen deficiency and the accumulation of dampness, which can eventually lead to liver cancer.

3. The role of Chinese medicines and their active compounds in liver cancer treatment

3.1. Chinese medicines and their active compounds for preventing liver cancer

From a TCM point of view, a good doctor should prevent and cure potential disease in the initiating stage. "Treating before getting illness" is one of the preponderant thoughts of TCM in dealing with disease and health. It is important to prevent the occurrence of liver cancer by keeping healthy diet and lifestyle according to the TCM theories. As we have discussed earlier, spleen deficiency may cause the occurrence of liver cancer. Symptoms such as ascites and abdominal distention are all related to spleen deficiency. According to the relationship among the TCM five internal organs (heart, liver, spleen, lungs and kidneys), the spleen and the liver can influence on each other. Therefore, spleen deficiency can also restrict the liver function. In order to strengthen spleen health and protect liver function, people should avoid taking too much spicy and "cold" food such as pepper, green beans and cold water. Alcohol beverage can also induce spleen deficiency by aggravating the dampness in the body. But moderate drinking are beneficial for preventing liver diseases such as liver cancer according to TCM theories [12].

Many Chinese medicines (CMs) and its active compounds are effective in reducing inflammation as confirmed by modern science [13, 14]. Recent studies have demonstrated that inflammation is a major stimulus for hepatic carcinogenesis and some CMs may prevent liver cancer by inhibiting inflammation in liver. Xiao Chai Hu Tang (XCHT) is an herbal medicine formula used in some Asian countries for treating chronic viral liver diseases. According to the TCM theories, XCHT can modulate Qi activity and balance between Yin and Yang. Recent studies found that XCHT can prevent chronic hepatitis C-related liver cancer by suppressing inflammation and inhibiting fibrosis in the liver [15]. Shi Quan Da Bu Tang (SQDBT) is a classic TCM herbal diet formula that was documented in the "Tai Ping Imperial Grace Formulary" in Song dynasty. In TCM, SQDBT were used to regulate Qi and treat Yang deficiency. Modern scientific research show that SQDBT can relieve chronic viral liver diseases by reducing inflammatory processes and controlling serum alanine transaminase (ALT) levels, thus it may prevent liver cancer development [16]. Other TCM herbal extracts or isolates such as the Salvia Miltiorrhiza extracts, Schisandra chinensis extracts, silymarin, glycyrrhizin, baicalein and baicalin may prevent liver cancer by relieving chronic liver diseases associated hepatic steatosis and fibrosis [17–21].

3.2. Chinese medicines and their active compounds for inhibiting liver cancer development

Invigorating Qi and strengthening the spleen; relieving Qi stagnancy in liver, clearing heat and detoxifying, activating blood circulation to dissipate blood stasis, supplementing Qi and nourishing yin are the main principles in treating primary liver cancer with TCM. Inhibiting tumor growth, suppressing metastasis and preventing recurrence with TCM is the key to restrain liver cancer development. According to a large-scale cohort study in Taiwan, Jia Wei Xiao Yao San (JWXYS) and Chai Hu Shu Gan Tang (CHSGT) are the most common TCM prescriptions for liver cancer treatment. These TCM formulae can significantly inhibit tumor development and improve survival in patients with primary liver cancer [22]. JWXYS are used for invigorating the spleen and nourishing blood, it is effective for relieving Qi stagnancy in liver. Besides its antihepatoma effects, JWXYS can also inhibit colon cancer and breast cancer [23, 24]. CHSGT are also used for dispersing the Qi stagnancy in liver. Different from the JWXYS that focuses on invigorating the spleen, CHSGT is mainly applied for activating Qi movement and relieving pain. Both of these formulae have been safely used in liver cancer treatment for patients in China, Taiwan and Hong Kong, with few side effects being reported. Some pharmacological studies also revealed that a lot of CMs extracts or isolates could inhibit liver cancer growth or metastasis both *in vitro* and *in vivo*. This includes but not limited to Coptidis Rhizome extracts, Radix Bupleuri extracts, Radix Salvia Miltiorrhiza extracts, silymarin, berberine, Wogonin, bufalin and curcumin [25–28].

3.3. Chinese medicines and their active compounds for improving the quality of life and reducing the side effects of conventional therapy in liver cancer patients

As most of the liver cancer patients are diagnosed with late-stage cancer, only 20% patients may have the chance to receive curative treatment. In this case, improving the quality of life and reducing the side effects of conventional therapy are very important for liver cancer patients. The common side-effects of conventional therapies, such as nausea, vomiting, fever, abdominal pain, loss of appetite, alopecia and myelosuppression may lead to noncompliance of treatment and thus affect treatment outcomes and reduce the quality of life. According to a series of randomized clinical trials, CMs are effective in extending survival time, improving quality of life, and reducing side effects of conventional therapies for liver cancer patients [29]. For example, Ophiopogonis Radix and Galli Gigerii Endothelium Corneum (Ji Nei Jing) are most commonly used CMs for appetite improvement; Astragali Radix is widely used for alleviating fatigue; Artemisiae Scopariae Herba is recommended for abating jaundice; Toosendan Fructus and Corydalis Rhizoma are effective in relieving abdominal pain; Pericarpium Arecae, Polyporus, Poria can be used to treat ascites [26].

4. The molecular mechanism on liver cancer treatment by Chinese medicines and their active compounds

4.1. Traditional Chinese medicines and its active compounds for inhibiting the proliferation and inducing cell death in liver cancer cells

Jie Du Xiao Zheng Yin (JDXZY) is a typical TCM formula for liver cancer treatment. Recent studies have found that JDXZY can suppress the proliferation of liver cancer cells in a dose- and time-dependent manner [30]. *In vivo* studies also confirmed that JDXZY could increase the tumor apoptotic index and reduce tumor size in nude mice. Mechanism studies showed that JDXZY may induce human hepatoma HepG2 cell apoptosis by mitochondrial-related pathway. Treatment with JDXZY can activate caspase-9 and caspase-3 as well as up-regulate the ratio of Bax/Bcl-2, which may partially demonstrate its antihepatoma effects. In addition, another study also found that JDXZY could inhibit the proliferation of HepG2 cells by arresting the cell cycle at the G0/G1 phase [31].

Bufalin is a digoxin-like agent isolated from Chansu which is a precious CMs extracted from parotoid glands of toads. Previous studies found that bufalin exhibited significant anticancer activities in many cancer cell lines *in vitro* and *in vivo*. A recent research showed that bufalin can suppress AKT-related signaling pathway in HepG2 and HCCLM3 cell lines. After bufalin treatment, the proliferation-related proteins in AKT/GSK3beta/beta-catenin/E-cadherin-signaling pathway were significantly inhibited [32]. Thus, bufalin may be a potential anti-hepatoma agent by inhibiting the proliferation of cancer cell.

Gekko swinhonis Guenther also called ShouGong in TCM; it was a widely used anticancer drug in China for hundreds of years. Modern science has demonstrated that one of the major active components in *Gekko swinhonis* Guenther is sulfated polysaccharide–protein complex (GSPP). Previous studies showed that GSPP can suppress the proliferation of liver cancer cells and arrest the cell cycle in SMMC-7721 cells with little direct toxicity [33]. In addition, Gepsin, the monomeric protein in GSPP also showed strong inhibition on the proliferation of hepatocarcinoma Bel-7402 cells [34].

Many researches have revealed the strong anticancer activity of berberine. The protective effects of berberine on liver diseases including liver cancer have been widely studied by our groups. The quaternary ammonium salt derived from Coptidis Rhizome (Huanglian in TCM) can induce both autophagy and apoptosis in hepatocellular carcinoma cells (HCC). Further mechanisms studies demonstrated that berberine could induce mitochondrial apoptotic signaling pathway in MHCC97-L and HepG2 cells via upregulating Bax expression. Furthermore, berberine could also induce autophagic cell death in HCC cells through inhibiting the activity of Akt and activating the p38 MAPK-signaling pathway [35].

4.2. Chinese medicines and their active compounds for inducing liver cancer cells differentiation

Panaxydol is one of the bioactive components in Panax Notoginseng (Sanqi in TCM). Panax Notoginseng is a famous hemostatic in TCM and it can also relieve other blood disorders, such as blood stasis or blood deficiency. Recent studies have shown that the panaxydol could induce cell differentiation in human HCC cell lines SMMC-7721 [36]. Ultrastructure morphology observation confirmed that there have obvious cell morphologic changes after panaxydol treatment. The activity of several differentiation related proteins such as alkaline phosphatase and albumin were increased, while AFP activity was significantly decreased after panaxydol treatment. These results showed that panaxydol may be a potential antihepatoma agent by inducing tumor cell differentiation.

Gepsin can also inhibit liver cancer development by inducing cancer cells differentiation. Studies showed that after gepsin treatment, the HCC cell line Bel-7402 presents ultrastructural morphology of differentiation. Western blot results revealed that the differentiation related proteins such as the AFP protein secretion significantly decreased, while ALB protein expression was obviously up-regulated on gepsin-treated cancer cells [34].

Ginseng is one of the most widely used herbs in TCM for thousands of years. Ginsenosides are the main bio-active components in Ginseng. There are many reports verified the anticancer effect of ginsenosides *in vitro* and *in vivo*. For example, ginsenosides-Rh2 (G-Rh2) can inhibit the proliferation of SMMC-7721 cells as well as induce the mature and normality of cell ultrastructure morphology. The expression of AFP, gamma-GT and heat-resistant ALP were also significantly decreased after 10 mg/ml G-Rh2 treatment [37].

4.3. Chinese medicines and their active compounds for averting the invasion and metastasis of liver cancer cells

Ardipusilloside I is a triterpene-saponin separated from the TCM herbs *Ardisia pusilla* A. DC. Recent studies have revealed its anticancer effects through inhibition invasion and metastasis of HCC cells [38]. Both *in vitro* and *in vivo* studies demonstrated that Ardipusilloside I may suppress migration of HCC cells partially by decreasing the expression of the metalloproteinase (MMP)-2 and MMP-9 proteins. In addition, Ardipusilloside I can activate Rac1 protein and further induce E-cadherin which may result in inhibition of cancer cells migration.

As we have discussed earlier, GSPP and its monomeric protein gepsin are effective in inhibiting the proliferation of HCC cells. Recent studies found that GSPP was also effective in suppressing the migration of HCC cells [33]. GSPP treatment remarkably decreased the concentration of intracellular calcium. Many studies have demonstrated that low intracellular calcium concentration is associated with reduced cancer migration. GSPP treatment could remarkably decrease the concentration of intracellular calcium. Thus, the antimigration effect by GSPP may be partially a consequence of downregulation of intracellular calcium concentration together with an upregulation of actin filaments polymerization in HCC cells.

The hepatic protective effects of Radix Salviae have been verified through its extensive use in TCM. Recent studies also found that aqueous extracts of Radix Salviae can inhibit the development of liver cancer by suppressing the metastasis and recurrence in animal models [21]. *In vitro* study showed that Radix Salviae treatment significantly decreased the expression of Intercellular Adhesion Molecule 1(ICAM-1) in SMMC-7721 cells. In addition, it could suppress the invasion of SMMC-7721 cell and make the fibronectin-attached cells exfoliated. The cell adhesion ability of HCC-HCC, HCC-lymphocyte and HCC-endothelial cell also decreased after Radix Salviae treatment. The tumor xenograft mice model also confirmed the antimetastasis effects of Radix Salviae on posthepatectomy liver cancer *in vivo*.

Curcumin, a polyphenol isolated from the rhizome of Curcuma longa (Jiang in TCM) has potential anti-cancer effects in many types of cancers. However, due to its poor aqueous solubility, the clinical application of curcumin has been limited. A recent study has used the polymeric nanoparticle formulation of curcumin to improve its solubility as well as anticancer activity [39]. The results showed that when used as a combination with sorafenib, the modified curcumin can suppress the proliferation and invasion of HCC cells *in vitro*. Furthermore, *in vivo* study also found curcumin could inhibit liver cancer growth and lung metastases. Mechanisms study found curcumin and sorafenib synergistically inhibited the expression of MMP9 by down-regulating NF-kappaB/p65-signaling pathway. Taken together, the polymeric nanoparticle formulation of curcumin may exhibit antitumor activity by inhibiting liver cancer metastasis.

4.4. Chinese medicines and their active compounds for inhibiting angiogenesis in liver cancer treatment

Angiogenesis is a physiological process during which new blood vessels are produced and developed based on the original vessels. As angiogenesis plays a crucial role in tumor growth and metastasis, the novel antitumor therapies targeting angiogenesis may provide new hopes for cancer treatment. Livistona Chinensis seeds (EELC) have been used for centuries in TCM for cancer treatment. HCC xenograft mice model confirmed that EELC can inhibit tumor angiogenesis through the Notch-signaling pathway [40]. After EELC treatment, *in vivo* results showed remarkable decrease in intratumoral microvessel density (MVD) in the HCC xenograft mice tumors. In addition, the angiogenesis-related proteins such as the VEGF-A and VEGFR-2 were significantly decreased after EELC treatment. The mechanism study demonstrated that the antiangiogenesis effect was related with the inhibition of the Notch pathway as the expression of Notch, Dll4 and Jagged1 were down regulated according to the real-time polymerase chain reaction (RT-PCR) results.

Yang Zheng Xiao Ji (YZXJ) is a commercial TCM product for supplementary treatment of advanced liver cancer. Some clinical trials indicated that YZXJ may improve the curative effect of interventional chemotherapy for advanced liver cancer patients. *In vitro* studies showed that YZXJ can inhibit the matrigel-based sandwich tubule formation and cell migration. Western blot results confirmed that inhibition of the activation of focal adhesion kinase may at least in part confer the YZXJ-induced inhibition of cell migration and tube formation [41]. These results indicated that YZXJ could be a potential antihepatoma TCM product via suppressing tumor angiogenesis.

Asparagus polysaccharide, the bioactive derivate from Asparagus, is a common TCM herbal diet that may exhibit anticancer activity according to previous researches. One study has explored the adjunctive effects of asparagus polysaccharide in liver cancer chemotherapy [42]. Their results showed that asparagus polysaccharide significantly suppressed liver cancer growth in combination with transcatheter arterial chemoembolization (TACE) therapy in orthotopic HCC rat model. Tumor angiogenesis may be the major target for asparagine gelatinous in liver cancer treatment. Several angiogenesis markers such as CD34 and VEGF significantly decreased after asparagine gelatinous treatment. The expression of MVD markers also remarkably reduced in asparagus polysaccharide treated liver tumors. These results suggested that asparagus polysaccharide with TACE could apparently inhibit the tumor angiogenesis *in vivo*; asparagus polysaccharide might be a potential adjunvant therapy for TACE in treating liver cancer.

4.5. Chinese medicines and their active compounds for enhancing immunological function in liver cancer patient

The TCM formula Songyou Yin (SYY) was developed by Professor Zhao-You Tang for liver cancer treatment. Recent studies have found that the antimetastasis and anti-recurrence effects by SYY may be correlated with its immunomodulation activity. SYY can significantly extend survival and inhibit the tumor growth and metastasis in tumor-burdened mice. SYY remarkably increased the ratio of CD4/CD8 in peripheral blood and decreased the serum TGF-beta1 activity as well as the percentage of Treg cells both in spleen and peripheral blood. Thus, the TCM product SYY may strengthen the immunity of liver cancer patient and prevent tumor recurrence [43].

Mylabris mixture is a popular anticancer TCM formula which mainly consists of the Mylabris extracts, Tangerine Peel and Millet Sprout. Recent studies found that Mylabris mixture could obviously suppress the growth of liver cancer H22 cells by improving the immunological function in mice model [44]. After Mylabris mixture treatment, the stimulation index of T-lymphocyte transformation and proportion of NK cells were apparently increased. The subpopulation percentage of T lymphocytes also significantly increased after Mylabris mixture treatment. Up-regulation on the secretion of interferon-gamma and interleukin-4 by T lymphocytes also confirmed the immunoloregulation effects by Mylabris mixture.

A recent study has explored the immunoloregulation effects of ultrasound-guided intratumoral injection of TCM formula "Star-99" in HCC in mice model. Star-99 can improve the cellular immunity and induce HCC cell apoptosis by increasing the level of plasma IL-2 and TNF-alpha. The cytokines IL-2 can be considered as an immunological response modifier. It can improve the activity of lymphocyte and the anti-tumor effects of NK, CTL and LAK cells as well as cytokine secretion. In addition, another experiment also found that many lymphocytes can be observed in the tumor tissues after the Star-99 treatment [45]. The electron microscope results observed that the microvilli on the surface of the lymphocytes attacked the cancer cells. The membrane of tumor cell in contact with the sensitized T lymphocyte became broken with the organelle and the nucleus dissolved and the vacuolation of the cytoplasm as well. This phenomenon further illustrate that the Star-99 could stimulate and induce the cellular immunity function of the organism.

Previous studies revealed the TCM herbal product Kanglaite (KLT) which mainly consists of Jobstears Seed oil exhibits anticancer and immunoregulation activities. According to a clinical study, KLT treatment can improve the immunological function via increasing the proportion of T cells and NK cells in the blood of HCC patients [46]. *In vivo* study in tumor-bearing mice showed that KLT enhanced the immune system by increasing the secretion of several cytokines such as the IFN-gamma and IL-2, and up-regulate the proportion of CD4+ T cells in mice. These events further improved the killing activity of NK cells and CD8+ T cells against the HepG2 cells. KLT treatment also up-regulate the mRNA level of some NF-kappaB responsive genes in CD4+ cells. In conclusion, KLT may have immunomodulatory activity at least partially through the activating of NF-kappaB mediated gene transcription in CD4+ T cells.

4.6. Chinese medicines and their active compounds for reversing drug resistance in liver cancer treatment

Astragaloside is a saponin isolated from Radix Astragali, one of the popular TCM herbs. Astragaloside has been reported to be an effective agent in reversing multidrug resistance (MDR) of cancer treatment. A recent study found that astragaloside can modulate the expression of P-glycoprotein in human hepatic cancer cells Bel-7402 and reverse 5-fluorouracil resistance in chemotherapy. As P-glycoprotein majorly is responsible for the drug efflux in cancer treatment, the down-regulation of P-glycoprotein will inhibit P-glycoprotein-mediated drug efflux and improve the efficacy of chemotherapies [47]. Thus, astragaloside may be a potential anticancer drug for reversing drug resistance in liver cancer treatment.

Polyphyllin D is a saponin derived from a TCM herb Paris Polyphylla. The herb of Paris Polyphylla has been used for liver cancer treatment in China for thousands years. Previous study showed that polyphyllin D can induce apoptosis in multi-drug resistant HepG2 cells [48]. Further mechanism study demonstrated that polyphyllin D may elicit mitochondrial fragmentation in HCC cells. When treating polyphyllin D directly to the isolated mitochondria, the mitochondria exhibited strong swelling with deep transmembrane depolarization. In addition, significant apoptosis-inducing factor release could be observed from the multidrug-resistant HepG2 cells. These results suggest that polyphyllin D may be a potential anti-cancer agent targeting drug resistance in HCC cells by inducing mitochondrial damage.

Piper betel leaves (PBL) are enriched with medication properties in TCM for many centuries. Modern researches have proven that PBL has antioxidation activity and may inhibit gene mutation. Recent study has found that PBL extract can inhibit total Glutathione S-transferase (GST) and alpha class of GST (GSTA) in HepG2 cells [49]. Further study showed PBL could enhance the sensitivity of HCC cells to chemotherapy. The results revealed that the cytotoxicity of cisplatin was apparently increased in cell with PBL treatment, with the mechanism related to the inhibition of multidrug resistance protein 2. These results indicated that PBL extract may reduce drug resistance and improve the efficacy of chemotherapy in liver cancer treatment.

5. Future prospect of liver cancer treatment by Chinese medicines and their active compounds

CMs and its active compounds have a long history for anticancer treatment in China. In recent decades, many TCM formulae, herbal extracts or isolates have been developed to treat liver cancer, especially for patients with advanced-stage liver cancer. According to both clinical studies and basic researches, CMs have less toxicity and exhibit multitarget anticancer activity. In China, the antihepatoma effects of several TCM products have been verified by clinical trials, such as the Songyou Yin and Kanglaite injection. Many studies have proven that CMs had beneficial effects in relieving fatigue and pain, preventing respiratory tract infections and alleviating gastrointestinal symptoms in liver cancer patients.

However, there are also some problems with CMs in current cancer treatment that should be considered seriously. First of all, most of the CMs are extracted from plants or animals, their pharmacological active components are still unknown CMs. Second, the adverse effects, contraindications and corresponding clinical data of CMs are rarely indicated by TCM doctors or CMs manufacturers. Third, the frequent occurrence of fatal accidents such as allergy and phlebitis has been observed during TCM treatment especially in TCM injection treatment. Finally, although there are many clinical trials on CMs for liver cancer treatment, none of them were large multicenter trials with strict and standard criteria CMs. In this case, it is difficult to give an accurate conclusion about the effects of CMs for liver cancer treatment when conducting a meta-analysis. Therefore, large-scale multicenter clinical trials with strict and standard criteria are urgently needed for the development of TCM in liver cancer treatment. According to the previous studies, combination of CMs and its active compounds with surgery, TACE or chemotherapy may protect liver function, enhance the patients' immune response, and reduce the side effects and complications of conventional therapy as well as prolong lifespan. With the rapid development of modern scientific research, the combination therapy with TCM will be definitely promising for future liver cancer treatment.

Acknowledgements

This research was partially supported by the research council of the University of Hong Kong 8 (Project Code: 104001764 & 104002320) and donations of Modern oncology of Chinese Medicine (Project code: 20006276) and the Gaia Family Trust, New Zealand (Project code: 20007008).

Author details

Ming Hong, Ning Wang and Yibin Feng*

*Address all correspondence to: yfeng@hku.hk

School of Chinese Medicine, Li Ka Shing Faculty of Medicine, The University of Hong Kong, Pok Fu Lam, Hong Kong, China

References

[1] Nault, J.C. Reports from the international liver cancer association (ilca) congress 2014. *Journal of Hepatology* 2015, *62*, 477-482.

[2] MacLachlan, J.H., Cowie, B.C. Liver cancer is the fastest increasing cause of cancer death in Australians. *The Medical Journal of Australia* 2012, *197*, 492-493.

[3] Zhang, X.F., Bian, J.C., Zhang, X.Y., Zhang, Z.M., Jiang, F., Wang, Q.M., Wang, Q.J., Cao, Y.Y., Tang, B.M. Are polymorphisms of n-acetyltransferase genes susceptible to primary liver cancer in Luoyang, China? *World Journal of Gastroenterology: WJG* 2005, *11*, 1457-1462.

[4] Wang, J.H., Kuo, Y.H., Wang, C.C., Chen, C.L., Cheng, Y.F., Hsu, H.C., Lu, S.N. Surgical resection improves the survival of selected hepatocellular carcinoma patients in Barcelona clinic liver cancer stage c. *Digestive and Liver Disease : Official Journal of the Italian Society of Gastroenterology and the Italian Association for the Study of the Liver* 2013, *45*, 510-515.

[5] Kudo, M. Surveillance, diagnosis, treatment, and outcome of liver cancer in Japan. *Liver Cancer* 2015, *4*, 39-50.

[6] Benckert, C., Bruns, C. The role of liver resection in the treatment of hepatocellular cancer. *Der Chirurg; Zeitschrift fur alle Gebiete der operativen Medizen* 2015, *86*, 803.

[7] Kelley, R.K. Adjuvant sorafenib for liver cancer: wrong stage, wrong dose. *The Lancet. Oncology* 2015, *16*, 1279-1281.

[8] Woo, H.Y., Heo, J. Sorafenib in liver cancer. *Expert Opinion on Pharmacotherapy* 2012, *13*, 1059-1067.

[9] Kudo, M., Izumi, N., Ichida, T., Ku, Y., Kokudo, N., Sakamoto, M., Takayama, T., Nakashima, O., Matsui, O., Matsuyama, Y. Report of the 19th follow-up survey of primary liver cancer in Japan. *Hepatology Research: The Official Journal of the Japan Society of Hepatology* 2016, *46*, 372-390.

[10] Wang, A., Lin, L., Wang, Y. Traditional Chinese herbal medicine penthorum chinense pursh: A phytochemical and pharmacological review. *The American Journal of Chinese Medicine* 2015, *43*, 601-620.

[11] Zhang, W.B., Wang, G.J., Fuxe, K. Classic and modern meridian studies: A review of low hydraulic resistance channels along meridians and their relevance for therapeutic effects in traditional Chinese medicine. *Evidence-based Complementary and Alternative Medicine: eCAM* 2015, *2015*, 410979.

[12] Ji, G., Wang, L., Zhang, S.H., Liu, J.W., Zheng, P.Y., Liu, T. Effect of Chinese medicine qinggan huoxuefang on inducing hsc apoptosis in alcoholic liver fibrosis rats. *World Journal of Gastroenterology : WJG* 2006, *12*, 2047-2052.

[13] Wen, Y., Zhan, Y., Liu, H., Zhao, T., Yang, L., Zhang, H., Dong, X., Li, P. Yi qi qing re gao formula ameliorates puromycin aminonucleoside-induced nephrosis by suppressing inflammation and apoptosis. *BMC Complementary and Alternative Medicine* 2015, *15*, 155.

[14] Wei, Y., Luo, Q.L., Sun, J., Chen, M.X., Liu, F., Dong, J.C. Bu-shen-yi-qi formulae suppress chronic airway inflammation and regulate th17/treg imbalance in the murine ovalbumin asthma model. *Journal of Ethnopharmacology* 2015, *164*, 368-377.

[15] Miyanishi, K., Hoki, T., Tanaka, S., Kato, J. Prevention of hepatocellular carcinoma: Focusing on antioxidant therapy. *World Journal of Hepatology* 2015, *7*, 593-599.

[16] Rino, Y., Tarao, K. Anti-inflammatory drugs reduce the risk of hepatocellular carcinoma development. *ISRN Oncology* 2011, *2011*, 390676.

[17] Zhu, S.Y., Dong, Y., Tu, J., Zhou, Y., Zhou, X.H., Xu, B. Silybum marianum oil attenuates oxidative stress and ameliorates mitochondrial dysfunction in mice treated with d-galactose. *Pharmacognosy Magazine* 2014, *10*, S92-99.

[18] Park, H.J., Lee, S.J., Song, Y., Jang, S.H., Ko, Y.G., Kang, S.N., Chung, B.Y., Kim, H.D., Kim, G.S., Cho, J.H. Schisandra chinensis prevents alcohol-induced fatty liver disease in rats. *Journal of Medicinal Food* 2014, *17*, 103-110.

[19] Wang, E., Bussom, S., Chen, J., Quinn, C., Bedognetti, D., Lam, W., Guan, F., Jiang, Z., Mark, Y., Zhao, Y., *et al.* Interaction of a traditional chinese medicine (phy906) and cpt-11 on the inflammatory process in the tumor microenvironment. *BMC Med Genomics* 2011, *4*, 38.

[20] Dhiman, R.K., Chawla, Y.K. Herbal medicines for liver diseases. *Digestive Diseases and Sciences* 2005, *50*, 1807-1812.

[21] Sun, J., Zhou, X., Liu, Y. Study on preventive and therapeutic effect of radix salviae miltiorrhizae on recurrence and metastasis of liver cancer. *Zhongguo Zhong xi yi jie he za zhi Zhongguo Zhongxiyi jiehe zazhi = Chinese Journal of Integrated Traditional and Western Medicine/Zhongguo Zhong xi yi jie he xue hui, Zhongguo Zhong yi yan jiu yuan zhu ban* 1999, *19*, 292-295.

[22] Liao, Y.H., Lin, C.C., Lai, H.C., Chiang, J.H., Lin, J.G., Li, T.C. Adjunctive traditional Chinese medicine therapy improves survival of liver cancer patients. *Liver International: Official Journal of the International Association for the Study of the Liver* 2015, *35*, 2595-2602.

[23] Lai, J.N., Wu, C.T., Wang, J.D. Prescription pattern of Chinese herbal products for breast cancer in Taiwan: A population-based study. *Evidence-Based Complementary and Alternative Medicine: eCAM* 2012, *2012*, 891893.

[24] Chao, T.H., Fu, P.K., Chang, C.H., Chang, S.N., Chiahung Mao, F., Lin, C.H. Evidence-based Chinese medicine research, G. Prescription patterns of Chinese herbal products for post-surgery colon cancer patients in Taiwan. *Journal of Ethnopharmacology* 2014, *155*, 702-708.

[25] Zhai, X.F., Qiao, C.X., Liu, Q., Chen, Z., Ling, C.Q. Quality assessment of clinical research on liver cancer treated by intra-arterial infusion of Chinese medicine. *Chinese Journal of Integrative Medicine* 2014, *20*, 870-875.

[26] Liu, X., Li, N. Regularity analysis on clinical treatment in primary liver cancer by traditional Chinese medicine. *Zhongguo Zhong yao za zhi = Zhongguo zhongyao zazhi = China Journal of Chinese Materia Medica* 2012, *37*, 1327-1331.

[27] Li, M., Qiao, C., Qin, L., Zhang, J., Ling, C. Application of traditional Chinese medicine injection in treatment of primary liver cancer: A review. *Journal of Traditional Chinese Medicine = Chung i tsa chih ying wen pan/sponsored by All-China Association of Traditional Chinese Medicine, Academy of Traditional Chinese Medicine* 2012, *32*, 299-307.

[28] Wu, M.C. Traditional Chinese medicine in prevention and treatment of liver cancer: Function, status and existed problems. *Zhong xi yi jie he xue bao = Journal of Chinese Integrative Medicine* 2003, *1*, 163-164.

[29] Li, X.Q., Ling, C.Q. Chinese herbal medicine for side effects of transarterial chemoembolization in liver cancer patients: A systematic review and meta-analysis. *Zhong xi yi jie he xue bao = Journal of Chinese Integrative Medicine* 2012, *10*, 1341-1362.

[30] Cao, Z., Chen, X., Lin, W., Zhao, J., Zheng, L., Ye, H., Liao, L., Du, J. Jiedu xiaozheng yin decoction inhibits hepatoma cell proliferation by inducing apoptosis via the mitochondrial-mediated pathway. *Molecular Medicine Reports* 2015, *12*, 2800-2806.

[31] Cao, Z., Lin, W., Huang, Z., Chen, X., Zhao, J., Zheng, L., Ye, H., Liu, Z., Liao, L., Du, J. Ethyl acetate extraction from a Chinese herbal formula, jiedu xiaozheng yin, inhibits the proliferation of hepatocellular carcinoma cells via induction of g0/g1 phase arrest in vivo and in vitro. *International Journal of Oncology* 2013, *42*, 202-210.

[32] Qiu, D.Z., Zhang, Z.J., Wu, W.Z., Yang, Y.K. Bufalin, a component in chansu, inhibits proliferation and invasion of hepatocellular carcinoma cells. *BMC Complementary and Alternative Medicine* 2013, *13*, 185.

[33] Chen, D., Yao, W.J., Zhang, X.L., Han, X.Q., Qu, X.Y., Ka, W.B., Sun, D.G., Wu, X.Z., Wen, Z.Y. Effects of gekko sulfated polysaccharide-protein complex on human hepa-

toma smmc-7721 cells: Inhibition of proliferation and migration. *Journal of Ethnopharmacology* 2010, *127*, 702-708.

[34] Wu, X., Chen, D., Xie, G.R. Effects of gekko sulfated polysaccharide on the proliferation and differentiation of hepatic cancer cell line. *Cell Biology International* 2006, *30*, 659-664.

[35] Wang, N., Feng, Y., Zhu, M., Tsang, C.M., Man, K., Tong, Y., Tsao, S.W. Berberine induces autophagic cell death and mitochondrial apoptosis in liver cancer cells: The cellular mechanism. *Journal of Cellular Biochemistry* 2010, *111*, 1426-1436.

[36] Wang, Z.J., Song, L., Guo, L.C., Yin, M., Sun, Y.N. Induction of differentiation by panaxydol in human hepatocarcinoma smmc-7721 cells via camp and map kinase dependent mechanism. *Yakugaku zasshi: Journal of the Pharmaceutical Society of Japan* 2011, *131*, 993-1000.

[37] Zeng, X.L., Tu, Z.G. Induction of differentiation by ginsenoside rh2 in hepatocarcinoma cell smmc-7721. *Ai zheng = Aizheng = Chinese Journal of Cancer* 2004, *23*, 879-884.

[38] Lou, L., Ye, W., Chen, Y., Wu, S., Jin, L., He, J., Tao, X., Zhu, J., Chen, X., Deng, A., *et al.* Ardipusilloside inhibits survival, invasion and metastasis of human hepatocellular carcinoma cells. *Phytomedicine: International Journal of Phytotherapy and Phytopharmacology* 2012, *19*, 603-608.

[39] Hu, B., Sun, D., Sun, C., Sun, Y.F., Sun, H.X., Zhu, Q.F., Yang, X.R., Gao, Y.B., Tang, W.G., Fan, J., *et al.* A polymeric nanoparticle formulation of curcumin in combination with sorafenib synergistically inhibits tumor growth and metastasis in an orthotopic model of human hepatocellular carcinoma. *Biochemical and Biophysical Research Communications* 2015, *468*, 525-532.

[40] Lin, W., Zhao, J., Cao, Z., Zhuang, Q., Zheng, L., Zeng, J., Hong, Z., Peng, J. Livistona chinensis seeds inhibit hepatocellular carcinoma angiogenesis in vivo via suppression of the notch pathway. *Oncology Reports* 2014, *31*, 1723-1728.

[41] Jiang, W.G., Ye, L., Ji, K., Frewer, N., Ji, J., Mason, M.D. Inhibitory effects of yangzheng xiaoji on angiogenesis and the role of the focal adhesion kinase pathway. *International Journal of Oncology* 2012, *41*, 1635-1642.

[42] Weng, L.L., Xiang, J.F., Lin, J.B., Yi, S.H., Yang, L.T., Li, Y.S., Zeng, H.T., Lin, S.M., Xin, D.W., Zhao, H.L., *et al.* Asparagus polysaccharide and gum with hepatic artery embolization induces tumor growth and inhibits angiogenesis in an orthotopic hepatocellular carcinoma model. *Asian Pacific Journal of Cancer Prevention : APJCP* 2014, *15*, 10949-10955.

[43] Zhang, Q.B., Meng, X.T., Jia, Q.A., Bu, Y., Ren, Z.G., Zhang, B.H., Tang, Z.Y. Herbal compound songyou yin and moderate swimming suppress growth and metastasis of liver cancer by enhancing immune function. *Integrative Cancer Therapies* 2016 Sep;15(3): 368–75.

[44] Zhou, A.G., Zhang, Y., Kong, D.Y., Wang, Y., Zhang, H.Z., Wang, S.J., Kui, G., Hong, S., Ge, H.L., Ren, Q.H., *et al.* Tumor inhibiting and immunoloregulation effects of mylabris

mixture on h22 cancer-bearing mice. *Zhong xi yi jie he xue bao = Journal of Chinese Integrative Medicine* 2006, *4*, 504-508.

[45] Lin, L.W., Sun, Y., He, Y.M., Gao, S.D., Xue, E.S., Lin, X.D., Yu, L.Y., Lin, X.F., Yang, Y.H. Percutaneous intratumoral injection of traditional Chinese herbal compound medicine star-99 in treatment of hepatocellular carcinoma of mice. *Hepatobiliary & Pancreatic Diseases International: HBPD INT* 2004, *3*, 49-54.

[46] Huang, X., Qin, J., Lu, S. Kanglaite stimulates anticancer immune responses and inhibits hepg2 cell transplantation induced tumor growth. *Molecular Medicine Reports* 2014, *10*, 2153-2159.

[47] Wang, P.P., Xu, D.J., Huang, C., Wang, W.P., Xu, W.K. Astragaloside reduces the expression level of p-glycoprotein in multidrug-resistant human hepatic cancer cell lines. *Molecular Medicine Reports* 2014, *9*, 2131-2137.

[48] Ong, R.C., Lei, J., Lee, R.K., Cheung, J.Y., Fung, K.P., Lin, C., Ho, H.P., Yu, B., Li, M., Kong, S.K. Polyphyllin d induces mitochondrial fragmentation and acts directly on the mitochondria to induce apoptosis in drug-resistant hepg2 cells. *Cancer Letters* 2008, *261*, 158-164.

[49] Young, S.C., Wang, C.J., Hsu, J.D., Hsu, J.L., Chou, F.P. Increased sensitivity of hep g2 cells toward the cytotoxicity of cisplatin by the treatment of piper betel leaf extract. *Archives of Toxicology* 2006, *80*, 319-327.

9

SHetA2, a New Cancer-Preventive Drug Candidate

Shengquan Liu, Guangyan Zhou,
Sze Ngong Henry Lo, Maggie Louie and
Vanishree Rajagopalan

Abstract

SHetA2 (NSC 721689) is a novel synthetic flexible heteroarotinoid that has promising cancer-preventive activity, and has exhibited growth inhibition on 60 cancer cell lines in vitro, along with ovarian, lung, and kidney cancers *in vivo*. It binds and interferes with the function of a molecular chaperone, mortalin, leading to mitochondrial swelling and mitophagy that induce apoptosis in cancer cells without harming normal cells. It showed minimal toxicity in preclinical studies and thus is now in Phase-0 clinical trial. This chapter summarizes its evolution, synthesis, structure-activity relationship, mechanism of action, pharmacokinetics, and potential clinical applications in last 12 years. It also provides insights into designing more potent and safer SHetA2 analogs for future cancer-preventive drug development.

Keywords: SHetA2, flexible heteroarotinoids, apoptosis, cancer prevention, ovarian cancer

1. Introduction

Cancer-preventive agents are biologics, dietary supplements, nutrients or marketed drugs used to reduce the risk of developing cancer or prevent the recurrence of cancer [1]. The cancer-preventive actions of these agents are mediated by a variety of proposed mechanisms, which include inhibition of oxidative and inflammatory stress, immunomodulatory action, induction of cell differentiation and apoptosis, and inhibition of cell growth and angiogenesis. Hundreds of natural and synthetic compounds have been shown to inhibit cancer cell growth including vitamins (vitamins A, D, and E), organosulfur compounds (brassinin, sulforaphane, and isothiocyanates), minerals (calcium and selenium), phytoestrogens (resveratrol), flavonoids (genistein and quercetin), synthetic compounds (retinoids, sulforamate, and prenylated flavonoid analogs) [2], and marketed drugs (tamoxifen, raloxifene, finasteride, aspirin, sulindac, difluoromethylornithine, and metformin) [3]. Drug development for cancer prevention imposes distinct challenges beyond those associated with drug development for cancer therapy. One of the challenges is that cancer preventive agents must have higher therapeutic index. Nevertheless, the potential to intervene prior to the cancer developing is an attractive strategy to fight cancers [4].

A novel class of anticancer agents that has demonstrated such qualities is the flexible heteroarotinoids (Flex-Hets). Flex-Hets, derived from the retinoids, have exhibited potential anticancer activities in various cancer cell lines, while displaying minimal toxicity to normal cells. Among these compounds, SHetA2 [(4-nitrophenyl)amino][2,2,4,4-tetramethylthiochroman-6-yl]amino]methane-thione) exhibited the greatest growth inhibitory efficacy and potency against various cancer cell lines and was chosen as a lead compound for further development [5–7]. SHetA2 has been shown to interfere with mortalin binding to p53 and p66 Src homologous-collagen homologue (p66shc) leading to apoptosis in cancer cells [8]. Furthermore, it has been shown to induce both intrinsic [9] and extrinsic apoptotic pathway [10], cause cell cycle arrest [11], induce differentiation [7], and inhibit angiogenesis [12] in cancer cells, while displaying negligible toxicity in animal models [13]. Hence, SHetA2 was regarded as a novel class of promising anticancer agent that selectively targeted the cancer cells. Consequently, it was evaluated in preclinical development for cancer prevention through the National Cancer Institute (NCI) Rapid Access to Intervention Development (RAID) and Rapid Access to Preventive Intervention Development (RAPID) program [6]. Studies in rats and dogs showed that no toxicity was observed in any of the tested dosage groups. The no-observed-adverse-effect-level (NOAEL) for SHetA2 was not established and was considered to be above 1500 mg/kg/day in dogs [13]. The therapeutic window for administrative safety with SHetA2 was determined to be 25- to 150-folds above *in vivo* effective doses. As a result, it is currently undergoing Phase-0 clinical trials through RAID [14]. This chapter will provide a comprehensive review of SHetA2, including its design and development, and possible molecular targets and mechanisms of action and its potential clinical applications, based on the literature published thus far.

2. History of retinoid development

2.1. Retinoids

Retinoids, including natural retinoic acid (RA) and its synthetic derivatives, are a group of promising anticancer agents that have shown both chemotherapeutic and chemopreventive potential in both animals and humans [15–17]. They exhibit therapeutic properties by activating the retinoic acid receptors (RARs) and the retinoid X receptors (RXRs) [18]. Each receptor has three subtypes (-α, -β, -γ), and they belong to a family of proteins that regulate the transcription of genes responsible for a variety of metabolic, developmental, and differentiation pathways in cells and tissues [19]. Retinoids have been shown to inhibit growth, and induce differentiation and apoptosis of cancer cells both *in vitro* and *in vivo* [20, 21]. Naturally occurring retinoids, all-*trans*-retinoic acid (ATRA, **Figure 1, 1**), 9-*cis*-retinoic acid (**Figure 1, 2**), and 13-*cis*-retinoic acid (**Figure 1, 3**) have been shown to display significant anticancer activities [22]. Synthetic retinoids, such as *N*-(4-hydroxyphenyl) retinamide (4HPR, fenretinide, **Figure 1, 4**), are also effective inducers of apoptosis [23]. However, the use of retinoids as chemotherapeutics has been hampered by their local and systemic toxicities and side effects. Chronic retinoid treatment can lead to teratogenicity and toxicities to the skin, mucus membranes, hair, eyes, gastrointestinal system, liver, endocrine system, kidneys, and bone [24]. These toxicities are found to be associated with the activation of the nuclear retinoid receptors [25, 26].

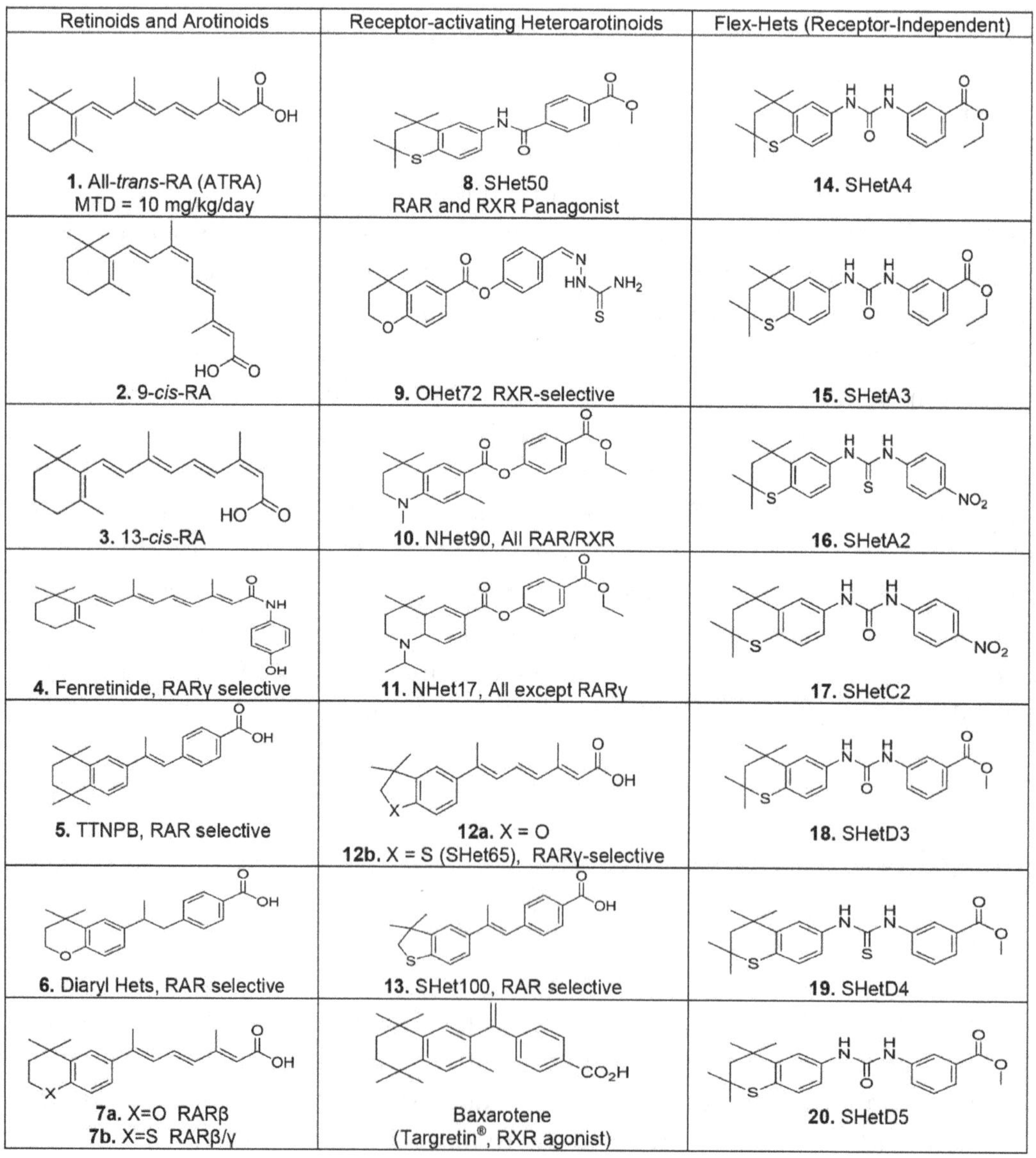

Figure 1. Chemical structures of retinoids, heteroarotinoids, and flexible-heteroarotinoids.

2.2. Arotinoids

Recognizing the potential chemopreventive and chemotherapeutic effects of retinoids, chemists have tried to design and synthesize new retinoid derivatives that express high cytotoxic potential with lower toxicity. The rationale is that by developing compounds that selectively activate only one retinoid receptor subtype, the associated toxicities could be reduced. For example, RXR-selective compounds were thought to have great potential for pharmacological use against tumors and other diseases due to a large number of ligand activated receptors whose activities involve dimerization with RXR receptors [19]. Bexarotene (Targretin®, with a one-carbon linker), is a selective RXR agonist and the first synthetic arotinoid approved for the treatment of all stages of cutaneous T-cell lymphoma [27]. RARγ, selectively expressed at high levels in the skin, has been shown to be the mediator of retinoid activity [28]. Early efforts to increase the therapeutic ratio of retinoids included increasing the structure rigidity by incorporating a double-bond between the two aromatic rings, leading to the development of arotinoids with two atom linker. For example, TTNPB (**Figure 1, 5**), an arotinoid with significant anti-tumor activity [29] was found to be selective for RAR receptors [30]. Unfortunately, intolerable toxicities observed in animal models limited its clinical utility [29].

2.3. Heteroarotinoids

Subsequent structural modifications involved the addition of one heteroatom (O, N, and S) in the cyclic ring of the arotinoids to block its oxidation into toxic metabolites. This resulted in the development of a new class of compounds called the heteroarotinoids (Hets, **Figure 1, 6–12**). These Hets exhibited similar biological activities to retinoids, but with significantly reduced toxicities [29, 31].

2.4. Flexible heteroarotinoids

Different linkers were placed between the two aryl groups of the Hets to increase their rigidity, providing a more specific fit into each receptor's binding pocket. Two-atom linkers, such as amide (**Figure 1, 8**) and esters (**Figure 1, 9–11**) were synthesized, and they showed varying degree of receptor selectivity. Interestingly, Hets with either the three-atom urea (**Figure 1, 14, 17, 18**) or thiourea (**Figure 1, 15, 16, 19, 20**) linker demonstrated significant anticancer activity without activating any of the retinoid receptors [6]. These compounds showed significant growth inhibitory activities against the ovarian cancer cell lines: Caov-3, OVCAR-3, and SK-OV-3, while exhibiting low activities against normal and benign cells. Moreover, due to the lack of RAR/RXR activation, these compounds did not exhibit the associated toxicities observed with other retinoids. Among these compounds, SHetA2 (**Figure 1, 16**) demonstrated the greatest potency against the aforementioned ovarian cancer cell lines at concentrations ranging from 0.2–3.7 μM. Since both urea and thiourea linkers are somewhat flexible in nature, these compounds were termed flexible heteroarotinoids (Flex-Hets). The evolution of SHetA2 is shown in **Figure 2**.

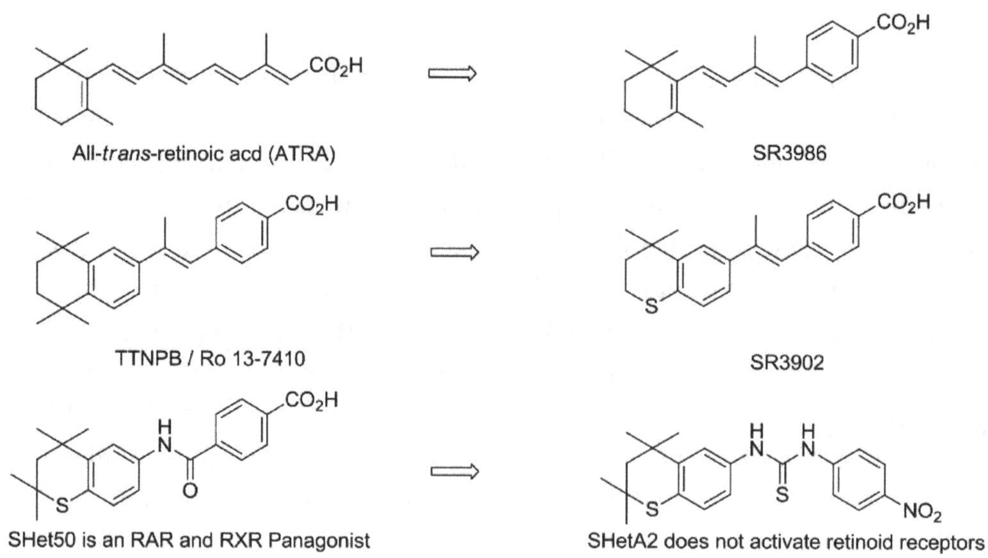

Figure 2. The evolution of SHetA2 from all *trans* retinoic acid (ATRA).

3. SHetA2, a Flex-Het

Flex-Hets have shown cancer-preventive activity by regulating apoptosis, cell growth, and differentiation in multiple types of cancer cell lines. They display significantly greater growth inhibition activities against ovarian cancer cells than both normal and benign ovarian cells [6]. Among the Flex-Hets, SHetA2 has shown to induce the highest levels of apoptosis in multiple cancer cell types, while retaining the differential resistance in normal cells [5]. SHetA2 functions independently of retinoid receptors [32] and therefore, lacks the toxicities associated with conventional retinoids. More importantly, SHetA2 differentially induces apoptosis in cancer cells while sparing normal cells [6]. All 60 cancer cell lines in NCI human tumor panel were sensitive to the growth inhibition activities of SHetA2 at micromolar concentrations [5] (**Table 1**). Despite this wide range of activity against cancer cells, normal and benign human ovarian, endometrial, and oral cultures were resistant to SHetA2-induced apoptosis and growth inhibition [6, 9]. In a recent study, SHetA2 was tested to be negative across three genetic toxicology assays, namely the *in vitro Salmonella-Escherichia coli* mutagenicity assay, Chinese hamster ovary cell chromosome aberration assay (CHO-CA), and *in vivo* mouse bone marrow micronucleus assay [34]. These assays are recommended by the International Conference on Harmonization (ICH), US Food and Drug Administration (FDA), and other regulatory agencies for the detection of mutagenicity by chemicals [35]. These negative results showed that SHetA2 was neither mutagenic nor genotoxic. In addition, SHetA2 exhibited no evidence of toxicity in animal models including dogs [13], and it did not induce skin irritation or teratogenicity [5, 36]. Encouraged by these promising results, SHetA2 was evaluated by NCI's RAID program for preclinical development as a cancer therapeutic agent (Application 196, Compound NSC 726189), and by RAPID program as a chemopreventive agent. Since SHetA2 showed no toxicity in preclinical studies, it is now in Phase-0 clinical trial.

GI_{50} Mean Graph for SHetA2 (NSC 726189) [33]

Cancer panel	Cell line	Log GI_{50} (SHetA2)	Log GI_{50} (ATRA)
Leukemia	CCRF-CEM	−4.9	−4.2
	HL-60(TB)	−4.5	−4.7
	K-562	−5.0	−4.3
	MOLT-4	−4.7	−4.3
	RPMI-8226	−4.5	−5.7
	SR	−4.9	−4.2
Nonsmall-cell lung carcinoma	A549/ATCC	−4.9	−4.3
	EKVX	−4.9	−4.0
	HOP-62	−4.7	−4.2
	HOP-92	−4.7	−4.0
	NCI-H226	−4.9	−4.3
	NCI-H23	−4.9	−4.2
	NCI-H322M	−5.0	−4.0
	NCI-H460	−4.6	−4.2
	NCI-H522	−5.0	−4.2
Colon cancer	COLO 205	−4.9	−4.2
	HCC-2998	−5.4	−4.2
	HCT-116	−4.8	−4.2
	HCT-15	−4.9	−4.2
	HT29	−4.6	−4.2
	KM12	−5.0	−4.3
	SW-620	−4.8	−4.2
CNS (gliomas)	SF-268	−4.6	−4.0
	SF-295	−5.0	−4.2
	SF-539	−5.0	−4.2
	SNB-19	−4.7	−4.2
	SNB-75	−4.8	−4.0
	U251	−5.0	−4.2
Melanoma	LOX IMVI	−4.9	−4.4
	MALME-3M	−5.6	−4.3
	M14	−4.7	−4.2
	MDA-MB-435	−4.9	−4.2
	SK-MEL-2	−5.0	−4.4
	SK-MEL-28	−4.8	−4.2
	SK-MEL-5	−5.0	−4.2
	UACC-257	−4.9	−4.2
	UACC-62	−5.0	−4.0
Ovarian cancer	IGROV1	−5.0	−4.0

	OVCAR-3	−5.0	−4.2
	OVCAR-4	−4.8	−4.0
	OVCAR-5	−4.8	−4.0
	OVCAR-8	−4.8	−4.2
	NCI/ACR-RES	−4.9	−4.4
	SK-OV-3	−4.8	−4.0
Renal cancer	786-0	−4.8	−4.2
	A498	−5.0	−4.0
	ACHN	−5.0	−4.2
	CAKI-1	−4.9	−4.2
	RXF 393	−4.7	−4.0
	SN12C	−5.0	−4.2
	TK-10	−5.0	−4.1
	UO-31	−4.9	−4.0
Prostate cancer	PC-3	−4.0	−4.3
	DU-145	−4.9	−4.2
Breast cancer	MCF7	−4.5	−4.4
	MDA-MB-231	−5.0	−4.3
	HS 578T	−4.6	−4.0
	BT-549	−4.9	−4.2
	T-47D	−4.8	-6.3

Lower values indicate greater inhibition of cell growth.

Table 1. Growth inhibition values (GI_{50}) of NCI's human tumor cell line panel expressed in log scale.

4. Synthesis of SHetA2

The synthesis of SHetA2 mainly involved the preparation of the intermediate, aminothiochroman (**Figures 3** and **4**). Early synthetic procedure (**Figure 3**) involved using Fe/HOAc to reduce the nitro group with a yield of 40% [6]. The nitration reaction was the problematic step with only a 26% yield, since many additional by-products were formed in this reaction. In order to address this issue, Tallent et al. employed a nitrogen-containing starting material (4-acetamidobenzenethiol) [37] (**Figure 4**). They used methyllithium instead of methylmagnesium bromide to form the intermediate carbinol. In the cyclization procedure to form the thiochroman, chlorobenzene was used as solvent with a 58% yield avoiding the use of flammable and noxious CS_2. This method circumvented the low-yielding nitration step and the subsequent reduction step to generate the amine group of aminothiochroman. The improved synthesis was shorter and afforded a 5-fold higher overall yield. The final product, SHetA2, was formed by reacting the aminothiochroman with 4-nitrophenyl isothiocyanate in tetrahydrofuran (**Figure 4**).

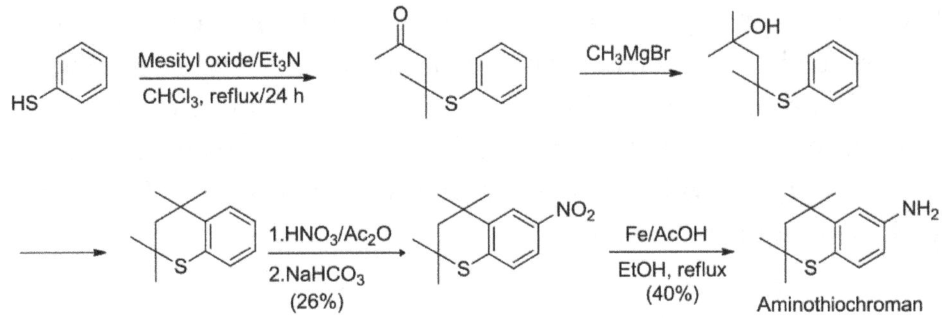

Figure 3. Synthesis of aminothiochroman.

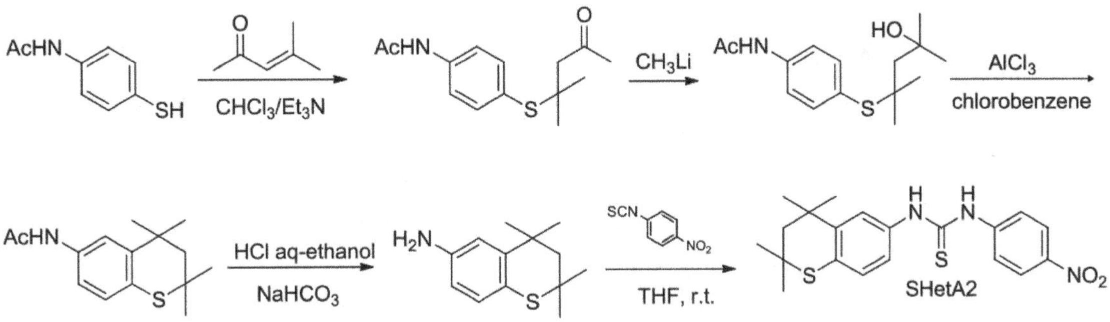

Figure 4. Improved synthesis of aminothiochroman and SHetA2.

5. Structure-activity relationship

Structure-activity relationship (SAR) of SHetA2 and its derivatives has been valuable to identify important structural modifications that have contributed to its anticancer potency and selectivity, and to guide the design of more potent and less toxic SHetA2 analogs. **Figure 2** illustrates the structural evolution of SHetA2 from ATRA. The goal was to increase the selectivity of retinoids towards RAR/RXR subtypes, so as to reduce the associated toxicities while retaining its anticancer activities. It has been shown that RAR-specific ligands can rescue *Raldh2*$^{-/-}$ embryos as effectively as ATRA, whereas RXR ligand showed no effect [36]. One strategy was to conformationally restrict the double-bonds of RA to allow a better fit into a specific receptor subtype by incorporating aromatic rings. For example, SR3986 (**Figure 2**) was developed with an aromatic ring from ATRA. Subsequently, TTNPB (**5**), the lead arotinoid, was modified with a diaryl group to increase its rigidity, and it was found to be selective for RAR receptors and 10 times more potent as compared to ATRA [38]. Unfortunately, this compound also exhibited a 10,000-fold increase in toxicity, which limited its clinical usage [29].

In order to reduce toxicity, a benzylic carbon in the tetrahydronaphthalene was replaced with a heteroatom (O, N, and S). The purpose was to prevent benzylic (metabolic) oxidation which could result in toxic metabolites. This single modification resulted in Hets (**Figure 1, 6–12**) with similar biological activities to RA but significantly reduced toxicities [29, 31]. An example was the diaryl heteroarotinoid (**Figure 1, 6**), a RAR-selective retinoid derivative. It differed from TTNPB by an oxygen heteroatom, but exhibited a significant decrease in toxicity, increasing the maximum tolerated dose (MTD) by 3000-fold as compared to TTNPB (**Figure 1, 5**) [39]. Other monoaryl heteroarotinods (**Figure 1, 7a, 7b**) were also evaluated, and revealed a 3-fold decrease in toxicity along with a decreased ability to activate the RAR receptors when compared to ATRA (**Figure 5**) [40, 30].

Compounds	Maximum Tolerated Dose (MTD)
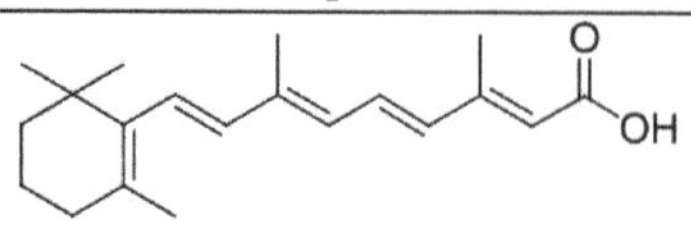 ATRA (**1**)	MTD = 10 mg/kg/day
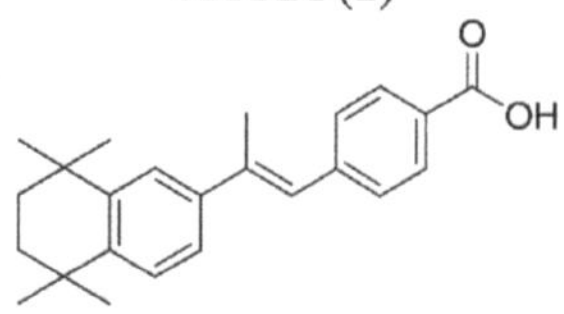 TTNPB (**5**)	MTD = 0.01 mg/kg/day
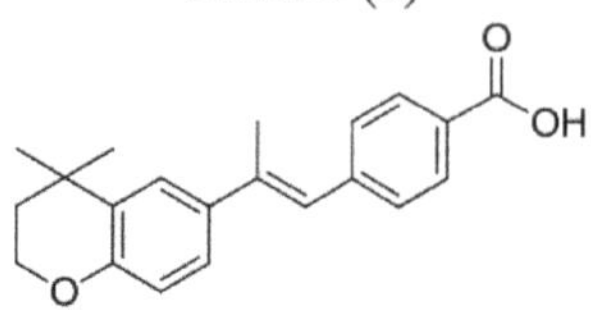 Diaryl Heteroarotinoid (**6**)	MTD = 9.4 mg/kg/day
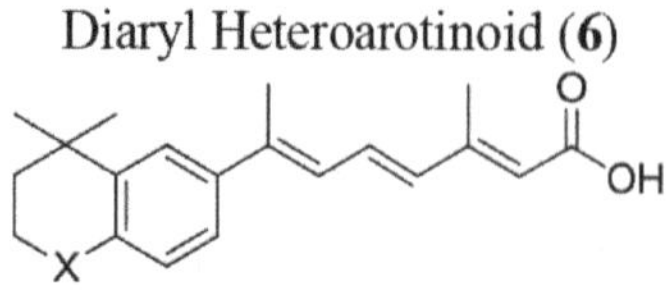 **7a.** X = O, **7b.** X = S	X = O MTD = 32 mg/kg/day X = S MTD = 34 mg/kg/day
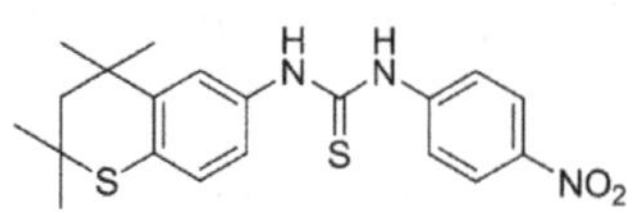 SHetA2 (**16**)	MTD > 1500 mg/kg/day

Figure 5. Maximum tolerated dose (MTD) for retinoids and their derivatives.

5.1. Thiochroman rings

SAR studies have identified structures containing six-membered ring (**Figure 1, 7a, 7b**) tend to confer increased RARβ selectivity over five-membered ring systems (**Figure 1, 12a, 12b**), while sulfur heteroatom confers a greater RARγ selectivity over oxygen atom [19]. The thiochroman ring system is flexible and has been shown to induce apoptosis to a greater extent than a rigid planar quinoline unit [41]. These findings highlight the important role played by the thiochroman ring in enhancing the activity of Flex-Hets. Therefore, the thiochroman ring forms one of the fundamental moieties of SHetA2 and its analogs (14–20).

5.2. Two-atom linkers

To further increase the selectivity for each RAR and RXR receptors, various linkers were placed between the two aryl groups of the Hets by modifying their structure rigidity. Two-atom linker compounds such as amide (**Figure 1, 8**) and ester (**Figure 1, 9**) were reported [42, 43]. Compound (**8**) was found to be a receptor panagonist, while compound (**9**) was RXR selective. Both showed significant growth inhibitory activities against head and neck cancer using a tumor xenograft mouse model [42]; however, only compound (**8**) induced apoptosis in ovarian cancer cells. This indicated that RXR activation is sufficient to inhibit tumor growth, while activation of both RAR and RXR are required for the maximum activity, at the expense of toxicity. Other two ester-linked compounds (**Figure 1, 10, 11**) were found to activate both RARs and RXRs [44]. On the other hand, these ester-linked Hets appeared to only induce growth inhibition but not apoptosis.

5.3. Three-atom linkers

Three-atom linkers have also been reported in the literature (**Figure 4, 21, 22**). It was suggested that the presence of a three-atom linker may increase RAR selectivity [45], and the ability for linkers to form hydrogen bonds may enhance RARγ selectivity [46]. As such, a series of urea/thiourea derivatives were synthesized and evaluated (**Figure 1, 14–20**) [6, 7]. Unlike conventional retinoids, these Flex-Hets were able to induce selective and potent apoptotic activity in cancer cells independent of RAR/RXR activation [44]. The only retinoid activity retained by Flex-Hets is the ability to induce differentiation and reverse the cancerous phenotype.

The X-ray crystal structure of the Flex-Hets showed that a unique lattice network formed through extensive intermolecular H-bonding between the NH and the oxygen of the highly polarized C=O urea linker in another molecule, whereas this was not observed in the C=S thiourea derivatives. It suggested that the urea derivatives may be more active than its thiourea counterpart. This observation is also supported by their *in vitro* growth inhibition activities where the urea derivative, SHetC2 (**17**), demonstrated to be slightly more potent (EC_{50}= 1.02 μM) than its thiourea counterpart, SHetA2 (**16**) (EC_{50}= 1.72 μM) [41].

Regardless, the fact remains that millions of dollars have been invested by the NCI RAID and RAPID programs in the preclinical development of SHetA2, and many studies involving animal models have shown that SHetA2 is a potent and selective inducer of apoptosis with no significant toxicities. While SHetC2 lacks these extensive studies, it does show potential as the next chemopreventive drug candidate following SHetA2. These results indicate that the inclusion of three-atom urea/thiourea linker is critical to induce potent anticancer activities independent of RAR/RXR activation as observed in these Flex-Hets. **Tables 2** and **3** summarize the effects of the structural modifications on the growth inhibition by these derivatives against various cancer cell lines reported to-date.

Compound	Cell growth inhibition													
	Renal (%)		Ovarian cancer (%)			NE EC$_{50}$ (μM)	Vulvar cancer (%)		Cervical cancer (%)				HN cancer (%)	
	Cancer	Normal												
	1	1	1	2	3	NE	1	2	1	2	3	4	1	2
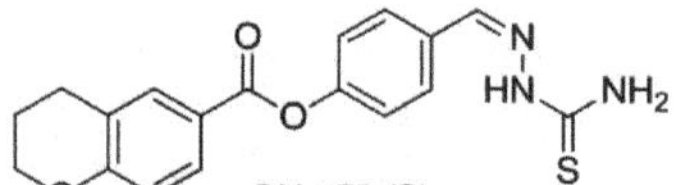 OHet72 (**9**)	–	–	–	–	–	–	–	–	–	–	–	–	19	18
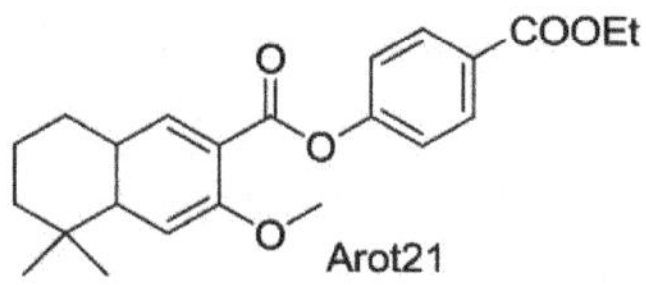 Arot21	–	–	–	–	–	–	–	–	–	–	–	–	15	12
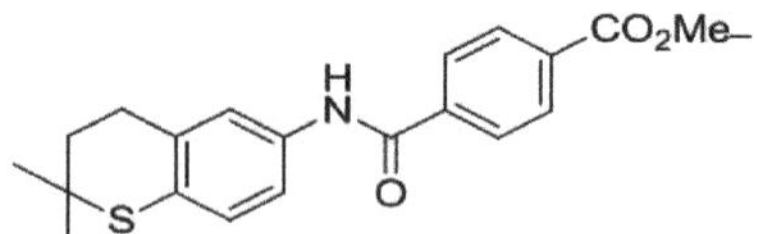 SHet50 (**8**)	–	–	–	–	–	–	–	–	–	–	–	–	64	37
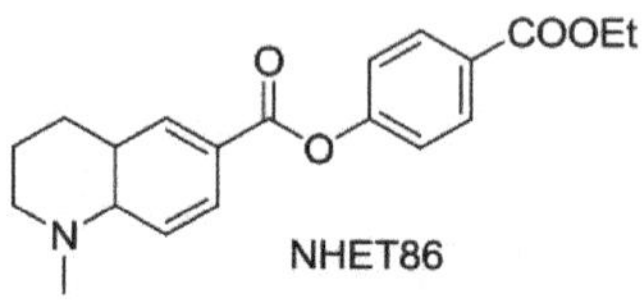 NHET86	–	–	0	–	1	–	34	14	40	25	–	–	12	13
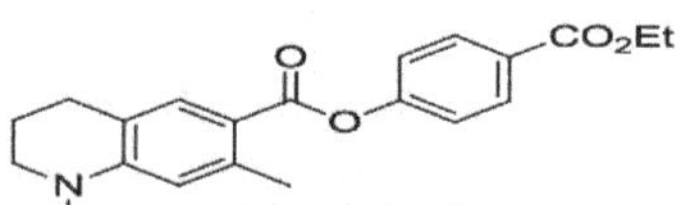 NHet90 (**10**)	–	–	5	–	0	–	81	84	26	16	–	–	9	7
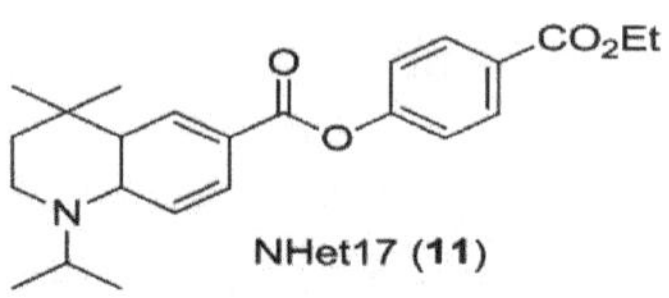 NHet17 (**11**)	–	–	6	–	2	–	47	25	25	13	–	–	5	15
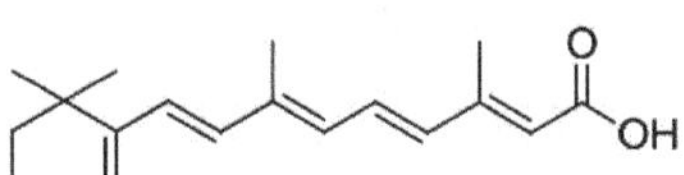 ATRA (**1**)	6.5	16	–	–	–	–	–	–	–	–	–	–	–	52
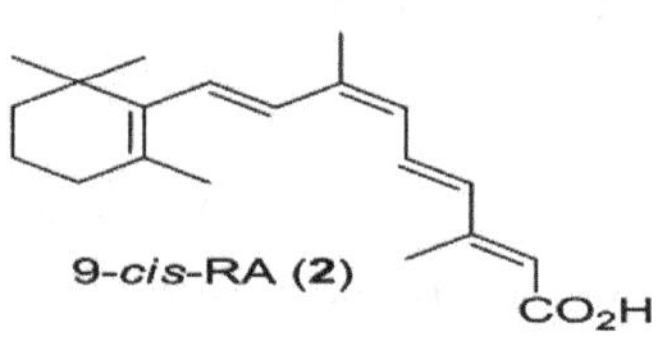 9-*cis*-RA (**2**)	–	–	25	–	31	>10	38	31	24	28	45	47	–	51
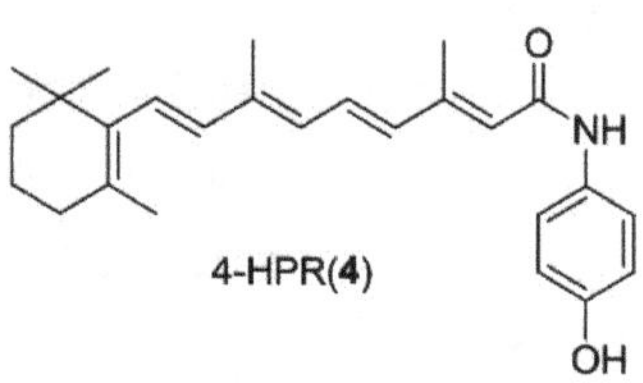 4-HPR(**4**)	–	–	62	43	65	>10	–	–	–	–	–	–	–	74

Compound	Cell growth inhibition						
	Renal (%)		Ovarian	NE	Vulvar	Cervical cancer	HN cancer
	Cancer	Normal	cancer (%)	EC_{50} (μM)	cancer (%)	(%)	(%)
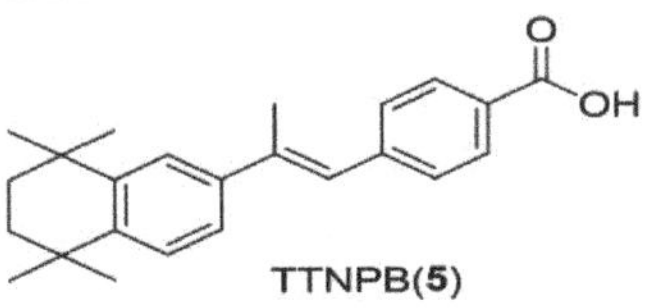 TTNPB(**5**)	–	–	11 – 19	–	34 19	– – – –	74 –

Growth inhibition (%) for renal cancer cell lines (1) Caki-1 and (2) 786-0; Normal renal cells (1) HK-2 and (2) RTC91696 [23]. Growth Inhibition (%) for ovarian cancer cell lines (1) CAOV-3, (2) OVCAR-3, and (3) SKOV-3 [6]. EC_{50} values for 50% growth inhibition for ovarian cancer cell line (4) A2780, and Normal endometrial cells (NE) [6, 41]. Growth inhibition (%) for cervical cancer cell lines (1) SiHa, (2) CC-1, (3) C33a, and (4) HT-3 [5]. Growth inhibition (%) for head and neck squamous cell cancer cell lines (HN) (1) SCC-2 [43], and (2) SCC-38 [32, 42]. Growth inhibition (%) for vulvar cancer cell lines (1) SW954 and (2) SW962 from Ref. [43].
"–" indicates no data available.

Table 2. Structural modifications of Hets, and their effects on cancer cell growth.

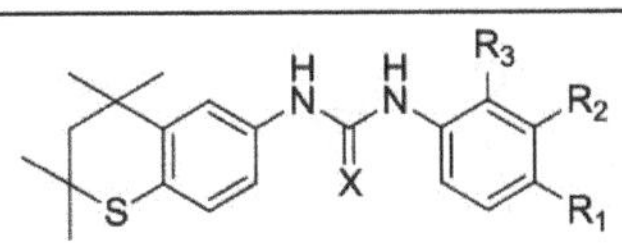

General Structure of Flex-Het

					Cell growth inhibition													
					Renal cancer (%)		Renal normal (%)		Ovarian cancer (%)				NE	Cervical cancer (%)				HN cancer (%)
									EC_{50}(μM)									
	X	R_1	R_2	R_3	1	2	1	2	1	2	3	4	NE	1	2	3	4	1
14	O	CO_2Et	H	H	69	45	26	40	40	69	47	2.8	4.5	67	59	85	76	42
15	S	CO_2Et	H	H	56	54	35	28	24	58	42	2.9	2.7	58	42	84	65	39
16	S	NO_2	H	H	84	72	51	37	55	67	45	1.7	3.0	68	58	87	92	81
17	O	NO_2	H	H	86	79	53	52	–	–	–	1.0	2.3	–	–	–	–	–
18	O	CO_2Me	H	H	57	62	26	46	–	–	–	–	–	–	–	–	–	–
19	S	CO_2Me	H	H	39	45	44	38	–	–	–	–	–	–	–	–	–	–
20	S	H	CO_2Me	H	34	42	48	–	–	–	–	–	–	–	–	–	–	–
SHetA19	S	NO_2	H	Me	–	–	–	–	32	65	51	–	–	–	–	–	–	68

Growth inhibition (%) for renal cancer cell lines (1) Caki-1 and (2) 786-0; Normal renal cells (1) HK-2 and (2) RTC91696 [23]. Growth Inhibition (%) for ovarian cancer cell lines (1) CAOV-3, (2) OVCAR-3, and (3) SKOV-3 [6]. EC_{50} values for 50% growth inhibition for ovarian cancer cell line (4) A2780, and Normal endometrial cells (NE) [6, 41]. Growth inhibition (%) for cervical cancer cell lines (1) SiHa, (2) CC-1, (3) C33a, and (4) HT-3 [5]. Growth inhibition (%) for head and neck squamous cell cancer cell lines (HN) (1) SCC-2 [43], and (2) SCC-38 [32, 42]. Growth inhibition (%) for vulvar cancer cell lines (1) SW954 and (2) SW962 from Ref. [43].
"–" indicates no data available.

Table 3. Structural modifications of Flex-Hets, and their effects on cancer cell growth.

Substitutions on the phenyl group have also been evaluated [7]. The nitro (NO_2) substitution (**Table 3, 16, 17**) consistently exhibited greater growth inhibitory and apoptotic activity than their methyl (**Table 3, 18–20**) or ethyl ester counterparts (**Table 3, 14, 15**). This suggests that the nitro substitution may have enhanced the overall activity of the compound. Collectively, for the Flex-Hets, the thiochroman ring and nitro substitution are important for enhancing the anticancer activity, while the thiourea linker is crucial for RAR/RXR independent and selective anticancer activities against cancer cells.

5.4. Three-atom linker with thiochroman ring replaced

In order to expand the potential clinical applications, we designed, synthesized, and evaluated nine *p*-nitrodiarylthiourea analogs in breast (MCF-7, T-47D, MDA-MB-453) and prostate (DU-145, PC-3, LNCaP) cancer cell lines for their anticancer activities. Majority of our compounds were able to inhibit the growth of these six cancer cell lines at low micromolar concentrations. Compound **23** (**Figure 6**) was found to be the most potent anticancer agent in this series with GI_{50} values of 3.16 μM for MCF-7, 2.53 μM for T-47D, 4.77 μM for MDA-MB-453 breast cancer lines and 3.54 μM for LNCaP prostate cancer cell line. These GI_{50} values were comparable to the parent compound, SHetA2 [47].

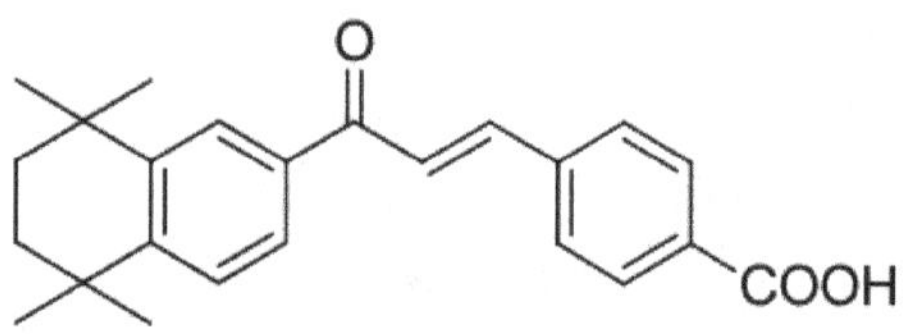

21. Chalcone-Linker

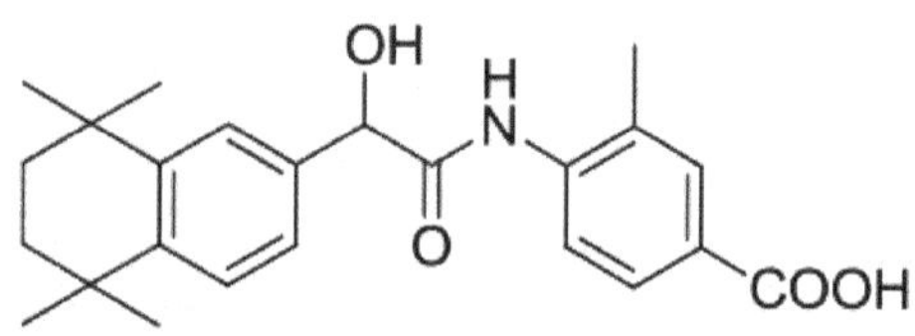

22. α-hydroxyamide-Linker

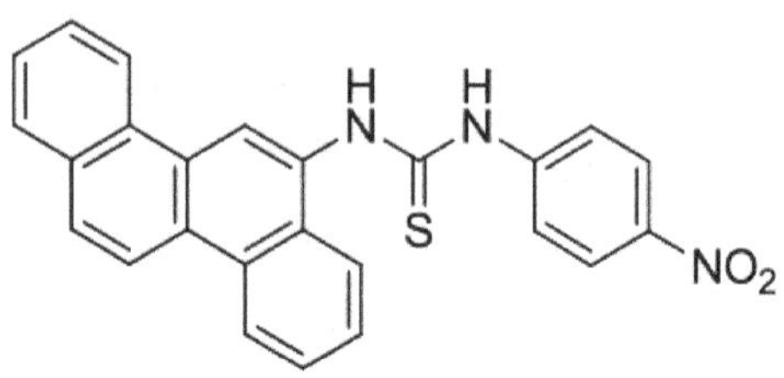

23. Compound 7- Liu

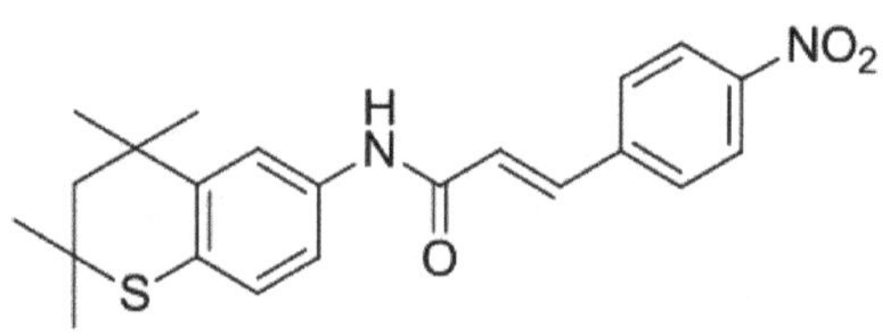

24. 18b- Bunce

Figure 6. Three- and four-atom linkers in retinoid derivatives.

5.5. Four-atom linker

Another approach to the structure modification of SHetA2 was to keep the thiochroman ring but replace the thiourea linker with a 4-atom acrylamide linker NC(O)C=C and various substitutions on the terminal aryl ring. When evaluated in a cytotoxicity assay of the human A2780 ovarian cancer cell line, results indicate that activity of 4-nitro phenyl analogs are comparable to that of SHetA2 with efficacies slightly reduced compared to SHetA2 [48]. The α,β-unsaturated acrylamide may contribute to its increase in potency and the compound **24** (**Figure 6**) is the example.

6. Mechanism of action

The biological targets and SHetA2's mechanism of action have been extensively studied. Coimmunoprecipitation experiments demonstrated that SHetA2 interfered with the binding of mortalin, a molecular chaperone to p53 and p66 Src homologous-collagen homolog (p66shc) in A2780 ovarian cancer cell line, leading to mitochondrial swelling and mitophagy and finally apoptosis [8]. SHetA2 is also involved in modulating other cellular processes including cell-growth, differentiation, and angiogenesis.

6.1. Induction of apoptosis

6.1.1. Intrinsic pathway

SHetA2 is shown to selectively induce apoptosis in various cancer cell lines by targeting the mitochondria [32]. Exposure of SHetA2 to squamous carcinoma cells resulted in a decrease in mitochondrial permeability transition, followed by the release of cytochrome *c* into the cytoplasm, activation of caspase-3, and the induction of intrinsic apoptotic pathway. Further studies proposed that SHetA2-mediated mitochondrial swelling involved lowering the levels of anti-apoptotic proteins such as Bcl-XL and Bcl-2 in A2780 ovarian cancer cell [9]. However, the pro-apoptotic Bax expression was unaffected by SHetA2, suggesting SHetA2 may regulate the levels of Bcl-2 to promote apoptosis [9]. On the other hand, exposure of SHetA2 to normal ovarian or endometrial cells was found to increase both Bcl-XL and Bcl-2 protein levels. The up-regulation of these anti-apoptotic proteins may provide the cytoprotective effects necessary to block SHetA2-induced apoptosis in normal cells [9].

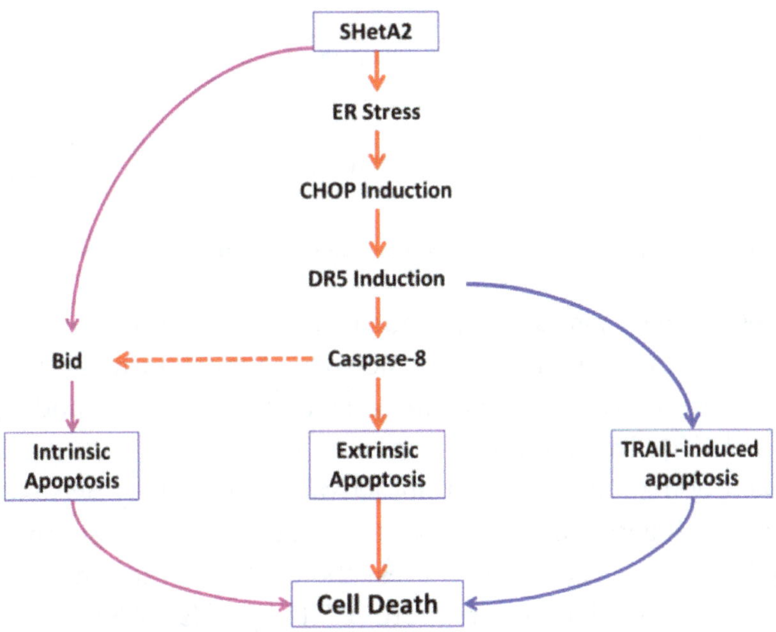

Figure 7. Pathways involving SHetA2-induced apoptosis.

6.1.2. Extrinsic pathway (death receptor pathway)

Exposure of non-small cell lung cancer cells (NSCLC) to SHetA2 revealed the induction of the extrinsic apoptotic pathway involving the death receptor 5 (DR5) [49]. It was shown that SHetA2-enhanced DR5 expression through the enhanced binding of CAAT/enhancer-binding protein homologous protein (CHOP) to its binding site located in the 5′-flanking region of the DR5 gene. Since CHOP is highly inducible during endoplasmic reticulum (ER) stress, this finding suggests that SHetA2 may act as an inducer of ER stress. The induction of DR5 expression leads to caspase 8-dependent apoptosis. Moreover, the induction of DR5 was shown to enhance tumor necrosis factor-related apoptosis-inducing ligand (TRAIL)-induced apoptosis (**Figure 7**). Further studies found that down-regulation of cellular FLICE-inhibitory protein (c-FLIP), and to a lesser extent of survivin, were involved in SHetA2-induced apoptosis, as well as enhancement of TRAIL-initiated apoptosis [50]. c-FLIP is a major inhibitor of the extrinsic apoptotic pathway [51], while survivin modulates both intrinsic and extrinsic apoptotic pathways [52].

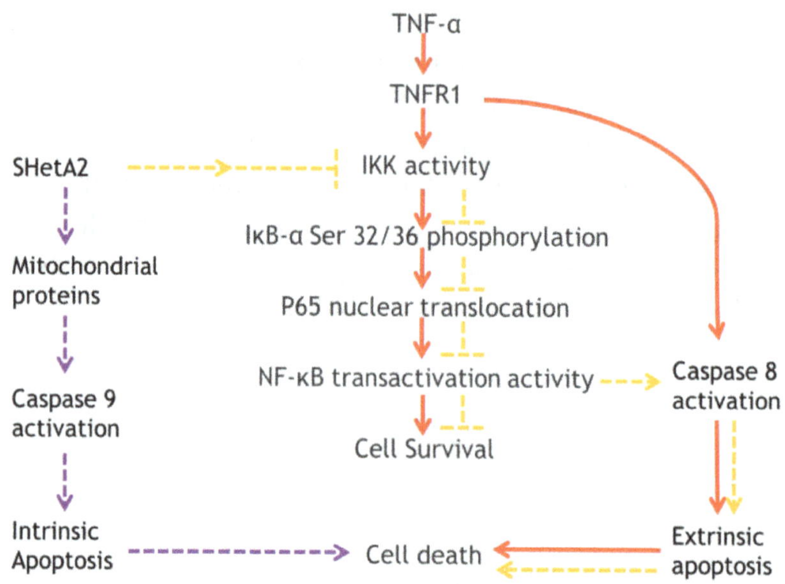

Figure 8. Working model for the apoptotic pathway involving NF-kB in ovarian cancer cells.

TRAIL and its receptors have also attracted much attention recently because TRAIL preferentially induces apoptosis in malignant cells while sparing most normal cells [53]. SHetA2 was found to sensitize ovarian carcinomas that are resistant to these DR ligands, without harming the normal cells [54, 55]. This suggests a possible synergistic effect Further investigation identified that downregulation of NF-kB transactivation activity by SHetA2 was involved in this sensitizing effect, triggering extrinsic apoptosis in cancer cells resistant to certain chemotherapeutics [55]. SHetA2 was shown to repress the upstream IkB kinase (IKK) activity that resulted in NF-kB downregulation. Apart from DR ligands, SHetA2 has also shown its chemosensitizing effects against cisplatin-resistant ovarian cancer through p53-independent pathways [6, 56]. However, such enhancement of sensitivities was not observed in resistant uterine cancer cell lines for a number of chemotherapeutics in combination with SHetA2 treatment (**Figure 8**) [57].

	Apoptotic pathways affected by SHetA2		
	Possible biological targets	Effect	Reference
Intrinsic	↓ GSH	Redox regulation	[7]
	↓ *Bcl-2*	Antiapoptotic	[9]
	↓ *Bcl-XL*	Antiapoptotic	[9]
	↓ Survivin	Antiapoptotic	[50]
	↑ Caspase-9	Proapoptotic	[49]
	↑ Caspase-3	Proapoptotic	[32]
	↑ Bid	Proapoptotic	[49]
Extrinsic	↑ Caspase-8	Proapoptotic	[10]
	↑ Bip/GRP78, IRE1α, ATF4, XBP1	ER stress	[49]
	↑ DR-5	Cell death	[55]
	↑ CHOP	Cell death	[49]
	↓ IKK	Cell survival	[55]
	↓ NF-kB	Cell survival	[50]
	↓ c-FLIP	Antiapoptotic	[50]
Cell cycle pathways			
	↓ Cyclin D1	G_1 arrest	[11]
	↓ AP-1	Cell-cycle progression	[62]
Differentiation induction pathways			
	↑ E-Cadherin	Differentiation	[7]
	↑ MUC1	Differentiation	[44]
Antiangiogenic pathways			
	↑ Thrombospondin (TSP-4)	Antiangiogenic	[12]
	↓ Thymidine Phosphorylase (TP)	Angiogenic	[12]
	↓ VEGF	Angiogenic	[12]
Signal transduction pathways			
	↓ KIT kinase (c-KIT)	Cell death	[63]

Table 4. Possible biological pathways affected by SHetA2 and its anticancer activities.

6.1.3. *ROS and GSH*

Increased reactive oxygen species (ROS) level was initially thought to be responsible for SHetA2-induced apoptosis. Multiple studies have documented the ROS generation along with mitochondrial swelling and the release of cytochrome *c* in various cancer cell lines [6, 32]. Studies have also shown that SHetA2 is able to form adducts with glutathione (GSH) [7, 58]. This was reflected by the generation of ROS as reported in several pharmacokinetic studies [58, 59]. GSH is essential for cell survival. Adduct formation with GSH causes GSH depletion, leading to accumulation of ROS resulting in oxidative mitochondrial damage, ultimately causing cell death [60]. Although the exact role of GSH depletion in apoptosis is still controversial, it remains an early hallmark in the progression of cell death in numerous cell types [61]. Therefore, adduct formation between SHetA2 and GSH could be vital to the induction of apoptosis, as indicated by the ROS generation. However, further studies suggested that ROS generation appeared to be a consequence of, and not a cause for, mitochondrial swelling and apoptosis induced by SHetA2 treatment [7, 9]. Addition of GSH did not attenuate SHetA2-induced apoptosis [55]. It was also noted that the cellular GSH level was in the μM range, while μM SHetA2 is sufficient to kill cells, indicating that GSH depletion and ROS accumulation are not the only mechanisms of action. These findings suggest that SHetA2 probably acts through several mechanisms of action to bring about its apoptotic effect, along with other anticancer activities, such as cell cycle arrest and induction of differentiation (**Table 4**).

6.2. Induction of cell-cycle arrest and differentiation

Apart from apoptosis, SHetA2 repression of NF-kB expression also initiates a series of events that can lead to cell-cycle arrest and cell differentiation. SHetA2-induced Cyclin D1 degradation in both Caki-1 renal cancer and normal HK-2 cell lines results in the accumulation of cells in the G_0-G_1 phase [7]. Cyclin D1 degradation alone has shown to be sufficient in inducing G_1 cell cycle arrest [11]. Cyclin D1 transcription can be induced by NF-kB through multiple NF-kB-binding sites in the Cyclin D1 promoter, which is consistent with the observed down regulation of Cyclin D1. Also, SHetA2 can induce cellular differentiation in kidney [7], as well as in ovarian cancer organotypic cultures and xenografts [5]. Treatment of these cancer cells shows that 1 μM SHetA2 is sufficient to reverse the cancerous phenotype depending on the status of the cells. However, at higher concentrations of SHetA2, apoptosis would dominate over differentiation. The mechanism for differentiation induction is likely to be associated with the upregulation of E-Cadherin in renal cancer cells observed with the repression of NF-kB [7]. Decrease or loss of nuclear E-Cadherin expression is associated with poor prognosis in kidney cancer, as it confers the ability to migrate and invade [64]. Therefore, up-regulation or restoration of E-Cadherin's function has been one of the therapeutic goals for anticancer treatments.

6.3. Antiangiogenic activity

Microarray analysis have suggested that SHetA2 treatment results in significant up-regulation of thrombospondin-4 (TSP-4), and down-regulation of thymidine phosphorylase (TP) in A2780 ovarian cancer cells. TSP-4 and TP protein levels followed those of the mRNA. TSP-4 was hypothesized to be antiangiogenic due to the presence of type-III repeats which is also found in TSP-1. The type-III repeats in TSP-1 has been reported to inhibit the binding of fibroblast growth factor-2 to endothelial cells, a process that leads to endothelial cell proliferation *in vitro* [65]. As for TP, it has found to be angiogenic through its ability to convert thymidine to thymine and the angiogenic 2-deoxy-D-ribose-1-phosphate, as well as its metabolite, deoxy-D-ribose. Protein levels of the angiogenic vascular endothelial growth factor A (VEGF) was also found to be downregulated despite its up-regulated mRNA level upon SHetA2 treatment. Interestingly, both mRNA and protein levels of the angiogenic basic fibroblast growth factor (bFGF) were also up-regulated, but its effect was deemed limited due to brief up-regulation of the gene only after hours of treatment with high concentration of SHetA2 [12]. Hence, the net effect of SHetA2 on these various proteins is antiangiogenic, and is supported by the decrease of endothelial tube formation observed in a number of cancer cell lines as well as human umbilical vascular endothelial cells (HUVECs) [12].

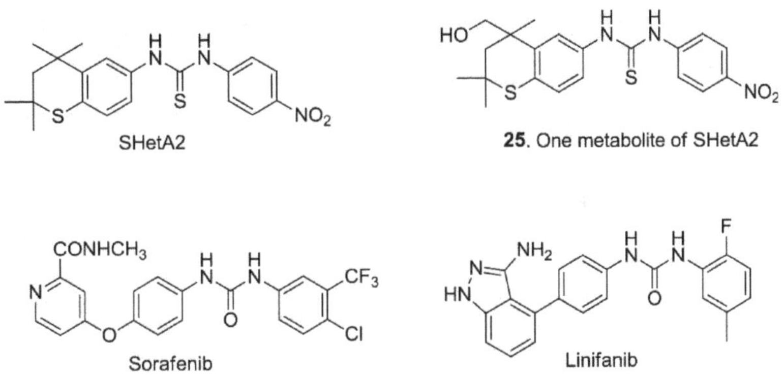

Figure 9. Structural comparison of SHetA2 and its metabolite with sorafenib and linifanib.

6.4. Kinase inhibitory activity

SHetA2 is also being evaluated for its ability to inhibit kinase activity based on its structural similarity to sorafenib and linifanib (**Figure 9**) [63]. Sorafenib is an FDA approved diarylurea multikinase inhibitor that inhibits tumor growth, while linifanib is a KIT-3 kinase inhibitor [66, 67]. All three compounds consist of a three atom urea or thiourea linker between two aromatic rings, of which this structural conformation is found to be vital for the formation of key H-bonds within the binding pockets of several kinases, including B-Raf, BCR-ABL, and KIT [63]. Upon evaluation with 442 different human kinases, SHetA2(**Figure 9**) has exhibited good binding affinity for KIT kinase (binding constant, Kd = 820 nM). This indicates that SHetA2 is a potential candidate for kinase inhibitor development. More importantly, one of the metabolites of SHetA2 (**Figure 9, 25**) has also shown comparable binding affinity for KIT kinase (Kd = 1200 nM) [63]. This suggests that other metabolites of SHetA2 may also be active, which could have acted via different mechanisms of action and contributed to the various anticancer effects observed, making it a versatile chemotherapeutic agent.

7. Metabolism of SHetA2

Using liquid chromatography and tandem mass spectroscopy, four GSH adducts were identified along with four mono- and dihydroxylated SHetA2 metabolites [58]. At least one of these metabolites (**Figure 9, 25**) has been deemed active against KIT kinase as mentioned earlier. Apart from the hydroxylated metabolites, other metabolites of SHetA2 were also detected *in vivo* [58, 59]. These metabolites may be produced upon formation of GSH adducts. The proposed mechanism for the formation of GSH adduct is shown in **Figure 10**. Subsequently, the GSH adduct could undergo further reactions that may result in the cleavage of the

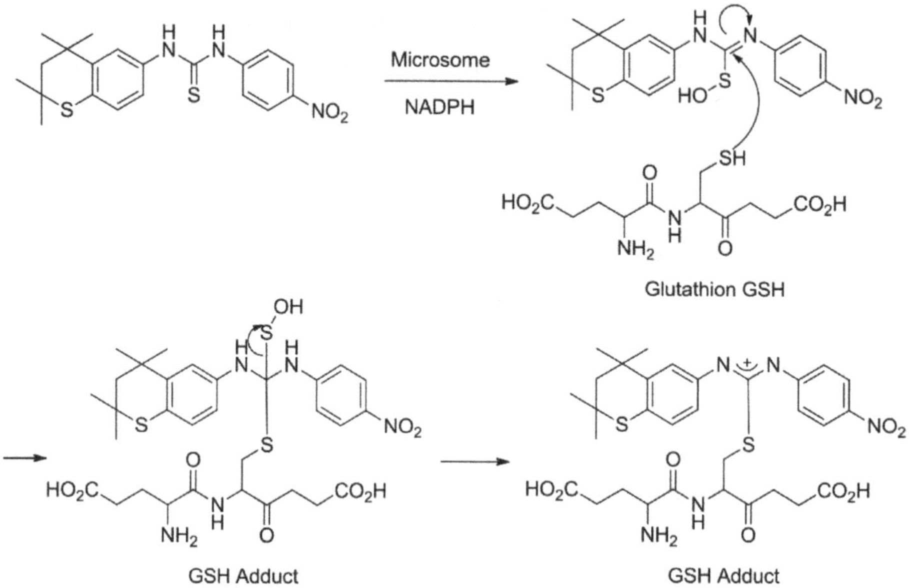

Figure 10. Proposed mechanism for the GSH adduct formation of SHetA2.

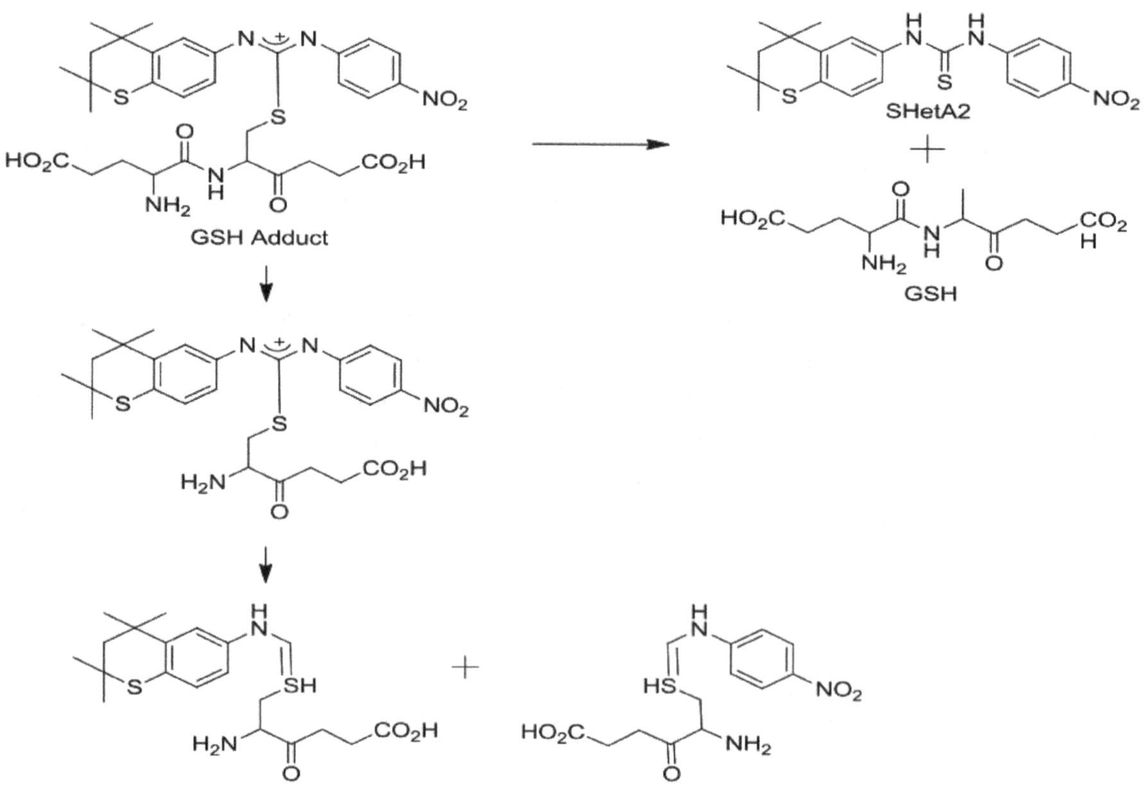

Figure 11. Proposed mechanism for the formation of metabolites following the formation of GSH adducts.

thiourea linker, yielding two metabolites that were also detected *in vivo* [58]. The proposed mechanism for the formation of these metabolites is shown in **Figure 11**.

Given that ShetA2 has several mechanisms of action involving various cellular targets, these findings suggest the possibility for SHetA2 to be metabolized into several active metabolites, each targeting a different molecular pathway. This is further supported by a recent *in vivo* study where the monohydroxy SHetA2 (**25**) was found to be the major metabolite of SHetA2 in rat plasma, and it was detected at a much higher concentration than the parent compound after oral and intravenous administration [13].

8. Pharmacokinetics

Pharmacokinetic studies using HPLC/UV of SHetA2 in mice(**Table 5**) have shown that pharmacokinetic profile of this compound is favorable for future development [59].

	PK	SHetA2
1	Oral bioavailability at 20 mg/kg	15%
	Oral bioavailability at 60 mg/kg	19%
2	Urinary excretion (%)	Not reported
3	Bound to mouse and human plasma proteins at μM concentrations	99.3–99.5%
4	Total body clearance (L/h/kg)	1.8
5	Volume distribution (L/kg) at steady state (*V*dss)	20.8
6	Half-life in mouse plasma	12.7 h
	Half-life in the mouse	Detectable after 60 h after IV administration
	Half-life in human plasma (once a day dosing proposed)	12 h
7	Peak time (plasma concentrations of 10 μM following i.v. bolus dose)	5 min
8	Peak concentration (IV 20 mg/kg dose of SHetA2 to mice)	10 μM after 5 min
	Maxima mean plasma concentration in the mouse (PO)	0.79 μM at 2 h
		2.35 μM at 3 h

Table 5. Pharmacokinetic data of SHetA2 [59].

9. Possible clinical applications

SHetA2 is now in Phase-0 clinical trial for ovarian cancer chemoprevention. However, since it inhibits growth of most cancers *in vitro* and *in vivo*, it may potentially be used for the prevention and treatment of other cancers which are listed in **Table 6**.

Cancer type	Findings	References
Ovarian cancer	G_1-phase cell cycle arrest through cyclin D1 degradation and apoptosis. Reduced cell survival, and increased sensitivity to TRAIL- and TNFα-induced apoptosis. Induced glandular differentiation reversed cancerous phenotype.	[14]
Uterine cancer • Endometrial carcinoma (HEC-1-A) • MMT (MES-SA) • uterine sarcoma (SK-UT-1)	SHetA2 decreased survival of all three cell lines, but did not increase sensitivities of cell lines to chemotherapeutic drugs.	[57]
Lung cancer (NSCLC)	Increased sensitivity to TRAIL-induced apoptosis through modulation of c-FLIP and upregulation of DR5. Inhibits growth, triggers ER stress.	[5, 49]
Head and neck cancer (HNSCC)	Apoptosis in 8 HNSCC cell lines.	[32]
Cervical cancer	Growth inhibition by micromolar concentrations.	[5]
Kidney cancer	Induced G_1 cell cycle arrest in Caki-1 and normal HK-2 cell lines; decreased cyclin D expression; induces apoptosis.	[7]

Table 6. Possible anti-cancer clinical applications of SHetA2 and documented results from different studies.

10. Conclusion

SHetA2 has exhibited anticancer activity in 60 NCI cancer cells and has shown favorable results in inhibiting various types of cancer growth *in vivo*, particularly ovarian cancer. It exerts various chemopreventive and chemotherapeutic activities through its ability to induce apoptosis and Differentiation, and inhibit angiogenesis and cell growth. It promotes mitochondrial swelling and mitophagy leading to apoptosis of cancer cells, while sparing normal cells. Once the targets are validated, tweaking of existing Flex-Hets or synthesis of newer related analogs may offer greater specificity and improved anticancer activity. Preclinical studies in animals have shown that SHetA2 has high efficacy with minimal toxicity and has a good pharmacokinetic profile. This provides the foundation for developing a novel class of more effective, chemo-preventive and anticancer drugs with a better therapeutic window.

Abbreviations

ATRA: All *trans* retinoic acid

c-FLIP: Cellular FLICE-inhibitory protein

DR5: Death receptor 5

EC50: 50% Effective concentration
FDA: US Food and Drug Administration
Flex-Hets: Flexible heteroarotinoids
GI50: 50% Growth inhibition
GSH: Glutathione
NCI: National Cancer Institute
MTD: Maximum tolerated dose
RA: Retinoic acid
RAR: Retinoic acid receptor
RAID: Rapid access to intervention development
RAPID: Rapid access to preventive intervention development
ROS: Reactive oxygen species
RXR: Retinoid X receptor
SAR: Structure activity relationship
SHetA2: [(4-Nitrophenyl)amino][2,2,4,4-tetramethylthiochroman-6-yl]amino]methane-thione
TP: Thymidine phosphorylase
TRAIL: Tumor necrosis factor-related apoptosis-inducing ligand
TSP-4: Thrombospondin-4
TTNPB: (E)-4-[2-(5,6,7,8-tetrahydro-5,5,8,8-tetramethyl-2-naphthylenyl)-1-propenyl] benzoic acid

Author details

Shengquan Liu[1*], Guangyan Zhou[1], Sze Ngong Henry Lo[1], Maggie Louie[1,2] and Vanishree Rajagopalan[1]

*Address all correspondence to: shengquan.liu@tu.edu

1 College of Pharmacy, Touro University, Vallejo, CA, USA

2 Department of Natural Sciences and Mathematics, Dominican University, San Rafael, CA, USA

References

[1] Perloff M, Steele VE: Early-phase development of cancer prevention agents: Challenges and opportunities. Cancer Prev Res. 2013; 6:379–383.

[2] Naithani R, Huma LC, Moriarty RM, McCormick DL, Mehta RG: Comprehensive review of cancer chemopreventive agents evaluated in experimental carcinogenesis models and clinical trials. Curr Med Chem. 2008; 15:1044–1071.

[3] Bode AM, Dong Z: Cancer prevention research – then and now. Nat Rev Cancer. 2009; 9:508–516.

[4] Kummar S, Doroshow JH: Phase 0 trials: Expediting the development of chemoprevention agents. Cancer Prev Res. 2011; 4:288–292.

[5] Benbrook DM, Kamelle SA, Guruswamy SB, Lightfoot SA, Rutledge TL, Gould NS, Hannafon BN, Dunn ST, Berlin KD: Flexible heteroarotinoids (Flex-Hets) exhibit improved therapeutic ratios as anti-cancer agents over retinoic acid receptor agonists. Invest New Drugs. 2005; 23:417–428.

[6] Liu S, Brown CW, Berlin KD, Dhar A, Guruswamy S, Brown D, Gardner GJ, Birrer MJ, Benbrook DM: Synthesis of flexible sulfur-containing heteroarotinoids that induce apoptosis and reactive oxygen species with discrimination between malignant and benign cells. J Med Chem. 2004; 47:999–1007.

[7] Liu T, Masamha CP, Chengedza S, Berlin KD, Lightfoot S, He F, Benbrook DM: Development of flexible-heteroarotinoids for kidney cancer. Mol Cancer Ther. 2009; 8:1227–1238.

[8] Benbrook DM, Nammalwar B, Long A, Matsumoto H, Singh A, Bunce RA, Berlin KD: SHetA2 interference with mortalin binding to p66shc and p53 identified using drug-conjugated magnetic microspheres. Invest New Drugs. 2014; 32:412–423.

[9] Liu T, Hannafon B, Gill L, Kelly W, Benbrook D: Flex-Hets differentially induce apoptosis in cancer over normal cells by directly targeting mitochondria. Mol Cancer Ther. 2007; 6:1814–1822.

[10] Moxley KM, Chengedza S, Benbrook DM: Induction of death receptor ligand-mediated apoptosis in epithelial ovarian carcinoma: The search for sensitizing agents. Gynecol Oncol. 2009; 115:438–442.

[11] Masamha CP, Benbrook DM: Cyclin D1 degradation is sufficient to induce G1 cell cycle arrest despite constitutive expression of cyclin E2 in ovarian cancer cells. Cancer Res. 2009; 69:6565–6572.

[12] Myers T, Chengedza S, Lightfoot S, Pan Y, Dedmond D, Cole L, Tang Y, Benbrook DM: Flexible heteroarotinoid (Flex-Het) SHetA2 inhibits angiogenesis in vitro and in vivo. Invest New Drugs. 2009; 27:304–318.

[13] Kabirov KK, Kapetanovic IM, Benbrook DM, Dinger N, Mankovskaya I, Zakharov A, Detrisac C, Pereira M, Martin-Jimenez T, Onua E, et al.: Oral toxicity and pharmacokinetic studies of SHetA2, a new chemopreventive agent, in rats and dogs. Drug Chem Toxicol. 2013; 36:284–295.

[14] Available from: https://projectreporter.nih.gov/project_info_description.cfm?projectnumber=1R01CA196200-01A1 [accessed: 07/18/2016].

[15] Evans TR, Kaye SB: Retinoids: present role and future potential. Br J Cancer. 1999; 80:1–8.

[16] Lotan R: Retinoids in cancer chemoprevention. FASEB J. 1996; 10:1031–1039.

[17] Leid M, Retinoids. In: Abraham DJ, editor. Burger's Medicinal Chemistry and Drug Discovery. Vol 4, 6th ed. John Wiley & Sons, Inc. Hoboken, NJ. 2003:317-358.

[18] Smith W, Saba N: Retinoids as chemoprevention for head and neck cancer: where do we go from here? Crit Rev Oncol Hematol. 2005; 55:143–152.

[19] Benbrook DM: Refining retinoids with heteroatoms. Mini Rev Med Chem. 2002(3); 277–283

[20] Gottardis MM, Lamph WW, Shalinsky DR, Wellstein A, Heyman RA: The efficacy of 9-cis retinoic acid in experimental models of cancer. Breast Cancer Res Treat. 1996; 38:85–96.

[21] Shalinsky DR, Bischoff ED, Lamph WW, Zhang L, Boehm MF, Davies PJ, Nadzan AM, Heyman RA: A novel retinoic acid receptor-selective retinoid, ALRT1550, has potent antitumor activity against human oral squamous carcinoma xenografts in nude mice. Cancer Res. 1997; 57:162–168.

[22] Gale JB: Recent advances in the chemistry and biology of retinoids. Prog Med Chem. 1993; 30:1–55.

[23] Dawson MI, Fontana JA: The peptidomimetic, 1-adamantyl-substituted, and flex-het classes of retinoid-derived molecules: structure-activity relationships and retinoid receptor-independent anticancer activities. Mini Rev Med Chem. 2010; 10:455–491.

[24] Silverman AK, Ellis CN, Voorhees JJ: Hypervitaminosis A syndrome: a paradigm of retinoid side effects. J Am Acad Dermatol. 1987; 16:1027–1039.

[25] Garattini E, Gianni M, Terao M: Retinoid related molecules an emerging class of apoptotic agents with promising therapeutic potential in oncology: pharmacological activity and mechanisms of action. Curr Pharm Des. 2004; 10:433–448.

[26] Sun SY, Lotan R: Retinoids and their receptors in cancer development and chemoprevention. Crit Rev Oncol Hematol. 2002; 41:41–55.

[27] Henney JE: From the Food and Drug Administration. JAMA. 2000; 283 (9):1131

[28] Chen S, Ostrowski J, Whiting G, Roalsvig T, Hammer L, Currier SJ, Honeyman J, Kwasniewski B, Yu KL, Sterzycki R, et al.: Retinoic acid receptor gamma mediates topical retinoid efficacy and irritation in animal models. J Invest Dermatol. 1995; 104:779–783.

[29] Dawson MI, Hobbs PD, Derdzinski K, Chan RL, Gruber J, Chao WR, Smith S, Thies RW, Schiff LJ: Conformationally restricted retinoids. J Med Chem. 1984; 27:1516–1531.

[30] Benbrook DM, Subramanian S, Gale JB, Liu S, Brown CW, Boehm MF, Berlin KD: Synthesis and characterization of heteroarotinoids demonstrate structure specificity relationships. J Med Chem. 1998; 41:3753–3757.

[31] Waugh KM, Berlin KD, Ford WT, Holt EM, Carrol JP, Schomber PR, Thompson MD, Schiff LJ: Synthesis and characterization of selected heteroarotinoids. Pharmacological activity as assessed in vitamin A deficient hamster tracheal organ cultures. Single-crystal X-ray diffraction analysis of 4,4-dimethylthiochroman-6-yl methyl ketone 1,1-dioxide and ethyl (E)-p-[2-(4,4-dimethylthiochroman-6-yl)propenyl]benzoate. J Med Chem. 1985; 28:116–124.

[32] Chun KH, Benbrook DM, Berlin KD, Hong WK, Lotan R: The synthetic heteroarotinoid SHetA2 induces apoptosis in squamous carcinoma cells through a receptor-independent and mitochondria-dependent pathway. Cancer Res. 2003; 63:3826–3832.

[33] NCI 60 cell line screen dose response data for compound NSC 726189. Available from: http://dtp.nci.nih.gov/dtpstandard/servlet/dwindex?searchtype=NSC&chemname-boolean=and&outputformat=html&searchlist=726189&Submit=Submit

[34] Doppalapudi RS, Riccio ES, Davis Z, Menda S, Wang A, Du N, Green C, Kopelovich L, Rao CV, Benbrook DM, et al.: Genotoxicity of the cancer chemopreventive drug candidates CP-31398, SHetA2, and phospho-ibuprofen. Mutat Res. 2012; 746:78–88.

[35] Cimino MC: Comparative overview of current international strategies and guidelines for genetic toxicology testing for regulatory purposes. Environ Mol Mutagen. 2006; 47:362–390.

[36] Mic F, Molotkov A, Benbrook DM, Duester G: Retinoid activation of retinoic acid receptor but not retinoid X receptor is sufficient to rescue lethal defect in retinoic acid synthesis. Proc Natl Acad Sci U S A. 2003; 100:7135–7140.

[37] Tallent CR, Twine CE, Risbood P, Seltzman HH: An improved preparation of 2,2,4,4-tetramethyl-6-amiothiochroman, a key intermediate to urea and thiourea heteroarotinoids for anticancer studies. Org Prep Proced Int. 2007; 39:96–101.

[38] Jong L, Lehmann JM, Hobbs PD, Harlev E, Huffman JC, Pfahl M, Dawson MI: Conformational effects on retinoid receptor selectivity. 1. Effect of 9-double bond geometry on retinoid X receptor activity. J Med Chem. 1993; 36:2605–2613.

[39] Benbrook DM, Madler MM, Spruce LW, Birckbichler PJ, Nelson EC, Subramanian S, Weerasekare GM, Gale JB, Patterson MK, Jr., Wang B, et al.: Biologically active heteroarotinoids exhibiting anticancer activity and decreased toxicity. J Med Chem. 1997; 40:3567–3583.

[40] Willhite CC, Jurek A, Sharma RP, Dawson MI: Structure-affinity relationships of retinoids with embryonic cellular retinoic acid-binding protein. Toxicol Appl Pharmacol. 1992; 112:144–153.

[41] Le TC, Berlin KD, Benson SD, Eastman MA, Bell-Eunice G, Nelson AC, Benbrook DM: Heteroarotinoids with anti-cancer activity against ovarian cancer cells. Open Med Chem J. 2007; 1:11–23.

[42] Zacheis D, Dhar A, Lu S, Madler MM, Klucik J, Brown CW, Liu S, Clement F, Subramanian S, Weerasekare GM, et al.: Heteroarotinoids inhibit head and neck cancer cell lines in vitro and in vivo through both RAR and RXR retinoic acid receptors. J Med Chem. 1999; 42:4434–4445.

[43] Dhar A, Liu S, Klucik J, Berlin KD, Madler MM, Lu S, Ivey RT, Zacheis D, Brown CW, Nelson EC, et al.: Synthesis, structure-activity relationships, and RARgamma-ligand interactions of nitrogen heteroarotinoids. J Med Chem. 1999; 42:3602–3614.

[44] Guruswamy S, Lightfoot S, Gold M, Hassan R, Berlin KD, Ivey RT, Benbrook DM: Effects of retinoids on cancerous phenotype and apoptosis in organotypic cultures of ovarian carcinoma. J Natl Cancer Inst. 2001; 93:516–525.

[45] Bernard BA, Bernardon JM, Delescluse C, Martin B, Lenoir MC, Maignan J, Charpentier B, Pilgrim WR, Reichert U, Shroot B: Identification of synthetic retinoids with selectivity for human nuclear retinoic acid receptor gamma. Biochem Biophys Res Commun. 1992; 186:977–983.

[46] Klaholz BP, Mitschler A, Belema M, Zusi C, Moras D: Enantiomer discrimination illustrated by high-resolution crystal structures of the human nuclear receptor hRAR-gamma. Proc Natl Acad Sci U S A. 2000; 97:6322–6327.

[47] Liu S, Louie MC, Rajagopalan V, Zhou G, Ponce E, Nguyen T, Green L: Synthesis and evaluation of the diarylthiourea analogs as novel anti-cancer agents. Bioorg Med Chem Lett. 2015; 25:1301–1305.

[48] Gnanasekaran KK, Benbrook DM, Nammalwar B, Thavathiru E, Bunce RA, Berlin KD: Synthesis and evaluation of second generation Flex-Het scaffolds against the human ovarian cancer A2780 cell line. Eur J Med Chem. 2015; 96:209–217.

[49] Lin YD, Chen S, Yue P, Zou W, Benbrook DM, Liu S, Le TC, Berlin KD, Khuri FR, Sun SY: CAAT/enhancer binding protein homologous protein-dependent death receptor 5 induction is a major component of SHetA2-induced apoptosis in lung cancer cells. Cancer Res. 2008; 68:5335–5344.

[50] Lin Y, Liu X, Yue P, Benbrook DM, Berlin KD, Khuri FR, Sun SY: Involvement of c-FLIP and survivin down-regulation in flexible heteroarotinoid-induced apoptosis and enhancement of TRAIL-initiated apoptosis in lung cancer cells. Mol Cancer Ther. 2008; 7:3556–3565.

[51] Irmler M, Thome M, Hahne M, Schneider P, Hofmann K, Steiner V, Bodmer JL, Schroter M, Burns K, Mattmann C, et al.: Inhibition of death receptor signals by cellular FLIP. Nature. 1997; 388:190–195.

[52] Altieri DC: Validating survivin as a cancer therapeutic target. Nat Rev Cancer. 2003; 3:46–54.

[53] Kelley SK, Ashkenazi A: Targeting death receptors in cancer with Apo2L/TRAIL. Curr Opin Pharmacol. 2004; 4:333–339.

[54] Moxley K, Chengedza S, Benbrook DM: Induction of death receptor ligand -mediated apoptosis in epithelial ovarian carcinoma: the search for sensitizing agents. Gynecol Oncol. 2010; 115:438–442.

[55] Chengedza S, Benbrook DM: NF-kappaB is involved in SHetA2 circumvention of TNF-alpha resistance, but not induction of intrinsic apoptosis. Anticancer Drugs. 2010; 21:297–305.

[56] Guruswamy S, Benbrook DM: Retinoids chemosensitize ovarian cancer cell lines to cisplatin independent of nuclear receptors and p53. Am J Pharmacol Toxicol. 2006; 1:87–93.

[57] Hyde J, Benbrook DM: Sensitivities of uterine adenocarcinoma, mixed mullerian tumor (MMT) and sarcoma cell lines to chemotherapeutic agents and a flex-het drug. Am J Pharmacol Toxicol. 2006; 1:83–86.

[58] Liu Z, Zhang Y, Hua YF, Covey JM, Benbrook DM, Chan KK: Metabolism of a sulfur-containing heteroarotionoid antitumor agent, SHetA2, using liquid chromatography/tandem mass spectrometry. Rapid Commun Mass Spectrom. 2008; 22:3371–3381.

[59] Zhang Y, Hua Y, Benbrook DM, Covey JM, Dai G, Liu Z, Chan KK: High performance liquid chromatographic analysis and preclinical pharmacokinetics of the heteroarotinoid antitumor agent, SHetA2. Cancer Chemother Pharmacol. 2006; 58:561–569.

[60] Trachootham D, Zhou Y, Zhang H, Demizu Y, Chen Z, Pelicano H, Chiao PJ, Achanta G, Arlinghaus RB, Liu J, et al.: Selective killing of oncogenically transformed cells through a ROS-mediated mechanism by beta-phenylethyl isothiocyanate. Cancer Cell. 2006; 10:241–252.

[61] Franco R, Schoneveld OJ, Pappa A, Panayiotidis MI: The central role of glutathione in the pathophysiology of human diseases. Arch Physiol Biochem. 2007; 113:234–258.

[62] Benbrook DM, Lightfoot S, Ranger-Moore J, Liu T, Chengedza S, Berry WL, Dozmorov I: Gene expression analysis of biological systems driving an organotypic model of endometrial carcinogenesis and chemoprevention. Gene Regul Syst Bio. 2008; 2:21–42.

[63] Nammalwar B, Bunce RA, Benbrook DM, Lu T, Li H-F, Chen Y-D, Berlin KD: Synthesis of N-[3,4-dihydro-4-(acetoxymethyl)-2, 2, 4-trimethyl-2 H-1-benzothiopyran-6-yl]-N′-(4-nitrophenyl) thiourea and N-[3, 4-dihydro-4-(hydroxymethyl)-2, 2, 4-trimethyl-2 H-1-benzothiopyran-6-yl]-N′-(4-nitrophenyl) thiourea, a major metabolite of N-(3, 4-dihydro-2, 2, 4, 4-tetramethyl-2 H-1-benzothiopyran-6-YL)-N′-(4-nitrophenyl) thiourea. Phosphorus Sulfur Silicon. 2010; 186:189–204.

[64] Howard EW, Camm KD, Wong YC, Wang XH: E-cadherin upregulation as a therapeutic goal in cancer treatment. Mini Rev Med Chem. 2008; 8:496–518.

[65] Margosio B, Rusnati M, Bonezzi K, Cordes BL, Annis DS, Urbinati C, Giavazzi R, Presta M, Ribatti D, Mosher DF, et al.: Fibroblast growth factor-2 binding to the thrombospondin-1 type III repeats, a novel antiangiogenic domain. Int J Biochem Cell Biol. 2008; 40:700–709.

[66] Wilhelm S, Carter C, Lynch M, Lowinger T, Dumas J, Smith RA, Schwartz B, Simantov R, Kelley S: Discovery and development of sorafenib: a multikinase inhibitor for treating cancer. Nat Rev Drug Discov. 2006; 5:835–844.

[67] Albert DH, Tapang P, Magoc TJ, Pease LJ, Reuter DR, Wei RQ, Li J, Guo J, Bousquet PF, Ghoreishi-Haack NS, et al.: Preclinical activity of ABT-869, a multitargeted receptor tyrosine kinase inhibitor. Mol Cancer Ther. 2006; 5:995–1006.

Permissions

AAll chapters in this book were first published in ACDNSC, by InTech Open; hereby published with permission under the Creative Commons Attribution License or equivalent. Every chapter published in this book has been scrutinized by our experts. Their significance has been extensively debated. The topics covered herein carry significant findings which will fuel the growth of the discipline. They may even be implemented as practical applications or may be referred to as a beginning point for another development.

The contributors of this book come from diverse backgrounds, making this book a truly international effort. This book will bring forth new frontiers with its revolutionizing research information and detailed analysis of the nascent developments around the world.

We would like to thank all the contributing authors for lending their expertise to make the book truly unique. They have played a crucial role in the development of this book. Without their invaluable contributions this book wouldn't have been possible. They have made vital efforts to compile up to date information on the varied aspects of this subject to make this book a valuable addition to the collection of many professionals and students.

This book was conceptualized with the vision of imparting up-to-date information and advanced data in this field. To ensure the same, a matchless editorial board was set up. Every individual on the board went through rigorous rounds of assessment to prove their worth. After which they invested a large part of their time researching and compiling the most relevant data for our readers.

The editorial board has been involved in producing this book since its inception. They have spent rigorous hours researching and exploring the diverse topics which have resulted in the successful publishing of this book. They have passed on their knowledge of decades through this book. To expedite this challenging task, the publisher supported the team at every step. A small team of assistant editors was also appointed to further simplify the editing procedure and attain best results for the readers.

Apart from the editorial board, the designing team has also invested a significant amount of their time in understanding the subject and creating the most relevant covers. They scrutinized every image to scout for the most suitable representation of the subject and create an appropriate cover for the book.

The publishing team has been an ardent support to the editorial, designing and production team. Their endless efforts to recruit the best for this project, has resulted in the accomplishment of this book. They are a veteran in the field of academics and their pool of knowledge is as vast as their experience in printing. Their expertise and guidance has proved useful at every step. Their uncompromising quality standards have made this book an exceptional effort. Their encouragement from time to time has been an inspiration for everyone.

The publisher and the editorial board hope that this book will prove to be a valuable piece of knowledge for researchers, students, practitioners and scholars across the globe.

List of Contributors

Linda-Lucila Landeros-Martinez, Daniel Glossman-Mitnik, Erasmo Orrantia-Borunda and Norma Flores-Holguin
NANOCOSMOS Virtual Lab, Department of Environment and Energy, Advanced Materials Research Center (CIMAV), Miguel de Cervantes 120, Complejo Industrial Chihuahua, Chihuahua, México

Satyajit Das, Jaydip Biswas and Soumitra Kumar Choudhuri
Department of In Vitro Carcinogenesis and Cellular Chemotherapy, Chittaranjan National Cancer Institute, Kolkata, India

Enke Baldini, Chiara Tuccilli, Salvatore Sorrenti, Domenico Mascagni, Stefano Arcieri, Angelo Filippini and Salvatore Ulisse
Department of Surgical Sciences, "Sapienza" University of Rome, Rome, Italy

Aurélien F.A. Moumbock
Department of Chemistry, University of Buea, Buea, Cameroon

Conrad V. Simoben and Wolfgang Sippl
Department of Pharmaceutical Chemistry, Martin-Luther University of Halle-Wittenberg, Halle, Germany

Ludger Wessjohann
Leibniz Institute of Plant Biochemistry, Halle, Germany

Stefan Günther
Pharmaceutical Bioinformatics, Albert-Ludwig-University Freiburg, Freiburg, Germany

Fidele Ntie-Kang
Department of Chemistry, University of Buea, Buea, Cameroon Department of Pharmaceutical Chemistry, Martin-Luther University of Halle-Wittenberg, Halle, Germany

Kalubai Vari Khajapeer and Rajasekaran Baskaran
Department of Biochemistry and Molecular Biology, School of Life Sciences, Pondicherry University, Pondicherry, India

Andreea Letitia Arsene
Department of General and Pharmaceutical Microbiology, Faculty of Pharmacy, University of Medicine and Pharmacy "Carol Davila", Bucharest, Romania

Cristina Manuela Dragoi and Alina Crenguta Nicolae
Department of Biochemistry, Faculty of Pharmacy, University of Medicine and Pharmacy "Carol Davila", Bucharest, Romania

Daniela Elena Popa and George T.A. Burcea-Dragomiroiu
Department of Drug Control, Faculty of Pharmacy, University of Medicine and Pharmacy "Carol Davila", Bucharest, Romania

Ion Bogdan Dumitrescu
Department of Pharmaceutical Physics and Informatics, Faculty of Pharmacy, University of Medicine and Pharmacy "Carol Davila", Bucharest, Romania

Olivia Carmen Timnea
Department of Medical Sciences, Faculty of Physical Education and Sports, Ecologic University of Bucharest, Romania

Denisa Ioana Udeanu
Department of Clinical Laboratory and Food Safety, Faculty of Pharmacy, University of Medicine and Pharmacy "Carol Davila", Bucharest, Romania

Jessica Castro, Marc Ribó, Antoni Benito and Maria Vilanova
Protein Engineering Laboratory, Department of Biology, Faculty of Sciences, University of Girona, Girona, Spain Institute of Biomedical Research of Girona "Dr. Josep Trueta" (IdIBGi), Girona, Spain

Ming Hong, Ning Wang and Yibin Feng
School of Chinese Medicine, Li Ka Shing Faculty of Medicine, The University of Hong Kong, Pok Fu Lam, Hong Kong, China

Shengquan Liu, Guangyan Zhou, Sze Ngong Henry Lo and Vanishree Rajagopalan
College of Pharmacy, Touro University, Vallejo, CA, USA

Maggie Louie
College of Pharmacy, Touro University, Vallejo, CA, USA Department of Natural Sciences and Mathematics, Dominican University, San Rafael, CA, USA

Index

www.ingramcontent.com/pod-product-compliance
Lightning Source LLC
LaVergne TN
LVHW060534210926
848485LV00005B/1194